Praise for *The Pure Cure*

"*The Pure Cure* is an insightful and powerful tool for those searching for meaningful health and healing. The authors expose the not-so-obvious and expound on the essentials in a way that empowers each reader to become a more responsive and responsible person.

In our stressful, busy world, most of us employ health-building methods in a cursory way, often neglecting the less obvious culprits that prevail. Most of us take our work and residential environments for granted. By lack of thought, we use cleaning products, building materials and even lighting methods that drain our health. We adorn our bodies with chemicals and chemically-treated fabrics that perpetuate disease. We eat chemically-laden food, drink chemically-treated water and breathe polluted air. And just when we think we have it all figured out, we remember our cell phone with its invisible wireless connectivity that links to computer, electronic books, iPods, and the big scary tower down the street. The authors leave no stone unturned. What I love most about this contribution is the nuance and detail that are central in health-building and conscious avoidance.

Tenuous, non-committal learned patterns are our greatest enemy. It is only wisdom and the application of truth that banishes these squelchers of human dignity. *The Pure Cure* is one of the most well researched and clearly composed works I have ever read. I strongly encourage you to do more than read this manuscript of truth. I encourage you to use it as a reference and to share this gift with those you love. It will help them and all of humanity to make necessary changes. I know you will be as deeply touched by the sincerity, authenticity, and revelations within it as I have been."

—Brian Clement, Ph.D., L.N. founder of the Hippocrates Health Institute

"Finally, two authors have put together a book that deals with the overwhelming toxic environment we live in. This outstanding book discusses everything from wireless toxins to toxic metals, to chemicals at home and in the workplace, to a whole host of everyday contaminants that are literally destroying human civilization. *The Pure Cure* is a must read. It provides real solutions for living in our toxic world."

—Stephen T. Sinatra, MD, FACC, CNS, coauthor of *Earthing*, and *The Healing Kitchen*

THE
PURE
CURE

A COMPLETE GUIDE
TO FREEING YOUR LIFE
FROM DANGEROUS TOXINS

SHARYN WYNTERS, ND
BURTON GOLDBERG, LHD

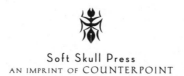

Soft Skull Press
AN IMPRINT OF COUNTERPOINT

Library of Congress Cataloging-in-Publication Data is available.

ISBN: 978-1-59376-500-2

Printed in the United States of America

Soft Skull Press
AN IMPRINT OF COUNTERPOINT
1919 Fifth Street
Berkeley, CA 94710

www.softskull.com
www.counterpointpress.com

Distributed by Publishers Group West

10 9 8 7 6 5 4 3 2 1

Dedication

This book is for those who yearn to be all they can be. It is for all those who acknowledge their innate connection with the earth and with nature. It is for every parent whose desire is to raise their children in a safe environment (physically, emotionally, and spiritually). It is for every health care practitioner whose mission is to be a catalyst for health, and it is for every person who yearns to be well.

It is dedicated with gratitude to the many teachers, friends, and loved ones who have inspired and supported the authors' journey through the years. It is also dedicated to their children and to all the children of the world. May they enjoy abundant health, and may they never forget the wonder of the sacred dance we call "life." The book is also dedicated to the memory of Wilk Wilkinson, who left this world September 27, 2006. He was an artist, a friend, a loving partner, and the perfect reflection of love.

EYE OF PASSION

Mid summer heat
A fleeting moment of spring beauty
Scented in the essence of
Feminine grace
Set in eternal bliss
A kiss away
As the summer winds of time
Blow forth
Like the mountain wild flowers
Radiant to all to see
Beyond the night flight
And so the dance of life
Touches the soul of those
Who
Participate in
Passion

Wilk Wilkinson (1998)

Contents

Foreword

THE PURE CURE

Years ago, when the Tree of Life Rejuvenation Center was in the planning stages, I envisioned a place where people could have an experience of conscious living—everything from organic gardens and life force-preserving food preparation, to buildings created from sustainable practices with clean sources of power. I envisioned a place where people could experience the healing energies of earth, air, water, sun, and cosmos; I referred to this experience as *holistic enlightened living*. Now, eighteen years later, *The Pure Cure* explains why *holistic enlightened living* is a must for everyone on the planet. I have looked at this book not only as a holistic physician, but also through Native American eyes as a sundancer, spirit dancer, and Lakota clan chief as well as a rabbi. These eyes are crying at the desecration of mother earth by a greed-oriented world. Not only is there a biblical teaching not to pollute the public commons, but also there are specific biblical teachings that we must not only preserve the ecology and feed the hungry with "good" food, but also have the moral and spiritual obligation to strongly protect our life force and health. These are the key points and teachings of this outstanding book that empowers us on all levels.

Sharyn Wynters and Burton Goldberg have created a masterful guide for those who are interested in conscious (enlightened) living. They have provided the background, the research and the reasons why we must look to non-toxic and sustainable options if we are to move forward as a liberated human community. The reader will find incentives to avoid foods grown on corporate farms, water treated in municipal treatment facilities, unseen electromagnetic fields from our electrical and wireless power grids, and chemicals found in clothing, personal care products, furniture, cleaning solutions, and building materials that contaminate the air we breathe. There is even a chapter on ways to overcome emotional and spiritual obstacles that are toxic in their own way.

Modern living has brought with it untold hazards many of which are cleverly hidden until someone points them out. *The Pure Cure, A Complete Guide to Freeing your Life from Dangerous Toxins* does a wonderful job of pointing them out. But the authors go beyond exposing the problems. Within the pages of *The Pure Cure,* you will find natural alternatives and sustainable options to help protect your health and preserve the Earth. You will gain a new appreciation for the bounty of life on this beautiful planet and you will want to participate in helping to restore balance.

I have always considered awareness and education to be cornerstones for change and optimal living. Much of what I do as a holistic medical doctor and as director of the Tree of Life Rejuvenation Center and Tree of Life Foundation is about educating those who come for assistance. *The Pure Cure* is a foundational work for providing education and the incentive to change. In a free society, we have choices. However, those choices are often made in ignorance—without full information they are not free choices. Those who may not have our best interests at heart and have chosen to rebel against the biblical injunction to "not pollute the public commons" often taint the act of free choice. *The Pure Cure* levels the playing field by giving us enough information to make authentic free choice by bringing awareness and education to those who are ready for change.

If everyone makes just a few changes at a time, we can begin the process of rebuilding our health, our home, and our bio-computer mind so we may rise above it and know the sovereign truth of who we are and our spiritual life purpose. We each have a birthright to live in a clean, balanced environment; to eat wholesome, nutritious food; to fill our lungs with fresh unpolluted air; to participate in honest, loving relationships; and to enjoy the bounty of our divine heritage. *The Pure Cure* will help you on the path to the realization of your birthright.

Eighteen years ago I envisioned a haven for those ready to experience enlightened living. Today, *The Pure Cure* brings the possibility of conscious (enlightened) living to your doorstep.

Rabbi Gabriel Cousens M.D., M.D.(H), D.D., Diplomat of Ayurveda, Diplomat of the American Board of Holistic Medicine – Founder and director of the Tree of Life Rejuvenation Center and the Tree of Life Foundation; author of: *There Is A Cure For Diabetes, Spiritual Nutrition, Rainbow Green Live-Food Cuisine, Depression-Free for Life, Conscious Eating, Torah as a Guide to Enlightenment,* and *Creating Peace by Being Peace.*

Introduction

Toxic chemicals from everyday products contaminate every person living in modern society today. Even if you don't live in the city, there are toxic chemicals in the air you breathe, in the water you drink, and in the soil from which your food is grown. Unfortunately, toxins have been discovered in the most remote and pristine parts of the world—the result of pesticide drift, industrial waste, and societal negligence.

Toxic chemicals are so pervasive that they infiltrate every aspect of our lives. Carpets, water bottles, shampoo, pots and pans, couch cushions, computers, toys, and baby bottles all emit toxic substances and other by-products that contaminate our living environment and our bodies. Today, newborn infants are born with dangerous levels of toxins, passed to them from their mothers while "safely" in the womb.

Of considerable concern is our food. The old adage, "An apple a day keeps the doctor away," has most people shaking their heads when they consider the fact that apples have become one of the most toxic of all fruits. Apples are sprayed with so many chemicals and pesticides—then often irradiated before they are placed on display—that unless they are organic, they can often be more harmful than healthful.

The human race has created chemicals for every purpose imaginable. In agriculture, there are chemicals to kill pests, to make foods ripen faster, to make foods grow bigger, and to lengthen their shelf life. In the food-processing industry, chemicals are used to bleach flour, to add colors to food, to preserve freshness, to line cans and boxes, and to trick your taste buds. The textile industry uses chemicals to make fabric. More chemicals are used to soften the fabric, to add color to it, to keep it from wrinkling, to make it fire retardant, to create resistance to stains, to keep it from collecting static, and to make it water resistant. In the personal care industry, chemicals are used to create suds; they remove grease, stiffen your hair, make your skin feel smooth, stop you from perspiring, change your hair color, lengthen your eyelashes, and make you smell good.

Unfortunately, the chemicals designed to make our lives easier are now being discovered to cause birth defects, hyperactivity, learning disabilities, attention deficit, early onset of puberty, and developmental problems for our children. Many of these chemicals are known to cause allergies, asthma, and other respiratory problems. Others are known to cause neurological disorders, sexual dysfunction, and cancer. Not only have environmental toxins been linked with a large number of existing diseases, but many scientists believe they are responsible for an entirely new group of disorders that involve multi-system symptoms, including chronic fatigue, food intolerances, autoimmune diseases, neurological diseases, multiple chemical sensitivity, and a variety of syndromes.

Beyond being at the root of many of our modern illnesses, environmental toxins contribute to a burden that we all bear—a burden that suppresses immune function and makes us too tired to enjoy the luxury of what we have created. Now that we have climbed to the pinnacle of technological advancement to become masters of our world, we are faced with the fact that we have nearly destroyed it—and ourselves—in the process.

Man-made substances do not degrade when placed back into the earth. Plastic bottles, polyester fabric, petroleum-based detergents, and solvents take decades to degrade—perhaps even centuries—all the while leaching toxins into the soil. Our landfills have become pockets of toxicity that cannot easily be incorporated back into the cycle of life. The same is true of our bodies. They were not designed to process or to remove synthetic chemicals. The enzymes intended to break down toxins have little capacity to work on man-made chemicals. Because of their durability, the foreign chemicals we breathe and ingest are deposited in tiny pockets in our bodies, destined to accumulate until they can no longer be contained.

But aren't we protected from toxic chemicals, by agencies designed to monitor and test them before they are sold as "safe"? The sad truth is we are not. The nation's toxic chemical regulatory law, the Toxic Substances Control Act, is in drastic need of reform. Passed in 1976 and never amended, the act is widely regarded as the weakest of all major environmental laws on the books today. When the act was originally passed, sixty-two thousand chemicals that were already on the market were declared to be "safe," even though little or no data were available. Since that time, another twenty thousand chemicals have been put into commerce—also with little or no data to support their safety.

All too often, the "facts" about chemical toxins are contingent on who is funding the research. In the past, research funding went to academic centers. Today it is contracted to for-profit research firms. How do research firms get ongoing funding if their studies are not crafted to support the products they research? When it comes to medicine, the pharmaceutical industry now finances 70 percent of the nation's clinical drug research. Unfortunately, many of the agencies designed to protect the public are in the back pocket of the huge corporations they are intended to police.

U.S. standards are so weak that even well-known toxins continue to find their way into food, water, air, and the products we use every day. Often, manufacturers of products containing known toxins are not required to list them. Whistle-blowers inside the Food and Drug Administration (FDA) and the Environmental Protection Agency (EPA) who have attempted to expose safety issues have been pressured, threatened with legal action, punished by their superiors, or discredited. Ultimately, it is up to *us* to become more aware and to make the conscious choices that will send messages to corporate America and that will also give us back our health. In spite of the enormity of the toxins that exist *around* us, and *in* us, it is not too late to make changes in our personal lives that will have a profound effect on our health and the health of our families. Sharyn Wynters's personal experience is a perfect example.

In her twenties, with everything going for her as a successful actress, Sharyn developed serious health problems. The medical profession could not help her. This opportunity was her chance to make changes that would affect the entire course of her life. Sharyn sought out alternative cancer researcher Dr. William Donald Kelley, and within a month her whole life had changed. She threw out toxic cosmetics and household cleaners, she had dental fillings replaced, and she completely altered her diet. Her quest for health became a passion. Ultimately, she accomplished what the established medical profession could not help her attain—vibrant health. At that point, Sharyn was determined to help others. She studied dozens of disciplines in wellness, body work, and spiritual attunement. She obtained a degree in massage therapy and a degree from Clayton School of Natural Healing as a naturopath. Since then, she has been able to help thousands of individuals on the pathway to a more healthy life.

And just as it is not too late to make changes in your personal life, neither is it too late to insist on legislation that halts the manufacture of dangerous toxins and that curbs our dependence on petrochemicals. This has been one of the torches carried by Burton Goldberg for many years. As the former publisher of *Alternative Medicine* magazine, he has championed many efforts to awaken the public to the health crisis in America. His efforts to promote public awareness, to support health care choice, and to endorse legislation that supports the environment have taken him into the halls of Congress to testify before the U.S. House of Representatives Committee on Government Reform.

Like many challenges the human race has encountered, our present circumstances represent an *opportunity*. It is easy to get caught up in fear, but that is not the purpose of this book. Its purpose is to encourage you to take personal action and to support your action with enough information to help you make empowering choices. It is not too late to take action. It is not too late to support efforts for reform. And it is not too late to teach your children to recycle, to honor the earth, and to understand that each one of us can make a difference.

If you are ready to take responsibility for your health, if you are eager to implement changes that will limit your exposure to toxic chemicals, and if you are willing to do what it takes to unburden your body (and in doing so to support the unburdening of the earth), then *now* is the time. This book is offered as a guide. It is divided into chapters that each address a specific area of concern—everything from toxins in air, water, food, clothing, cleaning agents, and personal care products; toxins in medical treatments (vaccines, radiology, and dental procedures); toxins in schools, airplanes, hotels, and restaurants; and even toxic thoughts and emotions. As you read, you will be introduced to many nontoxic alternatives. The *Sources* section at the end of each chapter is designed to get you started identifying products and companies that provide safer alternatives.

Because some toxins are so pervasive and because they are found in so many areas, there is some overlap of material in the book. For example: you will find formaldehyde in the chapter on air contaminants, but you will also find it in the chapter on clothing and fabrics and in the chapters on personal care products, home construction and remodeling, and vaccines. Wherever you see this symbol

you will be referred to other places in the book where there is additional information.

You may use the book as a reference or you may read it from cover to cover. Either way, we encourage you to begin by reviewing the chapter titles. This will help you to understand the scope of the book. We believe that once you have begun reading, you will want to complete the entire book—then to refer back to the information again and again. It is our hope that the book provides you with a desire to do your own research and to join with the growing number of individuals who are taking personal responsibility for their health and for the health of planet Earth.

Chapter 1

INDOOR AIR POLLUTION

✦

And what you can do about it

We were never intended to live in a perfect world. Our bodies have been granted the innate wisdom and the intelligence to deal with everything in our environment. Ultimately, the key is a healthy body, mind, and spirit. Helping you to maintain and/or to restore health on each of these levels is one of the goals of this book. With that in mind, it is also important to understand that we no longer live in a *natural* world. Much of what we find in our surroundings is synthetic, and many of the synthetic substances we have created contain chemicals and emit gases that are unnatural and harmful to our health. Maintaining balance is difficult in a toxic world—but not impossible.

Air pollution is usually associated with *outdoor* pollution—caused by automobiles and industrial wastes. However, according to the Environmental Protection Agency (EPA), *indoor* air pollution is an even greater concern. In 1990, The EPA classified indoor air quality as a high-priority public health risk, two to five times worse than outside air pollution. Over the last twenty years, builders have worked to improve the energy efficiency of buildings. These efforts have resulted in "tight buildings" that seal in air contaminants. The concentrated presence of these contaminants, combined with the fact that most of us spend about 90 percent of our time indoors, can cause substantial exposure to pollutants.

The immediate effects of indoor air pollution may show up as eye, nose, and throat irritation and are usually short term. Other, more serious health effects may show up after years of exposure. Thus, there is a need to improve indoor air quality in as many ways as possible—even if symptoms are not present. There are plenty of things you can do to improve the quality of the air you breathe indoors. The most important thing is to eliminate the sources of pollutants. This includes carefully selecting the cleaning agents and other chemicals you use in your home; maintaining/venting appliances properly;

and purchasing clothing, carpets, and furniture that do not emit volatile chemicals. Learning to eliminate the sources of indoor pollutants (even if you do this over a period of time) will offer you the greatest satisfaction and the greatest degree of control over your indoor breathing environment. Each time you purchase a cleaning agent or a home furnishing, make the choice with your health in mind.

Understanding the substances that influence indoor air quality is a key to improving the environment. This chapter identifies the major indoor air pollutants and their known sources. It also includes information on air-cleaning devices and other ways for improving the quality of the air in your home. Indoor air pollutants fall into the following categories:

Pollutant	Major Indoor Sources	Potential Health Effects
Environmental Tobacco Smoke	Cigarettes, cigars, and pipes	Respiratory irritation; bronchitis; pneumonia; emphysema; lung cancer; heart disease
Carbon Monoxide, Nitrogen and Sulfur Dioxides	Unvented or malfunctioning gas appliances, wood stoves, and tobacco smoke	Headache; nausea; fatigue; impaired vision and mental function; eye, nose, and throat irritation
Volatile Organic Compounds (VOCs)	Aerosol sprays, solvents, glues, cleaning agents, pesticides, paints, moth repellents, air fresheners, dry-cleaned clothing, formaldehyde, flame retardants, candles	Eye, nose, and throat irritation; headaches; loss of coordination; damage to liver, kidney, and brain; cancer
Biological Agents (mold, bacteria, viruses, pollen, animal dander, mites)	House dust, pets, bedding, poorly maintained air conditioners, humidifiers, and dehumidifiers, wet or moist areas	Allergic reactions; asthma; eye, nose, and throat irritation; humidifier fever; influenza and other infectious diseases
Heavy Metals (lead and mercury vapor)	Sanding or open-flame burning of lead paint; crafts; interior latex paint manufactured before 1990; some candles	Headache; fatigue; irritability; muscle cramps; abdominal discomfort; personality changes
Radon	Soil under buildings and ground water	Lung cancer

ENVIRONMENTAL TOBACCO SMOKE

Secondhand smoke or environmental tobacco smoke (ETS) contains more than four thousand chemical compounds, approximately forty of which are carcinogens (cancer causing) or suspected carcinogens. Secondhand smoke is classified as a Group A carcinogen—the classification for which there is *no safe level of exposure*. Secondhand smoke can cause immediate adverse effects: eye irritation, throat irritation, coughing, chest discomfort, and difficulty breathing. The effects of even brief exposure (minutes to hours) to secondhand smoke are nearly as severe as they are for chronic smokers. Long-term exposure to ETS is a proven cause of lung cancer.

Secondhand smoke is especially harmful for children. It causes between one hundred fifty thousand and three hundred thousand lower respiratory tract infections each year for children younger than eighteen months old.[1] Children subjected to ETS are also more prone to ear infections and asthma. Secondhand smoke may cause thousands of nonasthmatic children to develop asthma each year. Those already diagnosed are at even greater risk. Even though children and the elderly are the most susceptible, everyone who is exposed to secondhand smoke must bear the consequences.

> Cigarettes contain up to 600 additives. When these are set on fire, the smoke contains over 4000 chemicals. Over 40 of these are known to cause cancer.

The only effective way to eliminate ETS is to eliminate the smoke. Supporting a smoker's attempts to quit is in everyone's interest—just be careful not to use shame or guilt. These methods produce toxins of another nature, and the additional stress may truly cause more harm than good. Part of being able to thrive in a toxic world is being aware of how our actions affect the whole. As each individual acknowledges his/her contribution and seeks to make it positive rather than negative, we can make giant strides as members of the human race and enhance our quality of living (physically, emotionally, and spiritually). For the smoker and the nonsmoker, mutual understanding is more important than the smoke. Air purifiers may reduce secondhand smoke to a limited degree, but no air filtration or purification system can completely eliminate all the harmful constituents of secondhand smoke—and no device can "clear the air" if someone feels forced to quit smoking before they are ready. As a courtesy, smokers may be asked to smoke outside.

CARBON MONOXIDE, NITROGEN, AND SULFUR DIOXIDES

Carbon monoxide and other pollutants, such as nitrogen dioxide and sulfur dioxide, are released into the indoor environment by oil and kerosene heaters; by unvented gas stoves and ovens; and by back-drafting or malfunctioning gas furnaces, dryers, and water heaters. These pollutants can cause nausea, headaches, fatigue, impaired mental functioning, respiratory problems, and death. Since carbon monoxide poisoning can mimic flu symptoms, whole families that experience symptoms at the start of the heating season should be alerted. Annual inspections and cleaning will reduce pollution and save energy.

Oil and kerosene heaters are never a good option (except in emergencies) to supply supplemental heat in a home—they emit carbon monoxide, nitrogen dioxide, and sulfur dioxide gases that are not vented to the outdoors. Oil and kerosene heaters also create a serious fire hazard, and they are not energy efficient. Wood stoves and fireplaces are also less desirable (especially within city limits). In many areas, fireplace fires are restricted because they add to the already heavy burden of outdoor air pollution. For small areas, electric space heaters are much better alternatives. The new, far infrared heaters combine safety (they remain cool to the touch) with high efficiency and reduced heating costs. These are perfect for additional warmth in confined areas where small children are present (see sources).

One of the smartest things you can do is to install a carbon monoxide detector. These small devices are inexpensive (usually between $30 and $50). They sound an alarm when levels of carbon monoxide reach unsafe levels. Since nitrogen and sulfur oxides are usually produced at the same time carbon monoxide is produced, carbon monoxide detectors can also indicate the presence of nitrogen and sulfur oxides. The Consumer Product Safety Commission recommends a carbon monoxide detector on each floor of a home. At a minimum, a single detector should be placed on each sleeping level, with an additional detector in the area of any major gas-burning appliance, such as a furnace or water heater. In general, carbon monoxide detectors should be placed high (near the ceiling) for the most effective use (see sources).

VOLATILE ORGANIC COMPOUNDS (VOCs)
(Cleaning Agents, Formaldehyde, Pesticides, Paint, etc.)

Numerous studies conducted over the last twenty years have shown measurable levels of more than a hundred known carcinogens circulating in the air of modern homes and offices. Many of these compounds are referred to as volatile organic compounds (VOCs). Volatile means that a compound will vaporize, or become a gas, at room temperature. At higher temperatures or in humid environments, these compounds vaporize more rapidly. VOCs are emitted from cleaning agents, air fresheners, dry-cleaned clothing, aerosol sprays, adhesives, fabric additives, treated wood, paints, solvents, hobby supplies, and indoor pesticides. Even carpeting and furniture contains volatile compounds that release formaldehyde and other VOCs for months or years (called outgassing). Outgassing has been shown to cause cancer in laboratory animals, and it is believed to be a possible cause of cancer and other problems in humans. Breathing VOCs is widely known to cause headaches; eye, nose, and throat irritation; loss of coordination; nausea; and damage to the liver, kidneys, and central nervous system.

Adequate ventilation is the easiest and most effective way to maintain air quality when VOCs are present. This is particularly important when engaging in activities that generate these types of pollutants. Make sure solvents and paints are well sealed and stored outside the living area. Many air cleaning devices will remove VOCs (see sources).

Cleaning agents

Household cleaning agents are the number one source of toxins in the home—the vast majority of cleaners contain not one, but several VOCs. Most mainstream cleaning products contain petroleum-based surfactants and/or solvents that emit volatile gases, which have been linked to reproductive disorders, neurological problems, and cancer. Many household cleaners have not been thoroughly tested for their impact on human health, nor have they been tested for their impact on the environment. Chapter 6 is entirely devoted to a discussion of cleaning agents. It includes several home-made as well as eco-friendly alternatives. Today there are many available choices, so there is no need to use a cleaning agent that emits VOCs. The chemicals listed below are common VOCs in cleaning agents and other household products.

Acetone—Acetone is a solvent found in dishwashing detergents, glues, paints, lacquer removers, fingernail polish, and fingernail polish remover. It can cause irritation of the nose, throat, lungs, eyes, and skin. Repeated or prolonged exposure is toxic to the central nervous system. It may damage the kidneys, liver, and skin.

Alcohols—The alcohol family (including, butyl, ethyl, methyl, propyl, and isopropyl) includes harsh solvents that cause drying and cracking as well as premature aging of the skin. They also produce toxic fumes that can cause headache, muscle weakness, giddiness, confusion, nausea, and eye, skin, and throat irritation. Ethyl alcohol (also referred to as ethanol or grain alcohol) is not toxic in small amounts, but to be used in other products it must be denatured. The denaturing process is simply the addition of poisonous substances so that the alcohol cannot be consumed—a carryover from the days of prohibition that is still in force today. This means that if a product contains ethanol or ethyl alcohol, it also contains other poisons. These may include acetone, turpentine, and benzene, which can outgas VOCs.

Ammonia—Ammonia is a corrosive gas with a sharp odor. It is used to make household cleaners, fertilizers, fuels, and other chemicals. Low levels of ammonia cause irritation of the eyes, nose, and throat. Exposure to more concentrated levels can cause headaches, nausea, and intense burning of the eyes, nose, throat, and skin. Individuals with respiratory problems may be particularly sensitive to ammonia. Avoid cleaning agents that contain ammonia.

 (see Chapter 6: Cleaning Agents)

Benzene—Benzene, also known as Benzol, is a highly toxic solvent used in detergents, paints, styrene, nylon, synthetic fabrics, rubber products, dyes, pharmaceuticals, and pesticides. It is a known carcinogen. Once in the body, benzene moves through the blood and can be stored in bone marrow and fatty tissue. Chronic exposure to low levels of benzene causes headaches, loss of appetite, drowsiness, nervousness, psychological disturbances, and diseases of the blood system. Immunological and reproductive disorders have also been documented.[2] Despite the fact that benzene was banned as a solvent more than twenty years ago, indoor air may still be contaminated with benzene from products like glues, paints, furniture wax, and detergents. It will likely not be listed on a label of ingredients. There are safer cleaning agents and safer paints and varnishes.

 (see Chapter 6: Cleaning Agents)

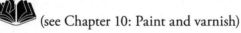 (see Chapter 10: Paint and varnish)

Trichloroethylene and perchloroethylene—Trichloroethylene (TCE), also known as Triclene and Vitran, and perchloroethylene (PCE), also known as tetrachloroethylene, are solvents with a wide variety of industrial uses. Both can be found in spot removers and aerosol sprays. During the use of an aerosol spray, PCE is released by evaporation, and 100 percent is emitted to the air.[3] PCE is also used in the dry cleaning industry as a solvent; dry-cleaned clothes may emit PCE vapors for many months. High concentrations of TCE and PCE (particularly in poorly ventilated areas) can cause dizziness, headache, sleepiness, confusion, nausea, and difficulty in speaking and walking. The National Institute for Occupational Safety and Health considers these chemicals to be potential carcinogens. Reduce or eliminate the use of aerosol sprays. Also limit the purchasing of clothing that must be dry-cleaned. Always wash permanent press fabrics before wearing.

 (see Chapter 9: Fabric treatments)

Xylene/toluene—Xylene and toluene are petroleum derivatives. They are used in cleaning agents as well as in paints and in the making of some plastics. These two chemicals are also common constituents in cosmetics—especially fingernail polish. Much research has been conducted on toluene because of its abuse as an inhalant. Chronic exposure has been shown to cause permanent damage to the central nervous system. It has also been linked with hearing and color vision losses. Chronic low-level exposure to toluene causes headaches, confusion, weakness, and loss of appetite.[4] Low-level exposure to xylene is suspected of causing nervous system damage and may lead to delayed growth in children.[5]

 (see Chapter 7: Common toxic chemicals in personal care products)

The Major VOCs and Their Common Sources

	Formaldehyde	Xylene/Toluene	Benzene	TCE/PCE	Ammonia	Alcohols	Acetone
Adhesives	X	X	X	X		X	
Carpeting	X					X	
Caulking	X	X	X			X	
Ceiling tiles	X	X	X			X	
Cleaning products					X		
Cosmetics	X					X	X
Draperies	X						
Dry-cleaned fabric	X			X			
Floor coverings	X	X	X			X	
Gas stoves	X						
Nail polish remover							X
Paints	X	X	X	X		X	
Paper towels	X						
Particleboard	X	X	X			X	
Photocopiers		X	X	X	X		
Plywood	X						
Shampoo	X						
Stains and varnishes	X	X	X			X	
Tobacco smoke	X		X				
Upholstery	X						
Wall coverings		X	X			X	

Indoor pesticides

Pesticides are intended to kill pests. Their vapors are poisonous and can seriously affect the quality of indoor air. Indoor pesticides in the form of aerosol ant and roach killers, impregnated strips, and foggers ("bug bombs") persist longer than outdoor pesticides because of the absence of wind, water, and sunlight to help remove or neutralize them. The immediate symptoms of exposure to pesticides may include headaches, dizziness, stomach cramps, fatigue, nausea, and skin and eye irritation. Pregnant women are particularly at risk; animal test data suggest that exposure to pesticides during pregnancy and early childhood may impair neurodevelopment. Studies have also linked the use of indoor pesticides with leukemia and other diseases.[6] There are several alternatives to toxic pesticides.

 (see Chapter 11: Pesticides)

Fire retardants (PBDEs)

In our modern world, most furniture, bedding, and electronics are treated with chemicals to make them flame resistant. Polybrominated diphenyl ethers (PBDEs) are the most common of a class of fire retardants known as brominated fire retardants. They are not chemically bound to the materials they treat. They leach into the air and are eventually found in food, water, and in our bodies. In animal studies, PBDE exposure causes neurological damage, behavioral changes, and memory loss. Exposure to PBDEs may also affect thyroid function and reproduction. Sweden was the first country to monitor humans for the build-up of PBDEs in breast milk. Scientists found that between 1972 and 1997, PBDE levels in human breast milk doubled every five years. Ask about PBDEs when purchasing furniture, bedding, and electronic equipment.

 (see Chapter 9: Flame retardants)

Formaldehyde

Formaldehyde is a chemical found in virtually all indoor environments. It is used in everything from carpets, furniture, and permanent-press fabrics to construction and building materials (paneling, insulation foam, and pressed-wood products). It is present in shampoo and in many paper products, including facial tissues, grocery bags, and paper towels, because it is used in the paper-processing industry. Urea-formaldehyde resins are used as stiffeners, wrinkle resisters, water repellents, fire retardants, and adhesive binders in floor coverings, carpet backings, and permanent-press clothing.

Formaldehyde irritates the mucous membranes of the eyes, nose, and throat. It is also a highly reactive chemical that combines with protein and can cause skin irritation and allergic contact dermatitis. The most widely reported symptoms from exposure to formaldehyde include headaches and eye irritation. Until recently, the most serious disease attributed to formaldehyde was asthma. However, recent research reports that long-term exposure to formaldehyde is strongly suspected of causing cancer and birth defects.[7]

Formaldehyde goes by many chemical and trade names. Some of the most common are:

- Formalin
- Methanal
- Methyl aldehyde
- Methylene oxide
- Morbicid acid
- Oxymethylene

When purchasing carpet, floor coverings, furniture, or drapes, avoid those that outgas formaldehyde. These include fabrics with stain repellents, brominated flame-retardants, and permanent-press treatments. Select carpets and furniture that are made of natural, untreated fibers. If you are moving into a new home or if you have recently redecorated, consider airing out your home for several weeks before you inhabit the residence. Especially avoid re-carpeting while pregnant; formaldehyde is suspected of being a reproductive toxin that can damage the developing fetus. This should also be a consideration when carpeting a room for a new baby. Infants are especially vulnerable to formaldehyde and other reproductive toxins.

 (see Chapter 10: Floor coverings)

Even clothing contains fabric finishes that will outgas formaldehyde. Some fabric finishes can be reduced by washing, but many are intended to remain in the fabric for the life of the clothing. When purchasing clothing, look for natural, organic fibers. These will contain fewer (if any) chemicals and they will support a more natural living environment.

 (see Chapter 9: Fabric treatments)

Candles

Candles are fast becoming one of the most common, unrecognized sources of indoor air pollution. Part of the candle craze may be due to new interest in aromatherapy, releasing natural fragrances into the air to provide pleasant aromas. Ironically, the very candles intended to freshen the atmosphere can cause serious health problems. As an alternative, put a few drops of an essential oil in a diffuser or into warm water when you want to freshen up the environment.

Common scented candles are made of paraffin wax, which is oil-based and can produce soot. This is a real problem for people who have asthma or for those with upper respiratory problems. Besides the soot, the smoke may contain VOCs. Soy candles make a great alternative to common paraffin candles. They offer many advantages. Soy candles are non-toxic, they burn clean, and they burn 50 to 60 percent longer than common candles. Soy candles are also easy to clean up—with hot water and soap—you'll never ruin another table or carpet. When soy candles are scented with natural essential oils they can provide long lasting ambiance for a variety of settings. The melting soy can be used as a moisturizer during massage (see sources).

 (see Chapter 1: Lead in candles)

BIOLOGICAL AIR POLLUTANTS
(Mold, Dust mites, Bacteria, Viruses, Pollen)

Biological air pollutants are found in every home. As a group, they represent some of the most prevalent and some of the most serious of the indoor air pollutants. They can cause allergies, infections, and hypersensitivity disorders. Sources of biological pollutants include outdoor air, which harbors pollen and insects; water reservoirs, such as humidifiers and air conditioners, which harbor mold and bacteria; and the household inhabitants themselves, which harbor bacteria, viruses, and pet dander. Many air pollutants can be overcome with indoor air filtration devices, and many allergies respond to changes in diet that include whole food nutrition.

 (see Chapter 19: Nutrition)

Mold

One of the worst of the biological air pollutants is molds. These are microscopic fungi that live on plant and animal matter. Warm and humid conditions encourage their growth. Humidity, even in arid climates, can build up inside the home environment—especially in places where water is used. Areas of the country that experience high humidity are even more prone to mold. Anywhere there is standing water or high humidity, mold will grow. Flooding, continually damp carpeting (which may occur when carpet is installed on poorly ventilated concrete floors), and inadequate ventilation in bathrooms and kitchens can be sources of major mold problems. Appliances, such as humidifiers, dehumidifiers, air conditioners, and drip pans under cooling coils (in refrigerators), also foster the growth of bacteria and mold; they can cause what has been referred to as *humidifier fever*.

 (see Chapter 1: Humidifier fever)

Most biological pollutants, including molds, can be filtered out of indoor air. The problem with mold is that it is very difficult (especially in the home environment) to maintain enough air movement to keep up with an ongoing source of mold. Air filtration devices are best placed in areas of concern and in areas where inhabitants spend considerable amounts of time (such as in bedrooms).

 (see Chapter 1: Air-cleaning devices)

The best level of control is the complete removal of any contaminated items. This often includes completely replacing wallboard, sheet rock, carpeting, or damaged wood. For minor instances, spray hydrogen peroxide (drugstore dilution), and allow these areas to dry completely. Keep relative humidity below 50 percent and keep equipment water reservoirs clean. Use exhaust fans in bathrooms and kitchens, and make sure clothes dryers are vented to the outside. Be sure there is no standing water in air conditioners, humidifiers, and dehumidifiers. Rigorous, daily, and end-of-season cleaning, coupled with disinfection, are the most effective measures for the control of mold.

Dust and dust mites

Dust mites are tiny insects found in every home. They are invisible to the naked eye. They don't burrow under the skin, they are not parasitic, and they do not bite. The concern with dust mites is that people sometimes experience allergic reactions. Body parts and feces from dust mites can trigger asthma and can cause asthma in children. Most often this occurs when individuals have been sensitized by other chemicals and when their immune system is already compromised. Symptoms associated with dust mite allergies include sneezing, itchy, watery eyes, nasal stuffiness, runny nose, respiratory problems, eczema, and asthma. Many people notice these symptoms when dust is stirred up during cleaning. But dust itself contains other allergens, including pet dander, cigarette ash, insect droppings, mold spores, and pollen.

Dust mites feed on human skin flakes. They are most commonly found in mattresses, pillows, carpets, upholstered furniture, bedcovers, clothes, and stuffed toys. To thrive, dust mites need warm temperatures (75–80° F) and high humidity levels (70–80 percent). When air temperatures are below 70° F and when humidity is below 50 percent, mite populations stop growing and die out. The best way to keep dust mite populations low is to keep temperature and humidity levels under control.

The use of an organic, cotton barrier cloth is also helpful for those with allergies to dust mites. The fabric used in barrier cloths is woven in a tight, overlapping pattern and has a higher thread count (usually 250+). These organic, toxin-free covers dramatically reduce dust mite populations by keeping skin flakes from penetrating the mattress where dust mites live (see sources). Another good way to minimize dust mite populations is to wash all bedding weekly. Laundering with very warm water (above 90° F) removes nearly all dust mite and allergens from bedding.

Dusting and vacuuming are also important to keep dust and dust mites under control. Regular, thorough vacuuming of carpets, furniture, textiles, and draperies will help. Dust furniture with a wet cloth *before* you vacuum to avoid scattering the dust. There are vacuums with high-efficiency particulate air (HEPA) filters designed for use by people with dust allergies. Hardwood floors with washable area rugs are ideal.

 (see Chapter 1: Vacuums)

Air filters with HEPA capacity are also effective for those allergic to dust and dust mites—especially in confined areas like the bedroom. Research at the University of Texas-Austin found HEPA filtration to be much more effective at removing dust than ion-generating air purifiers that cause particles to fall out of circulating air.[8]

 (see Chapter1: Air-cleaning devices)

Bacteria and viruses

Bacterial pollutants are everywhere. Most can be filtered from the air. The key is air *movement* so that indoor air gets filtered regularly. Bacteria can be neutralized in other ways. The use of essential oils is one way. Within each drop of essential oil, there are trillions of molecules. Some oils have antibacterial and antiviral properties.

 (see Chapter 1: Essential oils)

Pollen

Pollen is a tricky type of allergen that causes difficulty for many people. Pollen is easily airborne and can be tracked indoors by people, animals, or by a simple gust of wind. Since pollen is one of the smallest particles of concern in indoor air, it is an area of focus for many air cleaners. The best filtering systems to rid the air of pollen are HEPA filtering systems or electrostatic technology.

 (see Chapter 1: Air-cleaning devices)

HEAVY METALS

Lead vapor

The link between lead exposure and a number of severe health effects is well established. Long-term exposure in children can affect a child's growth. It can damage kidneys and cause learning and behavioral problems.[9] According to the American Academy of Pediatrics, an estimated three to four million children in the United States under age six have blood lead levels that could cause impaired development.[10] Lead poisoning via ingestion has been the most widely publicized cause. However, airborne lead is also a source of toxicity.

Even though indoor paint is now virtually lead-free, older homes and furniture built before 1978 may still be coated with leaded paint. Often, lead paint is exposed during renovation projects. Under these circumstances, lead dust and fumes can permeate the air inhaled by both adults and children.

AMF carries a line of coatings called Safecoat, made without toxic ingredients. These products create a "safe coating" with a unique molecular configuration designed to seal surfaces (including wood, metal, concrete, carpets, and many more), thus reducing outgassing and the release of toxins like lead. These products are great for new paint jobs and for sealing old, potentially harmful surfaces (see sources).

Additional sources of airborne lead include art and craft materials, from which lead is not banned, and some older scented candles. Significant quantities of lead are still found in many artistic paints and ceramic glazes, stained glass, and in some solder used in jewelry making. Other paints that are exempted from the ban on lead, and which require no warning label, include the lead-containing paint used for the backing on mirrors and metal furniture (other than children's furniture) that has a factory-applied paint. Check with manufacturers before purchasing.

> Do not buy lead-containing jewelry. If you are unsure, rub the piece of jewelry across a white cloth. If it leaves a mark, it likely contains lead.

Hazardous levels of atmospheric lead are also notoriously found at firing ranges. Make sure the indoor firing range you choose is clean and well ventilated, and always wear a respirator. Be careful to wash your hands and clothing before tracking lead dust back into your home.

Paint for artists

Lead has been one of the most toxic substances used by artists through the centuries. Once it is in the body, its effects are cumulative and can cause serious long-term health problems. In extreme cases, lead can cause irreversible brain damage, anemia, convulsions, and death. Paint for artists is exempted from the ban on lead. This means that artists' paint may contain lead, and no warning is required on the label.

Lead from pigments in paint can enter a painter's body if they get into the artist's mouth, if they penetrate the skin through cuts and scratches, or if the painter inhales vapors. Artists and their families are continually exposed to lead unless precautions are taken. The powdered nature of some pigments is the biggest hazard. It is suspected that several famous artists struggled with symptoms of lead poisoning.

Today, there are plenty of nontoxic artists' paints available. The CP (Certified Product), AP (Approved Product), and HL Health Label (Nontoxic) seals identify art materials that are safe and those that are certified to contain no materials in sufficient quantities to be toxic or to cause health problems. Artists who take a few simple precautions will make painting as safe as any other artist's activity.

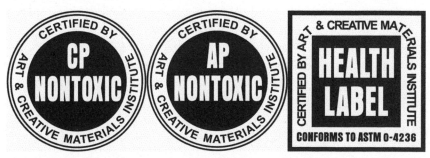

Tips for the Artist

1. Avoid lead-based paint and other lead-containing artists' supplies.
2. Wear a dust mask or respirator.
3. While working with powdered pigments, wear a long-sleeved smock, latex gloves, goggles, and a dust mask. Never leave the lid off a pigment container once you are finished with it.
4. Never heat pigments—they can give off toxic fumes.
5. Do not smoke, do not eat, and do not answer the phone until after you have washed your hands.
6. Protect open wounds. Wear gloves.
7. Make certain your work area is clean with lids fully secured before leaving your work area.
8. Dispose of lead-based products as you would dispose of other hazardous waste. Contact your local waste management facility for local guidelines.

Lead in candles

Some candle wicks are limp and tend to fall over into the wax, extinguishing the flame. Metal wicks keep candles burning longer, and they reduce *mushrooming* at the wick tip. But some older candles (made before 2001) contain lead, which is volatilized as the candle is burned. This contributes to high levels of lead in the air and on dust particles. Besides breathing lead fumes, occupants (especially children) are exposed to more lead that is eventually deposited on the floor, furniture, and walls.

In 1999, a study conducted by the University of Michigan School of Public Health examined the emissions from fifteen different brands of candles made in the United States, Mexico, and China. The study showed that lead emission rates ranged between 0.04 to 13.1 micrograms per cubic meter, which compares to the U.S. EPA upper recommendation of 1.5 micrograms per cubic meter for ambient air. After one hour, five of the fifteen candles tested had emitted unsafe levels of lead into the air. After five hours, the lead levels ranged from an estimated 0.21 to 65.3 micrograms per cubic meter. Candles produced in China and the United States released the highest levels of lead.[11] In 2001, candles with lead wicks were banned. However, many people still have candles purchased before that time. Discard older candles and don't use candles in jars when the candle leaves a soot ring on the jar's lip. Look for candles labeled to have lead-free wicks. Even better, select soy candles with 100% cotton wicks (see sources).

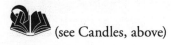 (see Candles, above)

Mercury vapor

Even tiny amounts of liquid mercury (just a few drops) can vaporize and reach levels that may be harmful to health. Mercury vapors may cause shortness of breath, nausea, vomiting, diarrhea, skin rashes, and eye irritation. Exposure to mercury vapors can also lead to damage of the central nervous system. Developing fetuses and young children are particularly vulnerable to the health effects of mercury.

Most thermometers these days are digital, but older mercury thermometers still exist. A broken mercury thermometer is a potentially serious exposure problem. Other common sources of mercury are blood pressure gauges, some thermostats, and even fluorescent light tubes. If you break one of these mercury-containing devices, DO NOT use a vacuum or a broom to clean up. These methods will distribute mercury vapors throughout the house.

 (see Chapter 10: Fluorescent lighting)

Mercury Clean-up

To clean up mercury, put on rubber gloves (never touch mercury with your bare hands). If the mercury is spilled on a hard surface or on a tightly woven fabric, use stiff paper to push mercury beads together. Use an eyedropper to suction mercury beads. Pick up any remaining beads of mercury with sticky tape. On a carpet or a rug, the mercury-contaminated section should be completely cut out and placed in a plastic bag with all the cleanup items. Vacuuming will contaminate the air for long periods of time. In a drain, mercury will get caught in the drain trap. Working over a tray, remove the drain trap and pour the contents into a plastic bag. After any clean up procedure, always label bags as mercury waste and call your state Pollution Control Agency for appropriate disposal.

Some paint may contain toxic levels of mercury. Interior latex (water-based) paint containing phenylmercuric acetate as a preservative was in use until 1990. Latex paints containing hazardous levels of mercury may still remain in some homes—left over after their initial use. Dispose of old interior latex paint manufactured prior to 1990.

RADON

Radon is a naturally-occurring, invisible, odorless, radioactive gas that comes from natural radioactive deposits in soil, rock, and water. It is harmlessly dispersed in outdoor air, but when trapped in buildings, it can reach toxic levels. All soils and rocks have radium, but some have much more than others.

During the winter, warm indoor air escapes through the top of the house. As a result, the pressure inside the house is lower than the pressure outside, so air is drawn into the house—this includes air from the soil around the house. Basements have a lot of surface area exposed to the soil, so radon can easily enter a basement. Basement concentrations are often more than twice as high as concentrations on upper floors. Areas in the Northern United States are considered to be at the greatest risk. However, depending on a variety of factors, small pockets in many areas of the country are at risk for radon.

Radon has a short half-life (four days) and decays into other solid, radioactive substances. These radioactive particles are inhaled and remain lodged in the lungs, causing continued exposure. Radon is thus the second leading cause of lung cancer after smoking. It accounts for fifteen thousand to twenty thousand cancer deaths per year in the United States alone.[12] A 1999 study found that even very small exposure to radon can result in lung cancer; There is no lower threshold below which radon levels are harmless.[13]

Many people think that radon concentrations can be accurately predicted from geologic information alone. Although this is a good place to start, geologic maps do not include soil permeability data, which is also a factor. The only way to determine if you have a radon problem—no matter what part of the country you live in—is to take radon measurements in your home. The amount of radon in the air is measured in "pico Curies per liter of air," or pCi/L. Average concentrations over 4 pCi/L are considered high. Outdoor radon levels are usually between 0.2–0.7 pCi/L.

Within the last year, some kitchen countertops made of granite have been found to be radioactive and to emit radon. Granite is a common source of both radioactivity and radon. Experts agree that most granite countertops emit radon at extremely low levels. Depending on what type of granite is installed and where it came from, kitchen countertops could be a problem. Some of the more exotic types of granite may be the worst. Red, pink, and purple colors appear to emit more radon than other colors.

A nuclear physicist at Rice University in Houston conducted preliminary testing on granite countertop materials. His initial findings indicated that most granite is safe but that there is cause for concern. A handful of samples showed radiation levels one hundred times above background levels.[14] This could be a problem—especially for pregnant women and young children who spend considerable time in the kitchen. According to experts, the only way to tell if your countertops are radioactive or releasing radon gas is to test them. Radon test kits are available at most hardware stores.

Radon exposure has no immediate symptoms. Lung cancers usually occur five to twenty-five years after exposure. Being aware of a potential problem is important. Even though radon is invisible, it's easy to measure. There are many inexpensive, do-it-yourself radon test kits available from retail outlets or through the Internet. Look for state-certified kits or those that meet the requirements of the National Radon Proficiency Program. You can also hire a trained contractor to do the testing for you. Radon information on a state by state basis is available at this Web site: http://www.epa.gov/iaq/whereyoulive.html.

A variety of methods can be used to reduce radon in homes. Sealing cracks and other openings in the foundation is a basic part of most approaches to radon reduction. In most cases, a system with vent pipes and fans is used to reduce radon. The right system depends on the design of your home and other factors. If you discover radon coming from granite countertops and cannot have them removed, ventilation is the next best solution. Open the windows as often as possible. A Home Buyers and Sellers Guide to Radon is available at this Web site: http://www.epa.gov/radon/pubs/hmbyguid.html. It includes what to do if you have a radon problem.

SICK BUILDING SYNDROME

The term "sick building syndrome" describes a circumstance where shared symptoms among building occupants appear to be linked to the amount of time spent in a building. There has been extensive speculation about the causes of sick building syndrome. Poor design, maintenance, and operation of ventilation systems may be at fault. Specific pollutants may be the cause—or at least they may contribute to the health effects. But most often, sick building syndrome is associated with newly constructed or remodeled buildings. This suggests that the chemicals used in construction products and furnishings are the major culprit. A 1984 World Health Organization report revealed that as high as 30 percent of new and remodeled buildings worldwide were the cause of complaints related to indoor air quality.[15]

 (see Chapter 10: Home Construction and Remodeling)

The following factors (alone or in combination) are likely to contribute to sick building syndrome:

- Inadequate ventilation
- Humidity (too low or too high)
- Chemical contaminants that enter the building through poorly located air intake vents

- Volatile organic compounds (VOCs), including synthetic fragrances in cleaning and maintenance products
- Environmental tobacco smoke
- Combustion by-products from unvented space heaters
- Molds and bacteria circulated in heating and air-conditioning systems
- Fluorescent lighting

 (see Chapter 10: Fluorescent lighting)

- Electromagnetic frequencies from computers and other electrical equipment

 (see Chapter 3: Electromagnetic Smog)

Typical symptoms of sick building syndrome include headaches, irritability, mood swings, inability to concentrate, anxiety, congestion, and a feeling of "spaciness." If you experience any of these symptoms on a regular basis, look for things you can do to improve ventilation, like opening windows or doors. Watch for the use of fragrances, cleaning agents, or air fresheners that can be eliminated. If these measures do not provide relief, gather evidence from other occupants of the building who may have experienced similar symptoms and meet with the owner of the building or with your local health department.

HUMIDIFIER FEVER

Humidifier fever is often confused with sick building syndrome. Unlike sick building syndrome, humidifier fever has a specific cause. Humidifier fever is caused by breathing water droplets from contaminated humidifiers (or from forced-air heating and air-conditioning systems, as well as from separate console units like those often used in homes), causing a variety of allergic reactions and respiratory symptoms. Humidifier fever has been reported more often in industrial buildings than in offices or public buildings, and it is a particular problem in printing establishments where humidity is high and paper dust provides nutrients for microbes.

The acute symptoms are like those of the flu—fever, cough, aching limbs, headache, tiredness, and lethargy—although the symptoms don't last as long as the flu. Symptoms usually develop on the first day back at work after the weekend or other break; they start only after a person has been back in the environment for several hours. Often, symptoms become more severe in the evening *after* a person has left work.

As with most other indoor air quality problems, controlling the source of the problem is the key. Be sure there is no standing water in air conditioners, humidifiers, and dehumidifiers. Regular replacement of filters, rigorous, daily, and end-of-season cleaning coupled with disinfection are the most effective methods of control.

ALLERGIES

Allergies to airborne pollutants are often the first sign of immune system deficiency. They present an opportunity to address chemical exposure *before* symptoms progress to more serious problems. Eyes, nose, throat, and sinuses are particularly vulnerable to chemical damage because they are usually the first to be exposed to pollutants. Mucus membranes are more porous and they absorb pollutants easily. Air purifiers placed in the bedroom or in the work area are extremely helpful for those with allergies.

 (see Chapter 1: Air-cleaning devices)

Allergies often respond to detoxification programs and to changes in diet. In fact, many (if not most) health problems respond to these programs. Organic, whole food nutrition will support the immune system and help to lower the body's burden of toxic chemicals. Some vitamins and minerals (vitamin C and magnesium) actually act as natural antihistamines. When taken as a part of a whole food diet, they can help bring balance to the immune system and they can provide support for many of the body's other functions.

 (see Chapter 19: Detoxification)

 (see Chapter 19: Nutrition)

MULTIPLE CHEMICAL SENSITIVITY

The National Institute of Environmental Health Sciences has defined multiple chemical sensitivity (MCS) as a "chronic, recurring disease caused by a person's inability to tolerate an environmental chemical or class of foreign chemicals." MCS is an adverse reaction to low levels of chemicals found in modern environments. This condition has also been referred to as toxic injury and environmental illness. There is no single stimulus, and at this time there is great debate over whether MCS symptoms result through immunologic, neurological, or psychological means (or a combination). Those who suffer from MCS complain of nonspecific symptoms from exposure to tiny levels of chemical, biological, or physical agents. Symptoms include headaches, itchy eyes, runny nose, sleepiness, heart palpitations, nausea, anxiety, aching joints and/or muscles, and scratchy throat.

A person with MCS somehow becomes sensitized to a chemical or class of chemicals. Subsequent exposure to even tiny amounts of the same chemical can bring about severe symptoms. The MCS sufferer usually becomes sensitive to a broad range of toxic chemicals—even though the initial sensitization may only have been to a single chemical. This suggests an immune reaction, which becomes generalized over a range of toxins. It also suggests that those with weakened immune systems are at the greatest risk. Healthy individuals usually experience no symptoms—even though they may be repeatedly exposed to the same toxins.

Many healthcare practitioners do not recognize MCS. For this reason, it is not possible to assess the number of people who actually suffer from it. More women than men claim to have MCS, and it appears to occur most often in people between the ages of 30 and 50 years. MCS can be so debilitating that a person cannot function outside of a tiny, well-guarded set of environmental conditions. Some individuals become homebound, but there are ways to break free. Sometimes MCS can be as simple as discovering and treating a parasitic infection or candida (yeast) overgrowth. Often, improved health does not manifest until a person acknowledges the emotional and spiritual connections with MCS. Emotions and beliefs can play a huge role in overcoming illnesses.[16]

 (see Chapter16: Toxic Thoughts and Emotions)

Numerous organizations and support groups exist for those with MCS. A very helpful online workshop can be found at: http://www.nap.edu/openbook.php?isbn=0309047366.

AIR-CLEANING DEVICES

Air-cleaning devices can provide great relief for those who are sensitive to indoor air pollutants. They often end up helping those who didn't realize they were sensitive. Many people find that when they begin using an air-cleaning device in their bedroom or at the office, their sinuses clear up or they sleep better. Although they can be extremely helpful, air-cleaning devices should not be used as a way to avoid taking care of the source of a potentially deeper problem. Getting to and removing the source of the problem is still the best solution.

The subject of air-cleaning devices can be complex. The following section is intended to give you an overview of the variety of devices available and how they work. It is not intended to be all-inclusive. Air-cleaning devices are designed to remove pollutants in one of three ways: particle removal, gaseous removal, and pollutant destruction.

Particle removal

Both mechanical and electronic air cleaners remove particulate matter from the air. Mechanical air cleaners remove particles by capturing them on filters. This type of air cleaner includes everything from everyday furnace filters to high-efficiency particulate air (HEPA) filters. Electronic air cleaners such as electrostatic precipitators use a process called electrostatic attraction to trap charged particles. They draw air through an ionization chamber where particles obtain an electrical charge. The charged particles then accumulate on a series of charged plates called collectors. Air ionizers work in a similar way but without a collector. Ionizers release charged particles into the air. The charge is attracted to airborne particles, causing them to attach to nearby surfaces or to settle faster; this keeps them out of the breathable air. A 2005 study showed that HEPA filtration was more efficient at removing particles from the air than were ionizers.[17] However, ionizers offer other benefits, as described later in this chapter.

 (see Chapter 1: Efficiency ratings)

 (see Chapter 1: Air ionizers)

Gaseous removal

Gas-phase air filters remove gases and many VOCs by using materials called sorbents. Sorbents, such as activated carbon, absorb gaseous pollutants. Some air-cleaning devices with gas-phase filters may remove a portion of the gases and VOCs; however, none are capable of removing all of the gaseous pollutants present in a typical home. Carbon monoxide is one such gas; it is not readily captured using gas-phase filtration.

Pollutant destruction

Some air cleaners use ultraviolet (UV) light technology to destroy indoor pollutants. These air cleaners are called ultraviolet germicidal irradiation (UVGI) cleaners and photocatalytic oxidation (PCO) cleaners. Ozone generators that are sold as air cleaners intentionally produce ozone gas to destroy pollutants. These are not recommended. (There are currently no standards for the measurement of the effectiveness of UVGI or PCO air cleaners.)

- **UVGI cleaners** use ultraviolet radiation from UV lamps to destroy airborne biological pollutants such as viruses, bacteria, allergens, and molds. They can be used with, but not as a replacement for, filtration systems.
- **PCO cleaners** use a UV lamp along with a substance called a catalyst that reacts with the light. They are intended to destroy gaseous pollutants by converting them into harmless products. Like the UVGI cleaners, they are not designed to remove particulate pollutants. If used, they should be used with air filtration systems.
- **Ozone generators** use UV light or an electrical discharge to intentionally produce ozone. Ozone generators have a great capacity to remove particles, gases, and biological pollutants. However, because ozone is a strong oxidant and also a lung irritant, ozone generators are not recommended for home environments unless residents are outside the home during and immediately following operation. Ozone generators are an excellent way to clear odors and contaminants after flooding or fire, but they are not recommended as a routine, in-home air cleaner.

Air-Cleaning Devices and the Pollutants They Control

	Air-Cleaning Device	*Pollutants Controlled*
Filtration	Air filters	Particles
	Gas-phase filters	Gases
Other Air Cleaners	UVGI	Biologicals
	PCO	Gases
	Ozone generators	Particles, gases, and biologicals

In-duct particle removal

Air-cleaning devices are designed to either function from the existing ductwork in heat, ventilation, and air-conditioning (HVAC) systems or as portable air cleaners. Most mechanical air filters are good at capturing larger airborne particles such as dust, pollen, dust mite and insect allergens, some molds, and animal dander. However, because these particles settle rather quickly, air filters are not very good at completely removing them from indoor areas. Although human activities such as walking and vacuuming can stir up particles, most of the larger particles will resettle before an in-duct air filter can remove them.

Besides placing an air filter in your HVAC system, you can also install filters to individual vents in each room throughout the house. This added protection traps lint, dust, and pollen particles. This type of filtration media is available in most hardware stores and it can easily be cut to fit each vent.

Efficiency ratings

Consumers can select a particle removal air filter by looking at its efficiency rating. Efficiency is measured by the minimum efficiency reporting value (MERV) for air filters installed in the ductwork. MERV ratings range from a low of one to a high of twenty. Some residential HVAC systems may not have enough fan or motor capacity to accommodate higher-efficiency filters. HVAC manufacturer's information should be checked prior to upgrading filters.

- **Flat or panel (low-efficiency) air filters** with a MERV of one to four are commonly used in residential furnaces and air conditioners. They are used to protect the HVAC equipment and are not intended for direct indoor air quality control. They have low efficiency on small airborne particles (viruses, bacteria, some mold spores, a significant fraction of cat and dog allergens, and a portion of dust mite allergens).
- **Pleated or extended surface filters** with a MERV rating between five and thirteen are considered medium-efficiency filters. These are reasonably efficient at removing small to large airborne particles. Filters with a MERV rating between seven and thirteen are nearly as effective as true HEPA filters at controlling most indoor airborne particles. Medium-efficiency air filters are less expensive than HEPA filters and allow higher airflow rates.
- **High-efficiency filters** with a MERV rating of fourteen to sixteen, sometimes misidentified as HEPA filters, are similar in appearance to true HEPA filters which have MERV values of seventeen to twenty. True HEPA filters are normally not installed in residential HVAC systems; installation of a HEPA filter in an existing HVAC system would require professional modification of the system because the filters require an increase in airflow.

> To qualify as a true HEPA filter, a filter must be able to capture at least 99.97 percent of all particles that are 0.3 microns in diameter or larger.

In-duct gaseous pollutant removal

Gas-phase filters are much less commonly used in homes than particle air filters. The useful lifetime of gas-phase filters can be short because the filter material can quickly become overloaded and typically needs to be replaced often. There is also a concern that, when full, these filters may release trapped pollutants back into the air. For most residential in-duct systems, gas-phase filters are not feasible.

In-duct pollutant destruction

UVGI and PCO cleaners used in in-duct applications may have limited effectiveness in killing bacteria and molds, simply because the pollutants do not always move through ductwork. These filters are usually more effective as portable units used where they are needed.

Portable air cleaners

Portable air cleaners offer the advantage that they may be moved from room to room and used when localized air cleaning is needed. They are most often used in the bedroom to provide clean air during the night. Some of the best portable air cleaners contain a fan to help move the air, and they use a combination of the air-cleaning methods discussed above.

Austin Air makes an exceptional line of portable air cleaners that use a combination of activated charcoal to trap some gasses, true HEPA filtration for 99.7 percent of particulate removal, and granular carbon/zeolite to remove mold. Some models also remove formaldehyde and ammonia. These units are constructed with 360-degree intake and three-speed fan motors. All include a five-year warranty with filters that last a full five years (see sources).

AIR IONIZERS

Ions are small particles with an electrical charge (either positive or negative). In nature, there are between a few hundred and a few thousand ions per cubic centimeter of air. The natural balance is nearly equal, with slightly more positive than negative ions. At times, the outdoor balance can shift, causing a predominance of positive ions that coincides with asthma attacks and other respiratory problems. The Santa Ana winds in Southern California are a good example. In contrast, the air by the ocean or adjacent to waterfalls has an unusually high concentration of negative ions, often associated with feelings of exhilaration and a heightened sense of well-being.

The negative ion count in fresh, country air is 2,000–4,000 ions per cubic centimeter. At Yosemite falls, the negative ion count is considerably greater (over 100,000 per cubic centimeter). On a Los Angeles freeway during rush hour, the negative ion count may be as low as 100 per cubic centimeter.

An organism receiving pure air for breathing is condemned to death if the air does not contain at least a small quantity of air ions.[18] Without ions, we cannot absorb oxygen, and the fewer ions there are, the lower the efficiency of our minds and bodies. The effect of ions on respiration has been known since the 1950s. Negative ion generators have been used in U.S. submarines. They are also used in military aircraft because they are known to improve alertness and response time for pilots.

In 1958, U.S. experimenters gave sixteen volunteers an overdose of positive ions for just twenty minutes; all of them developed dry throats, husky voices, headaches, and itchy or obstructed noses. Five of the volunteers were tested for total breathing capacity, and it was found that positive ions reduced breathing capacity by 30 percent.[19]

In 1966 at a hospital in Jerusalem, thirty-eight infants between the ages of two and twelve months old who were suffering from respiratory problems were divided into two groups. One group was given negative ion–enriched air; the other group was treated with traditional medications. Researchers reported that the group of children receiving negative ions recovered more rapidly and was less prone to relapses. They also found that babies receiving negative ions didn't cry as much.[20]

More recently in Britain, two Oxford University statisticians conducted a study among one hundred participants with asthma, bronchitis, and hay fever, chosen from a list of people who had purchased negative ion generators. They found that eighteen of twenty-four asthmatics, thirteen of seventeen bronchitis sufferers, and eleven of twelve with hay fever reported that negative ion generators had noticeably improved their conditions. A few even claimed the generator had cured them.

Forced-air heating and air conditioning systems set up friction resulting in the loss of ions from indoor air. What finally comes out of most heating or air conditioning outlets is overloaded with positive ions, which can upset the mental and physical equilibrium of everyone, and not just those who are sensitive.

Negative ion generators put negative ions back into the indoor air environment. They can support numerous respiratory conditions, and they are a recommended as part of any air treatment program. Ion generators also help to remove positively-charged dust particles and other particulate matter from the air.

Some of the first ion generators produced a significant amount of ozone, but newer models do not produce enough to be harmful unless the generator is placed directly in someone's face. The industry is well regulated. Bionaire sells an excellent line of negative ion generators, some in combination with HEPA filtration. These can be found at most department stores.

CAUTION: If you use a negative ion generator in your bedroom at night, be aware that the negative ions will keep you alert and may lessen the quality of your sleep. Some ion generators are combined with air filters and have an on/off switch for negative ion generation so that you can use just the filter at night.

Air Exchangers

Air exchangers are not air cleaners. They have a dual purpose: to recover heating or cooling energy and to improve indoor air quality by bringing in outside air on a consistent basis. Air exchangers, also called air-to-air exchangers, draw in air from a port to the outside of the building. The air is passed through a chamber (the exchanger), which is surrounded by indoor air. Highly conductive metal or other materials remove the energy (heat) from the warmer air and pass it on (exchange it) to the cooler air. Fresh air is then ducted into the house, and the indoor air is sent outside. Up to 80 percent of the energy can be exchanged, and moisture from humid air can be pumped outside.

Air exchangers are meant to completely exchange the air in a home about six times a day. In some states, air exchangers fulfill new construction code requirements for improving indoor air quality. However, if they are not well maintained, they can be an additional source of air pollution. This article found on the wikipedia Web site discusses the concept of air exchangers in greater detail:
http://en.wikipedia.org/wiki/Heat_recovery_ventilation

Duct Cleaning

Since conditions in every home are different, it is impossible to generalize about whether air duct cleaning might be beneficial. Generally, if no one in your household suffers from allergies or unexplained symptoms, and if you see no indication that your air ducts are contaminated with excessive dust or mold, having air ducts cleaned is probably not necessary. It is normal for the return registers to get dusty, but this is not an indication that your air ducts need to be cleaned. Consider having air ducts cleaned if:

- There is visible mold inside ducts or on other components of your heating and cooling system.
- Ducts are infested with insects.
- Offensive odors are coming from the ductwork, and/or if the ducts are actually releasing particles into the home.

If family members are experiencing unusual or unexplained symptoms, air duct cleaning could be one of several things you could do to improve the quality of the air in your living environment. However, *never* allow chemicals to be sprayed into the duct system. Some chemicals are so toxic that they can make a building uninhabitable.

VACUUMS

Carpets are a major reservoir for allergens, and although vacuum cleaning is one of the most common ways of attempting to manage the problem, studies show that the benefits are limited. Traditional vacuuming does little to relieve the irritations of carpet dust and mites. Vacuums with two- or three-layer bags perform better than those with a single-layer bag. The Allergy Buyers club provides ratings on a variety of vacuums: http://www.allergybuyersclubshopping.com/vacuumcleaners.html.   HEPA filters do a better job but the Rainbow vacuum (see below) appears to outperform them all.

HEPA filtered vacuums

Vacuums with HEPA filtration and higher airflow ratings will pull and contain more allergens—especially from bedding, carpets, and upholstery. If you purchase a HEPA-filtered vacuum, make sure that the HEPA filter is positioned in a sealed unit within the vacuum.

Rainbow vacuum

The Rainbow vacuum rivals the very best vacuums on the market. It utilizes a different concept in cleaning, and it is the only vacuum to also be certified as an air cleaner. The vacuum deposits dirt into a water reservoir, where a separator filters dirt from the air and returns water-washed air back into the home. Water filtration captures 99.997 percent of household dirt—then a HEPA neutralizer ensures that 100 percent clean air is returned to the home.

In a small trial of twenty families with asthma or allergy sufferers, the Rainbow vacuum outperformed other vacuums and provided relief of allergy/asthma symptoms that other vacuums could not.[21] It received the seal of approval from the California Orange County Mothers Against Allergies and Asthma in the Home (see sources).

Essential Oils

The antibacterial properties of plant-derived essential oils have been recognized for hundreds of years—some have antibacterial effects even greater than traditional antibiotics.[22] A recent study conducted at the University of California, Irvine, determined that the vapor from an essential oil blend called Breath Great (see sources) was capable of inhibiting the growth of all five bacteria tested[23] (E coli, Staphylococcus aureus, Staphylococcus epidermidis, Klebsiella pneumoniae, and Proteus vulgaris). These bacteria are responsible for pneumonia and other serious infections.

Essential oils can sometimes provide a much better source of protection than traditional antibiotics. They are easily absorbed into the bloodstream and can have almost immediate effects on blood pressure, bronchiole dilation, hormones, mental clarity, and stress. Unlike overexposure to pharmaceutical antibiotics, exposure to natural oils does not weaken your immune system, and subsequently bacteria do not build resistance to the oils.

> Essential oils were the inspiration for the creation of antibiotics. Their natural antibiotic properties have been extracted, synthesized, and altered to form the antibiotics of our day.

There are many ways to disperse essential oils into the breathing environment of your home or office. These include electric diffusers, steam pumps, and candle lamps. There are also several ways to concentrate the effects of essential oils for individual use. Essential oils of tea tree, rosemary, lavender, niaouli, palmarosa, ravensara aromatica, and eucalyptus are excellent for respiratory ailments, as well as for the elimination of bacterial and viral infections.

CAUTION: Those who suffer from asthma or those who are sensitive are cautioned to introduce their exposure to oils slowly.

Steam tents

Steam tents are an effective way to deliver essential oils to the respiratory tract. For this method, warm a pot of water in a stainless steel or glass container. Add two to three drops of an appropriate oil or oil blend. Cover your head with a towel, and, keeping your eyes shut, breathe the warm air vapor rising from the pot of water for about five minutes at a time. (Oils will evaporate quickly in hot water.) You can do this several times a day to clear sinuses or to help fight bacterial or viral infections. Steam tents are an effective way to ward off a cold. They are a good preventive when you have been exposed to sick people.

Nose cone

The nose cone method of introducing essential oils can be used almost anywhere for rapid results. To make a nose cone, double the thickness of a tissue and cut a two to three inch square. Place two drops of an appropriate blend of oils on the tissue and roll it up to fit in one nostril. Place the dry end in the nostril and breathe for about twenty minutes.

Steam baths

Steam baths are a wonderful way to introduce essential oils. Heat and water help the essential oils to penetrate the skin faster. Inhaling them while in the bath provides rapid respiratory benefits. Run your bath water as warm as you can tolerate. Add between five and fifteen drops of essential oils to the water; up to twenty-five drops can be added for larger bathtubs.

CAUTION: Be careful with citrus oils, as they can irritate the skin; two to four drops is plenty in a bathtub. For additional benefits, add one-half cup of sea salt, one-quarter cup of Epsom salt, and one-quarter cup of baking soda. These salts absorb toxins and prevent them from being reabsorbed into the body. The use of a steam bath is also a wonderful way to stimulate the lymphatic and circulatory systems, and to support detoxification.

 (see Chapter 19: Detoxification baths)

SALT LAMPS

When the sun heats up the largest natural salt solution, the ocean, it generates a natural energy vibration that permeates the planet. Our biology has naturally attuned itself to vibrations and frequencies such as these for thousands of years. They soothe our nervous system and they help us maintain balance in a variety of other ways. Salt lamps create the same natural energy field. They are a strikingly beautiful source of negative ions and balancing vibrations.

The nature of crystalline salt enables it to change back and forth from a crystalline to a liquid state. Gentle heat creates a higher surface temperature than the surrounding air, and tiny amounts of water condense on the crystal's surface. This enables the salt to split into positive (sodium) and negative (chloride) ions. When the water molecules evaporate again, the salt returns to its crystalline form. This natural ionization takes place millions of times each second as negative ions are released into the air. Negative ions become dust collectors, attaching themselves to positively charged dust particles and to other particulate matter.

Tests on hyperactive children with concentration and sleeping disorders have shown that the use of salt lamps reduces the symptoms after only one week—when the lamps were removed, symptoms returned.[24] Studies have also shown that salt lamps can increase the negative ion count. Negative ions benefit asthma patients, those with chronic lung illnesses, and allergy sufferers. They also help improve learning, memory, and emotional well-being (see sources).

 (see Chapter 1: Air ionizers)

Plants

In 1989, when considering ways to provide clean air aboard orbiting space stations, NASA conducted research to determine whether common house plants could reduce indoor air pollutants. Ten common house plants were evaluated for their ability to reduce levels of formaldehyde, benzene, and other airborne contaminants. According to the report, philodendron, spider plant, and golden pothos were the most effective plants for removing formaldehyde. Flowering plants such as gerbera daisy and chrysanthemums were rated superior in removing benzene from the atmosphere.[25] Further work indicated that it may have been the soil-born microorganisms associated with the plants that were responsible for the reduction in airborne pollutants.[26] Subsequent research in office environments has proven inconclusive, but many people still advocate the use of plants to help neutralize indoor toxicants. Whether or not house plants can significantly reduce indoor pollutants, they are aesthetically pleasing, they provide additional oxygen to an often depleted indoor environment, and they are a refreshing way to bring a bit of nature to the indoors.

SOURCES (in the order they appear in the chapter):

Soy candles:
http://www.wyntersway.com/soy-candles.html

Far infrared heaters:
http://edenpureus.us/

Carbon monoxide detectors:
http://www.kiddeus.com/
http://www.firstalert.com/

Barrier cloths:
Heart of Vermont: http://www.heartofvermont.com/

Paint and varnish:
Safecoat http://www.afmsafecoat.com/

Air cleaners:
Austin Air: available from American Environmental Health Foundation (AEHF) www.aehf.com and many other outlets

Rainbow vacuum:
http://rainbowsystem.com/

Essential oils:
Bio Excel, LLC. www.bioexcel.com

Salt lamps:
http://www.natural-salt-lamps.com/
http://www.pacificspiritcatalogs.com/product.php?productid=1425
http://wyntersway.com/salt_crystal_lamps.html

Chapter 2

WHAT TO DO ABOUT WATER

✦

Water contaminants—Water solutions

The eighteenth century poet Samuel T. Coleridge described the fate of a seaman in the poem, *The Rime of the Ancient Mariner*: "Water, water everywhere, Nor any drop to drink." Modern man finds himself in a similar situation—surrounded by water, but unable to find a suitable drop to drink.

And yet, drink we must! Hydration is a key to the proper functioning of our immune systems. It is also a factor in the function of *every* process in the human body. Even the slightest decrease in hydration can have major consequences: fatigue, impaired mental capacity (brain fog), constipation, dry skin, increased blood pressure, and headaches. Many of these symptoms are considered "normal" in today's world—possibly because much of the population is chronically dehydrated.

Chronic dehydration has been linked to many (if not all) of our modern diseases.[27] Daily replacement of the water we use for biological functions is an absolute must if we are to maintain health and vitality. Water is the primary source of energy in our bodies. It is also a carrier—responsible for taking nutrients to the cells. Water is a key factor in the circulation of blood; it lubricates joints, it softens the skin, it reduces the effects of stress, and it stabilizes the DNA.[28] Staying properly hydrated has the potential to enhance your quality of life in many ways.

The 8 X 8 Water Rule

The "8 X 8" water rule refers to the widely established recommendation for eight 8-ounce glasses of water every day. Interestingly, there is no scientific basis for this recommendation. Attempts to uncover its origin have failed. Every individual has a unique need for water that varies according to gender, age, height, weight, and level of activity. Men require more water than women; overweight individuals need more than those who are thin; both the young and the elderly (for different reasons) require more water; and our level of activity changes the requirement for water on an hourly basis.

A 2004 report from the Institute of Medicine found that women who were adequately hydrated consumed about 91 ounces of fluids/day; men consumed about 125 ounces. Eighty percent of their fluid intake was from drinking water and other beverages.[29] Based on this finding, the best guideline to follow is to drink half your body weight (measured in pounds) in ounces of water every day. This means that a person weighing 150 pounds ought to drink about 75 ounces (just over half a gallon) of water under normal circumstances. Men should drink more. Remember that this amount of water needs to come from pure water—not processed fruit juices, soda, coffee, or other beverages.

The most important times to drink water:

1. First thing in the morning. This is perhaps the single most important time to drink water.
2. At least 10 to 20 minutes before meals. This practice "primes" the digestive organs for better digestion. It is much better to drink water before meals and not with them. Water taken along with solid food slows the digestive process.
3. Before, during, and after exercise. Exercise requires water for muscle function as well as to remove the lactic acid from tissues following exercise

Drinking plenty of water is important. However, drinking contaminated water can often do more harm than good. Since water is meant to flush the toxins and waste materials from our bodies, drinking contaminated water can add to the toxic burden. Unfortunately, the average U.S. citizen faces numerous threats from the water that flows from the tap. Depending on where you live and depending on the effectiveness of your municipal water treatment, any number of contaminants can be present in the water that is supposedly safe to drink.

Chemicals from industrial waste, pesticides, fertilizers, and other sources eventually end up in the soil. From there, they find their way into the ground water. Across the nation about 50 percent of drinking water comes from ground water, which is currently contaminated with a variety of pesticides, fertilizers, and other wastes. According to the EPA's Groundwater Cleanup Cross-Program Task Force, "groundwater contamination is usually very difficult to characterize and clean up, often requiring decades of treatment and monitoring."[30] And if your source of water isn't from ground water, don't think you are any better off. Other sources of water are often worse, with industrial wastes, disinfectants, and even pharmaceuticals that make their way into municipal water supplies.

Ultimately, protecting rivers, streams, and wetlands is our best defense against water pollution. Every individual makes decisions each day that can make a difference. Choose *not* to use garden pesticides and fertilizers, which run off or seep into groundwater. Dispose of leftover paint and automotive and household chemicals through your community's hazardous waste collection program—don't pour them down the drain. Use biodegradable cleaning agents and detergents, and buy food that is organically grown in accordance with watershed-protecting farming practices.

 (see Chapter 6: Cleaning agents)

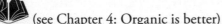 (see Chapter 4: Organic is better)

What are the alternatives to drinking tap water? What are the factors that determine "safe" water quality? And how can you be sure that the water you and your loved ones are drinking is safe? This chapter discusses the common contaminants in water and the best ways to remove them. It includes information on water purification systems and on the health hazards of the containers that water is often sold in. It also includes a discussion of the significance of minerals in water and a brief overview of the unique properties of water—properties that, when enhanced, can provide additional benefits to the water you drink.

WATER CONTAMINANTS

In a review of more than 22 million tap water quality tests, 260 water contaminants were found to be routinely served to the public. More than half of these contaminants are unregulated—public health officials have not set safety standards, and testing for them is currently not required.[31] A national tap water atlas published by the Environmental Working Group shows tap water testing results from forty thousand communities around the country. View the results at http://www.ewg.org/sites/tapwater/

Water Contaminants and Their Sources

Contaminants	Major Sources
Inorganic	Dissolved gasses, heavy metals, fluoride, nitrates and nitrites, hard water minerals
Organic	Pesticides, VOCs, pharmaceuticals, plastics, solvents, disinfectant by-products
Biological	Bacteria, virus, protozoans

INORGANIC CONTAMINANTS
(gasses, heavy metals, fluoride, and hard water minerals)

Most dissolved gases are normal in water (oxygen, carbon dioxide, nitrogen). Several, like chlorine, chloramines, hydrogen sulfide, and radon can cause problems. A discussion of the problematic gasses follows.

Chlorine

The addition of chlorine to drinking water began in the late 1800s. Even though our modern technology has identified safer, more effective methods to disinfect water, chlorine is still the standard in water treatment. Simply stated, chlorine is a pesticide. It was used as a chemical weapon in World War II. Its purpose as a drinking water additive is to kill living organisms. When you consume water containing chlorine, it also destroys cells and tissues inside your body.

The long-term dangers of drinking chlorinated water have been recognized for many years. When chlorine is added to water, it combines with organic compounds to form carcinogenic by-products called trihalomethanes or THMs. Although concentrations of these carcinogens are low, scientists believe they are responsible for many human cancers. High levels of THMs may also have an effect on the growing fetus during pregnancy.

More than twenty years ago, Dr. Joseph M. Price demonstrated the connection between the practice of chlorinating water and arteriosclerosis. He noticed an unusually high level of arteriosclerosis among soldiers in Vietnam, where very high concentrations of chlorine were routinely added to the water to prevent diarrhea and other intestinal problems. These young servicemen were found to have a high predisposition to arteriosclerosis— evidenced by extremely elevated cholesterol levels. Dr. Price's theory was that high levels of chlorine in the water was the cause. To substantiate his theory he conducted a controlled experiment using chickens. Two groups of several hundred birds each were observed throughout their life span. The group without chlorinated water grew faster and displayed more vigorous health. During the winter, the group with chlorinated water showed outward signs of poor circulation, drooped feathers, and a reduced level of activity. When autopsied, every specimen in the group that was raised on chlorinated water showed some level of heart or circulatory disease. The group without chlorine showed *no* incidence of disease.[32]

Heart disease is not the only disease that chlorinated water is suspected of causing. In 2007, a research team in Spain documented a two-fold increase in bladder cancer for those who drank chlorinated water.[33] Chlorinated water has also been linked with colon and rectal cancers.

The chlorine in water enters our bodies in more than just the water we *drink*. Over half of our harmful exposure to chlorine may be due to absorption through the skin and to inhalation while showering or bathing. Inhalation is a much more harmful means of exposure because the chlorine gas goes directly into our blood stream. In a closed, steamy room, chlorinated water creates a virtual gas chamber. The steam we inhale can contain many times the level of chemicals over ingestion because chlorine and most other contaminants vaporize much faster than water. The inhalation of chlorine is a suspected cause of asthma and bronchitis, especially in children. These respiratory problems have increased 300 percent in the last twenty years.

 (see Chapter 2: Shower filters)

> Chlorine robs the skin and hair of moisture and elasticity.
> A warm shower opens up the pores of the skin, allowing
> for accelerated absorption.

It is clear that chlorine represents a serious danger to our health. However, thinking that it will be removed in the near future is unrealistic. The good news is that chlorine is one of the easiest substances to remove from water. Even the least expensive, carbon-based home filtration systems will remove chlorine and most chlorine by-products.

 (see Chapter 2: Municipal water disinfection and treatment)

 (see Chapter 2: Water filtration/purification methods)

Chloramine

Chloramine is a more recent water treatment additive that is now being used in many water treatment facilities. It is a combination of gasses (chlorine and ammonia) used in addition to or in place of chlorine because its effects are longer lasting. However, numerous difficulties have been identified with the use of choramine as a water disinfectant:

- Chloramine remains in the water longer than chlorine—it does not evaporate when left in the open as chlorine does.
- Chloramine is toxic to fish, and it cannot be removed by boiling.
- Chloramine reacts with (deteriorates) certain types of rubber hoses and gaskets, such as those on washing machines and hot water heaters.
- Chloramine reacts with lead and lead solder in plumbing, causing toxic levels of lead to be released into drinking water.
- Chloramine is potentially lethal to kidney dialysis patients.

The use of chloramine as a water disinfectant can lead to the generation of iodoacid by-products—the most potent genetic toxin of mammalian cells. This was discovered recently by research scientist Michael Plewa.[34]

> When chloramines were put into use in Washington DC, lead levels 3,200 times EPA's "action level" were found in drinking water.
>
> When several cities in California switched to the use of chloramine, kidney dialysis patients suffered serious consequences.

Replacing chlorine with chloramine is like jumping from the fire into the frying pan, yet many large cities have already made the switch. You can read more about the public outcry against chloramine in this *American Free Press* article online:

http://www.americanfreepress.net/html/chloraminated_water.html

Carbon filters have a very limited capacity for chloramine removal—it takes much more carbon and much more contact time to do the job. If you were to use a simple carbon filter to remove chloramine, you would have to replace your filter so often that it would not be economically feasible. A reverse osmosis (RO) system cannot be counted on to remove chloramine either. The filtration membranes in a typical RO system do not filter out chloramine. Most RO systems have a carbon pre-filter, but that will not last long in the presence of chloramine.

Chloramine removal requires a special type of catalytic carbon filter. Most of these devices are tanks designed to filter the incoming water for the whole house. Vitamin C has also been shown to neutralize chloramine,[35] but this method is only realistic for smaller applications such as shower filters or countertop systems. The above methods are the only methods available at this time to remove or neutralize chloramine.

Hydrogen sulfide

Hydrogen sulfide is a naturally-occurring gas that imparts a rotten egg odor to water. It is more common in wells than surface water. Hydrogen sulfide is corrosive to plumbing fixtures even at low concentrations. Chlorine is currently used to eliminate it. Activated carbon filtration must then be used to remove the excess chlorine.

A better solution for removing the sulfur smell and corrosive effects from water that contains hydrogen sulfide lies in the use of magnetic or electromagnetic fields. These devices have received dubious reports over the last fifteen years as a variety of technologies have been marketed. However, in 1998, the U.S. Department of Energy released a report designed to speed the adoption of these energy-efficient technologies. One of the benefits of the technology (aside from the reduction of hard water deposits and scale on heating and cooling equipment) is a reduction of corrosion and the reduction of algae and hydrogen sulfide odors. The twenty-three-page report on the use of magnetic devices for the reduction of scale can be found at: http://www.etpwater.com/Reports/FTA/FTA.pdf

 (see Chapter 2: Magnetic water conditioners)

Radon

Radon is a radioactive gas that comes from the natural breakdown (radioactive decay) of radium. The primary source of radon in homes is from the underlying soil and bedrock. However, radon can also be found in the water supply, particularly if the house is served by a private well or by a small community water system. Since radon is a gas, it can be inhaled during showers or while bathing. It is easily removed by carbon filtration.

 (see Chapter 1: Radon)

HEAVY METALS

Heavy metals (lead, mercury, aluminum, cadmium, and arsenic) are dangerous in water even at extremely low concentrations.

Aluminum

The solubility of aluminum in water is so low that it is seldom a concern in municipal or industrial water systems. Aluminum in drinking water comes from the use of aluminum sulfate (alum) as a coagulant in water treatment plants. Reverse osmosis will reduce the aluminum content by over 98 percent. Distillation will reduce aluminum by more than 99 percent.

Arsenic

Arsenic and its compounds are used in pesticides and various metal alloys. When found in a water supply, they usually come from mining or metallurgical operations or from runoff in agricultural areas. Arsenic is highly toxic and has been classified by the EPA as a carcinogen. Filtration through activated carbon will reduce the amount of arsenic in drinking water by 40 to 70 percent. Reverse osmosis has a 90 percent removal rate. Distillation will remove 98 percent.

Cadmium

Cadmium makes its way into water supplies as a result of the deterioration of galvanized plumbing, industrial waste, or fertilizer contamination. Reverse osmosis removes 95 to 98 percent of the cadmium in water.

Lead

Lead is a highly toxic metal and a major health concern. Lead in the body can cause serious damage to the brain, kidneys, nervous system, and red blood cells. Lead in drinking water is primarily from the corrosion of the lead solder used to put together copper piping. Lead is released from plumbing when chloramine is used as a disinfectant in the water supply. Activated carbon filtration can reduce lead, to a certain extent. Reverse osmosis can remove 94 to 98 percent of lead in drinking water at the point of use. Distillation will also remove lead from drinking water.

Mercury

Mercury is unique among metals. It can evaporate when released to water or soil. Activated carbon filtration is very effective for removal of mercury. Reverse osmosis will also remove 95 to 97 percent of mercury.

FLUORIDE

Fluoride is a trace mineral found in varying concentrations in food and in water. Fluoride ions come from the element fluorine, an abundant natural element in the earth's crust and in the oceans. Small amounts of fluoride are present in all water sources. However, naturally-occurring fluoride is much different than the fluoride compounds used in toothpaste and to fluoridate water.

> **Fluoride in drinking water is an industrial waste product!**
>
> Ninety percent of the fluoride added to drinking water is hydrofluorosilicic acid—a compound that is a chemical by-product of aluminum, steel, cement, phosphate, and nuclear weapons manufacturing. It is an industrial waste product, passed off on the public as a "nutrient." It benefits manufacturers to the tune of about ten billion dollars every year.

Christopher Bryson's book, *The Fluoride Deception,* exposes the misrepresented science that has successfully promoted water fluoridation.[36] His book and many other articles and publications[37] expose the fact that fluoride is a poison. Before fluoride was sold as a cavity fighter, it was used as an insecticide and rat poison—and it still is. Fluoride accumulates in bones and tissues, not just teeth.

The National Medical Library has more than forty articles on the toxicity of fluoride. Half of the articles indicate that fluoride promotes cancer. The toxicity of fluoride has caused many countries to rethink allowing fluoride to be added to water. Those countries now banning fluoride are Sweden, Norway, Denmark, West Germany, Italy, Belgium, Austria, France, and the Netherlands.

Water fluoridation for the prevention of dental cavities is still a hotly contested subject. However, those who are willing to look beyond the politics and the money will find a vast array of evidence against fluoridation. In 1990, *Newsweek* magazine advised the public that "political decisions [about fluoridation] were at odds with expert advice" and that "fluoride from your tap may not do much good—and may cause cancer."[38]

 (see Chapter 2: Fluoride)

> **The online Fluoride Action Network provides actions anyone can take to help stop water fluoridation and other unnecessary fluoride treatments.**
> http://www.fluoridealert.org/action.htm

CAUTION: Carbon filtration does not remove fluoride. Reverse osmosis will remove 93 to 95 percent. If your water is fluoridated, you should consider purchasing a special fluoride filter but be careful because many point of use fluoride filters hve been determined to be ineffective or only effective for a short period of time.[39]

NITRATES AND NITRITES

Nitrates and nitrites are nitrogen-oxygen chemical units that combine with various organic and inorganic compounds. Because they are highly soluble and do not bind to soils, nitrates/nitrites migrate to ground water. When nitrate/nitrite levels are elevated, the surrounding area is often heavily developed, used for agricultural purposes or subject to heavy fertilization. The presence of nitrate and nitrite generally indicates that the activity producing the nitrate/nitrite is very recent or very nearby.

Excessive levels of nitrate in drinking water have caused serious illness—especially for infants. This is due to the conversion of nitrate to nitrite by the body, which can interfere with the oxygen-carrying capacity of the blood. Symptoms include shortness of breath and a blue tint to the skin. The EPA has approved ion exchange (similar to water softening) and reverse osmosis treatment as methods for removing nitrates/nitrites.

HARD WATER MINERALS

Calcium and magnesium ions in drinking water can be beneficial when they are biologically available. However, in the form of calcium carbonate and magnesium oxide (found in most hard water) they are not only biologically *un*available but they cause scaly deposits on faucets and in pipes and water heaters. They can do the same inside your body. Hard water minerals can be removed by a variety of water-conditioning techniques.

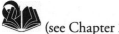 (see Chapter 2: Minerals)

Ion exchange water softeners

Traditional water softeners work on the principle of ion exchange where hard water minerals are exchanged for sodium. Although this eliminates hard water deposits and reduces wear and tear on equipment, you cannot drink the water. For this reason, water softening units should deliver soft water only through the hot water line so that water from the cold line can be consumed. The other problem with traditional water softeners is pollution. Tons of salt from water softeners are emptied back into water supplies every year, creating water treatment nightmares. Water softeners that use potassium rather than sodium are much more environmentally friendly and much better for your skin. These are available from many water treatment companies. Magnetic water treatment is another way to deal with hard water minerals.

Magnetic water conditioners

Magnetic technology has developed to the point where magnetic and electromagnetic devices can successfully reduce or eliminate the hard water problems in a home and in a commercial setting. According to a Department of Energy publication, these technologies can be used as a replacement for most water-softening equipment.[40] They are a one-time purchase (often they cost less than a water softener) typically installed on the outside of the incoming water line. There is no maintenance, they are environmentally friendly, and they can provide health benefits by structuring the water.

 (see Chapter 2: Water structure)

Magnetic water conditioners work based on the physics of the interaction between a magnetic field and a moving electric charge (the ions in the water). When ions pass through a magnetic field, they are forced to spin. Hard water minerals collide more often and more forcefully. Large particles break up, forming a different kind of precipitate that is less likely to adhere to pipes or equipment. Hard water minerals are not exchanged as they are when using a water softener; they are not physically removed from the water. However, because they do not collect in pipes and on equipment, there is a considerable savings on heating and cooling costs, as well as easier clean-up of sinks and tubs. The effects on skin in the shower and bath are also noticeable.

Reverse osmosis

Although reverse osmosis (RO) will remove 95 to 98 percent of the calcium, magnesium, and other hard water minerals in water, RO is not a recommended solution for hard water. Hard water will significantly shorten the life of any RO membrane. Many families with hard water (especially where the source of water is a well) use both a water conditioner and a purification system. This removes hard water minerals and maximizes the life of the RO unit.

ORGANIC CONTAMINANTS

Organic compounds are those that contain the carbon atom. They are usually associated with living matter (or matter that was once living) such as leaves and other debris that make their way into water. However, a growing list of *synthetic* organic compounds is being produced by modern technology. Many of these end up in water. They include pesticides, volatile organic compounds (VOCs), trihalomethanes (THMs), pharmaceuticals, and others. Organic compounds (especially those that are synthetic) comprise the longest list of potential water contaminants—in the thousands.

Many of these organic contaminants in water are presumed to increase the risk of various cancers in humans—often after many years of low-level exposure. Others may affect the nervous system, increasing the incidence of diseases like Parkinson's disease and Lou Gehrig's disease; some can cause hormonal disruptions, including infertility and impotency. Still others can cause autoimmune syndromes such as lupus and fibromyalgia. Organic contaminants are even suspected of having a relationship to emotional and sociopathic disorders.

Pesticides

Pesticides are common synthetic, organic contaminants in water. They reach surface and well water supplies from the runoff in agricultural areas. Some pesticides decompose and break down as they perform their function. However, many take years to break down. There is no EPA maximum contamination level for pesticides as a total; each substance must be considered separately. Most go unregulated in water. Activated carbon filtration will remove most pesticides. Reverse osmosis will remove 97 to 99 percent of pesticides.

Volatile organic compounds

VOCs, including benzene, carbon tetrachloride, and vinyl chloride (PVC), are known carcinogens. VOCs are man-made. Therefore, the detection of any of these compounds indicates that there has been a chemical spill or other incident. VOCs regulated under the Safe Drinking Water Act of 1986 are listed below. However, there are others that are not currently regulated.

- Trichloroethylene
- Tetrachloroethylene
- Carbon tetrachloride
- Trichloroethane
- Dichloroethane
- Vinyl chloride
- Methylene chloride (dichloromethane)
- Benzene
- Chlorobenzene
- Dichlorobenzene
- Trichlorobenzene
- Dichloroethylene

 (see Chapter 1: Volatile organic compounds)

The best choice for removing VOCs from water is activated carbon filtration. The adsorption capacity of the carbon will vary with each type of VOC. Reverse osmosis will remove 70 to 80 percent of the VOCs in the water.

MTBE

MTBE (Methyl tertiary-butyl ether) is one of the common nonregulated VOCs found in water. It is a gasoline additive that has contaminated drinking water across the country. Made from methanol and from a by-product of the oil-refining process, it was added to gasoline in an attempt to maintain octane ratings during the phase-out of lead in gasoline. It was also intended to make gasoline burn cleaner, but studies show that it has had little effect on curbing air pollution. MTBE is very soluble in water, and it is resistant to biodegradation. It has been found to persist in groundwater for decades— and it has been found in the water in all fifty states.

Although there is no established drinking-water regulation, the EPA considers MTBE to be a potential human carcinogen. Limits have been advised, based on the fact that MTBE has an offensive taste and odor You can easily detect its turpentine-like smell—even at extremely low concentrations. If you have MTBE in your water, you will likely know it by the odor.

Carbon filtration is the best way to remove MTBE. However, the contact time for removal needs to be longer than for most contaminants. This means you will need a larger carbon filter, and you will need to pay particular attention to timely filter replacement.

Trihalomethanes (THMs)

When chlorine reacts with organic matter in water it produces hundreds of chemical by-products, several of which have been proven to be carcinogenic. Trihalomethanes (THMs) make up the bulk of these cancer-causing by-products. The level of THMs in water is usually greater in water systems where surface water is the source. Levels vary seasonally with the organic content of the water. THMs are associated with increased risk of bladder and rectal cancer. Even drinking water with low-level THM contamination over a forty- to fifty-year period may increase the risk of cancer. Currently, carbon filtration is the best way to remove THMs and other dangerous chlorine disinfection by-products.

Pharmaceuticals

Americans take a lot of prescription medications. They take even more over-the-counter drugs. The body absorbs some of these medications, but some of them pass through and are flushed away. Unfortunately, wastewater treatment facilities are not set up to remove drug residue. This means that if you are drinking tap water or using it to cook with, you may be exposed to other people's medications in your water. Even bottled water (often just filtered tap water) and water from wells may contain drug residues.

Pharmaceuticals in Water

Medications pose a unique danger because, unlike most pollutants, they are designed to act on the human body at extremely low concentrations. The EPA has set no safety limits for pharmaceuticals in water and admits that there are no sewage treatment systems specifically engineered to remove them.

A vast array of pharmaceutical drugs, including antibiotics; pain medications; anti-depressants; cholesterol-lowering drugs; and medications for asthma, epilepsy, mental illness, and heart problems, have found their way into the drinking water supplies of at least 41 million Americans, according to a 2008 Associated Press investigation.[41] Officials in Philadelphia said testing discovered fifty-six pharmaceuticals or pharmaceutical by-products in treated drinking water. Sixty-three pharmaceuticals or their by-products were found in the city's watersheds.[42]

A number of advanced water treatment technologies have been evaluated for their ability to remove or neutralize the most common pharmaceuticals from drinking water. Some drugs, including widely used cholesterol medications, tranquilizers, and anti-epileptic medications, are completely resistant to current municipal wastewater treatment processes. Chlorine is only marginally effective. In fact, there is evidence that the addition of chlorine makes some pharmaceuticals more toxic.[43] A combination of ozone and ultraviolet (UV) light is quite successful. Ultrafiltration and reverse osmosis offer the most promise for the complete elimination of pharmaceuticals.

BIOLOGICAL CONTAMINANTS

Bacteria

Pathogenic bacteria cause illnesses such as dysentery, gastroenteritis, infectious hepatitis, typhoid, and cholera. E. coli (Escherichia coli) is the bacterial organism that is most often tested for. Its presence indicates fecal contamination, which enters the water supply from human or animal wastes. The newspaper series "Tap Water at Risk" by the *Houston Chronicle* reported that in 1994 through 1995, there were 3,641 water purification utilities in the United States that were in violation of the federal health standards for fecal bacterial contamination.[44]

The most common and undisputed method of removing bacteria from water is chemical oxidation and disinfection. The injection of ozone into a water supply is one form of chemical oxidation and disinfection. Chlorination is another. Reverse osmosis will also remove more than 99 percent of the bacteria in a drinking-water system.

Viruses

There are more than a hundred types of enteric viruses. Enteric viruses include hepatitis A, Norwalk-type viruses, rotaviruses, adenoviruses, enteroviruses, and reoviruses. The major enteric viruses and their diseases are indicated:

- Enteroviruses (polio, aseptic meningitis, and encephalitis)
- Reoviruses (upper respiratory and gastrointestinal illness)
- Rotaviruses (gastroenteritis)
- Adenoviruses (upper respiratory and gastrointestinal illness)
- Hepatitis A (infectious)
- Norwalk-type (gastroenteritis)

The test for coliform bacteria is widely accepted as an indication of whether or not water is safe to drink. Therefore, tests for viruses are not usually conducted. As with bacterial contaminants, chemical oxidation or disinfection is the preferred treatment for viral populations in water. Chlorine, followed by activated carbon filtration, is the most widely used treatment. Ozone or iodine may be utilized as oxidizing agents. Ultraviolet sterilization and distillation are also effective methods for the removal of viruses.

Protozoans

Protozoans, cryptosporidia, and giardia are single-celled organisms that lack a cell wall. They form dormant cysts that are resistant to typical levels of chlorination. Cryptosporidia and giardia cause nausea, abdominal cramps, and low-grade fever. For people with compromised immune systems, an infection can be fatal. Filtration is the most effective treatment for protozoan cysts. Filters rated at 0.5 microns are designed for the removal of protozoans.

MUNICIPAL WATER DISINFECTION AND TREATMENT

Although chlorine is still the most widely used method of municipal water disinfection, other methods of water treatment are available.

Chlorination

Chlorine is a very effective way to kill germs and bacteria, but it is not without consequences. As safe as we are told chlorination is, aquarium fish will die within a matter of minutes if chlorinated tap water is used to fill the fish tank. Long-term human use has now been linked with numerous diseases and cancer.

 (see Chapter 2: Chlorine)

Besides the chlorine itself, by-products are created when chlorine is added to water. It is estimated that only 50 percent of these by-products have even been identified. Trihalomethanes are the most widely known; they are known to cause numerous health difficulties—especially when chlorinated water is consumed over many years.

Chloraminization

In an effort to sidestep the negative effects of chlorination, the EPA began promoting chloraminization in 1994. Many municipal water districts across the United States have switched from the use of chlorine to the use of chloramine—but, as with the use of chlorine, there have been unintended consequences.

 (see Chapter 2: Chloramine)

When the nation's capital changed from using free chlorine to chloramine in 2000, serious problems with lead leaching started to occur, causing toxic levels of lead in drinking water. After switching to chloraminized water, children in Washington DC ingested more than 60 times the EPA's maximum level of lead with each glass of water! When several cities in California switched to chloraminization, kidney dialysis patients suffered serious consequences. Water treatment with chloramine is obviously not the answer.

If you live in an area where chloramine is used for water treatment, check your water for unusually high levels of lead and check your plumbing for corrosive activity. Better yet, install a treatment system that removes chloramine before it enters your home.

Ozonation

Because of the known hazards of chlorine and chloramine, there has been a strong movement toward ozone in both municipal water treatment and in wastewater treatment. The technology for ozone application has made tremendous strides in effectiveness and cost reduction. Ozone is a strong oxidant, with a short life span. It consists of oxygen molecules with an extra oxygen atom to form O_3. When ozone comes in contact with bacteria or viruses, the third oxygen is released and oxidizes (kills) pathogens. Oxygen (O_2) is the only by-product.

A number of cities now use ozone to disinfect their water. But although ozonation is an effective disinfectant that does not produce harmful by-products, it breaks down quickly and cannot be used to maintain disinfection within the distribution system. Ozone does not stay in the water after it leaves the treatment plant, so it offers no protection within the water pipes during the time it takes the water to be delivered to residents. It is, however, an effective treatment for pools and spas, where the water does not have to be delivered long distances after disinfection. At this time, the most realistic municipal water treatment system is the use of ozone with very light amounts of chlorine for protection during dissemination.

Chlorine dioxide

Chlorine dioxide is a water treatment method that has been used, on a small scale, to treat municipal drinking water in the United States and Europe for more than fifty years. It is recognized as a superior water disinfectant and has become increasingly popular as a water purification treatment. Chlorine dioxide is approved for both the pretreatment and final disinfection of municipal water. It does not combine with organic wastes to form carcinogens. It also provides protection throughout the distribution system to reduce the subsequent growth of bacteria, viruses, and algae. Chlorine dioxide is ideal for industrial water systems and community purification plants. It is also ideal for smaller water supplies such as cisterns and hospital water systems. Besides being an effective disinfectant, it removes hard water components (iron and manganese), promotes flocculation, and aids in levels of water turbidity.

Although the chemical name implies that chlorine dioxide contains chlorine, there is no free chlorine in chlorine dioxide. The additional oxygen atom changes the chemistry and creates a completely different chemical behavior and by-products. Chlorine dioxide releases oxygen in a highly active form, oxidizing viruses, bacteria, and protozoa. The only by-products are chlorite and chlorate ions, which are easily removed.

Many consumers use chlorine dioxide for water purification while camping, hiking, and other such outdoor activities. It is the perfect preparedness water purifier. Research also shows chlorine dioxide is a valuable dental hygiene product, effective for reducing the bacteria that cause gingivitis and periodontal disease.[45]

Chlorine dioxide is an effective disinfectant at concentrations as low as 0.1 parts per million (ppm) and over a wide pH range. It disinfects according to the same principle as chlorine; however, there are no harmful effects on human health.

Two Ways to Know What Is in Your Drinking Water:

1. Read the annual water quality report from your municipal water company. Your water company is required by federal law to provide reports listing the measured levels of the most common and/or harmful water contaminants. A summary of how to interpret this report can be found on this Web site: https://engineering.purdue.edu/SafeWater/drinkinfo/WQ-33.htm .
2. Test your water. If you have a private water source (well, spring, or surface water), you are responsible for the safety of your home's water supply. For a relatively inexpensive water test visit: www.watercheck.com.

Water fluoridation

According to recent estimates, 67 percent of Americans now live in areas where fluoridated water is provided through the municipal water system. But that doesn't mean they all drink it. There are many reasons why you shouldn't.

Dr. William Marcus, formerly the chief toxicologist for the EPA's Office of Drinking Water, lost his job in 1991 after he recommended an unbiased evaluation of fluoride's potential to cause cancer. Marcus fought his dismissal in court, and an investigation documented that government scientists had been coerced to portray fluoride in a favorable manner. His original memo[46] exposed the fact that ten thousand annual cancer deaths were linked to fluoridation of water supplies.[47] This evidence was tested in the Pennsylvania courts and found scientifically sound after careful scrutiny.

What about tooth decay? According to the largest study ever conducted on fluoridation and oral health, there was no statistical difference in tooth decay rates between fluoridated and nonfluoridated cities. This study included thirty-nine thousand school children in eighty-four areas around the United States. The World Health Organization records from 1970 onward show that the incidence of decayed, missing, or filled teeth has been steadily declining in France, Germany, Japan, Italy, Sweden, Finland, Denmark, Norway, The Netherlands, Austria, Belgium, Portugal, Iceland, Greece, and the United States. Only one of those countries routinely adds fluoride to drinking water—the United States. The only reason for the decline in cavities is obviously not fluoride. More realistically, it can be attributed to better oral hygiene and improved dental care.

Not only does fluoride *not* prevent cavities, the irony is that when you get too much fluoride, your teeth can become discolored and crumble. It's called dental fluorosis—a mottling and deterioration of the enamel on teeth. In 1940, this mottling condition occurred in 10 percent of children's teeth. Today, it is as high as 55 percent.

Dental fluorosis is one of the first indications that the body is getting excess fluoride. Bones also collect fluoride and can develop skeletal fluorosis. Since 1990, numerous studies have reported an association between fluoridated water and hip fractures. Fluoridation is also known to increase osteoporosis (brittle bones).

> **Children under three should never drink fluoridated water. Mothers should never use fluoridated water to prepare baby formula. Children should not use fluoridated toothpaste.**
>
> 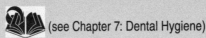 (see Chapter 7: Dental Hygiene)

In 1992, a U.S. study found a strong link between fluoridation and osteosarcoma, a bone cancer in young males. The rates of this malignancy were three to seven times higher in fluoridated areas of New Jersey.[48] Fluoride has been shown to enhance the brain's absorption of aluminum, which is found in elevated levels in the brains of most Alzheimer's patients. Studies in China show fluoride causes reduced IQ levels in children. Other effects include decreased concentration, memory loss, and confusion. Excessive fluoride damages the musculoskeletal and nervous systems, leading to limited joint mobility, ligament calcification, muscular degeneration, and neurological deficits. Studies also indicate that fluoride decreases levels of sperm production and testosterone.

Four Main Arguments Against Fluoridation:

1. Fluoridation does not prevent cavities. In fact, a growing body of recent scientific evidence shows that children in nonfluoridated areas have better dental heath and fewer cavities than those in fluoridated areas. At least four different publications from the United States, Canada, and New Zealand have reported similar or lower tooth decay rates in nonfluoridated areas as compared to fluoridated areas. One study showed decay was greater in the fluoridated area! Dental health all over Europe has improved since 1970 when the fluoridation of water stopped.
2. The chemicals used for fluoridation are not high purity, pharmaceutical quality products. Rather, they are by-products of aluminum and fertilizer manufacturing; they contain a high concentration of toxins and heavy metals—particularly lead. It has been found that the use of hydrofluorosilicic acid is associated with a significant increase of lead levels in the blood of children.
3. Fluoride may present unreasonable health risks at levels routinely added to tap water. Health risks include weakening of the architecture of bones, tooth discoloration, dental fluorosis (spotted and crumbly teeth), and lead poisoning. Besides making bones brittle and elevating the risk of fracture, scientists have been identifying connections between fluoridated water and neurological impairment, drops in IQ, depression of thyroid function, and suppression of the pineal gland. Most recently, a study was published out of Harvard that highlighted a connection between fluoridated water and a sevenfold increase in bone cancer in young boys.
4. Constitutional and civil liberty issues are in question regarding the forced mass medication of the population when alternative means of reducing cavities are available, such as tooth brushing.

If you live in an area where your water is fluoridated, use a water purification system that will effectively remove fluoride.

 (see Chapter 2: Fluoride)

What can you do about fluoridation?
Become active in your community's efforts to ban fluoride in drinking water.
Fluoride Action Network: http://www.fluoridealert.org/

WATER FILTRATION/PURIFICATION METHODS

Water filters use substances such as carbon that remove contaminants by keeping them from passing through a physical barrier. Purifiers (reverse osmosis, distillers, and ultraviolet devices), use methods other than filtration to reduce the level of contaminants in water. In our toxic environment, several of these methods are often used together in one system to produce multistage purification for the purest water possible.

Although there are many variations, the current filtration and purification methods for water are listed below. Singly, or in combination, they are incorporated in a wide variety of devices—everything from pitchers to faucet-mounted devices to under-the-counter and whole-home systems. At the very minimum, everyone should use a water purifier in their kitchen for drinking and cooking, and a shower filtration device in the bathroom. Install a whole-home filtration system on the incoming water line to your home, if possible. Maintain your unit on a regular basis and replace filters as recommended.

Ceramic filters

Ceramic water filters come as a cartridge that fits a filtration device. At the core of a ceramic filter is *diatomaceous earth*, a fossil substance, made up of tiny silicon shells left by microscopic, one-celled organisms called diatoms. Often, ceramic filters are used as prefilters to take out larger particles, sediment, and some bacteria. Ceramic filters generally remove particles that are 1 micron in size or larger (a human hair is 5 microns). They are ineffective against chemical contaminants.

Charcoal (carbon) filters

Carbon filters of many different kinds comprise about 95 percent of the filters in use domestically. Carbon filters effectively remove odors, chlorine, and chlorine by-products, VOCs, pesticides, radon, and most biological contaminants (bacteria, viruses, and protozoans). But they do not remove minerals—including fluoride. A carbon block filter is a pressed form of carbon. It will remove heavy metals and most particles down to 0.5 microns in size. Some carbon filters are enhanced by the use of activated nano-silver, which provides extra antibacterial protection. When looking for a carbon filter, make sure it is made of coconut shell carbon rather than carbon from coal. Some carbon filters made in China are made from coal and are contaminated with arsenic.

KDF filters

KDF filters use a granular media for eliminating chlorine and reducing bacteria and for precipitating some heavy metals, like lead. The KDF media works well with hot water and is often used in shower filters and in combination with activated carbon in household filtration systems.

Reverse osmosis (RO)

Reverse osmosis (RO) draws water through a fine membrane that acts like an extremely fine filter. Pressure must be applied to stop, and then reverse, the osmotic process. It generally takes a lot of pressure and is fairly slow. The RO process is recommended in situations where the water contains salts and heavy metals that cannot be reduced by activated carbon. A high-quality activated carbon filter should be part of a good RO system to reduce the VOCs not removed by RO. If you use RO for water purification, make sure you check and replace the filtration membrane as recommended. If there are chloramines in your water, purchase a chloramine filter or make sure to replace the carbon prefilter often. RO water is acidic and devoid of minerals. It is considered aggressive water that may rob the body of minerals when consumed long term.

 (see Chapter 2: Chloramine)

Distillation

Distillation rids water of nearly all impurities. However, the distillation process is very slow. Approximately five gallons of tap water are required to produce one gallon of distilled water.

In recent years, there has been a growing awareness of distilled water's effects on the balance of minerals in the body. Distilled water, like RO, is highly acidic and aggressive. It has been shown to pull minerals from the piping that water is delivered through. Significant evidence suggests that it does the same thing in the human body. A certain number of dissolved minerals in water serve an important function in supporting the body's metabolism. Long-term consumption of distilled water may not be in your best interest. If you use distilled or RO water, consider adding some form of ionized mineral complex to the water you drink.

 (see Chapter 2: Minerals)

Ultraviolet (UV) radiation systems

Ultraviolet (UV) systems use high-frequency light to irradiate water and to kill all living organisms. Although UV is an excellent sterilizing system, it is not recommended as a stand-alone water treatment because it does not reduce other harmful contaminants. It is a good option for providing additional protection when water is filtered by activated carbon or RO.

WHICH TYPE OF FILTRATION FOR YOU?

Once you know what is in your water, you can select the type of filtration technology for your needs. If you are looking for broad spectrum filtration, try an activated carbon filter. If bacteria are your concern, consider ultraviolet light. If you have concerns about contaminants that are very small (such as fluoride), purchase a fluoride filter or a reverse osmosis system. The very best units on the market today use a combination of technologies to remove as many different types of pollutants as possible. If you are unsure of what is in your water and are interested in an inexpensive water test visit:

www.aquaMD.com or www.watercheck.com.

Depending on your needs, there are a number of types of filtration systems available. When your water is either treated with chloramine or is fluoridated, pay special attention to get a system that will address these circumstances. Most filters will not routinely filter out these contaminants.

Pitchers

Pitcher-type water filters are popular and inexpensive—especially for apartment dwellers—but they are limited in what pollutants they can filter. This type of filter typically uses a simple carbon filter for a broad spectrum of contaminants. Some units offer multistage filtration and water enhancements (see sources).

Faucet-mount

Water filters that are designed to hook to the faucet are a little more convenient. They usually offer simple carbon filtration with a variety of enhancements, depending on the technology.

Countertop

Countertop units are a little more sophisticated and can offer multistage filtration for the removal of a wider variety of contaminants. The new Wellness Kitchen Filter released in October 2008 has received the highest National Sanitation Foundation certification ever given. It offers the most advanced technology with the capacity to remove even the most difficult contaminants. The Wellness Kitchen Filter also enhances the structure of the water for improved hydration; it adds bio-compatible minerals and other energetic enhancements that support cellular health. The Wellness filters use environmentally compatible components—they even offer a recycling program. Used filter cartridges are returned to the company at the time of replacement and are incorporated in the manufacture of agricultural water systems (see sources).

 (see Chapter 2: Water structure)

Under-the-counter unit
Under-the-counter filtration units require plumbing expertise to install in the plumbing line. These usually offer multistage filtration for the removal of many types of contaminants. The Wellness Kitchen filter (discussed above) can also be installed under the counter.

Whole-home system
Whole-home systems have the greatest potential to provide clean water throughout the house. They are recommended whenever possible. One of the biggest problems with a whole-house filter is neglect. The filtration components of these systems need to be replaced as recommended. Make sure you follow recommended filter changes and other maintenance.

Wellness Enterprises and Radiant Life both offer whole-home systems with many technological advances. Besides removing contaminants, they enhance the water to improve hydration (water structure) and to provide re-mineralization using biocompatible minerals (see sources).

Shower filters
With today's polluted water, taking long, hot showers can be a health risk. Showering and bathing in contaminated water lead to a greater exposure from toxic chemicals than drinking the water. Individuals can receive six to one hundred times more chemicals by breathing the air during a hot shower or bath. Most shower filters only remove chlorine, chlorine by-products, and a few contaminants. Only those that use vitamin C are capable of neutralizing chloramine (see sources).

 (see Chapter 2: Chloramine)

Bath filters

If you absorb a lot of chlorine standing in a shower, imagine how much more you absorb when you are immersed for twenty minutes in a hot bath. For those who prefer bathing over showering, you can purchase vitamin C tablets for your bathtub. Each 1000 mg tablet de-chlorinates up to a hundred gallons of water; it also provides benefits for skin, hair, and nails (see sources). Vitamin C will also neutralize chloramine.

Products referred to as Crystal Balls or Bath Balls also remove more than 90 percent of the chlorine from bath water. The balls hang from the bath faucet so that water pours over or through the ball on its way into the tub. These products are designed for use in any bathtub, Jacuzzi, or spa. They typically contain quartz crystals for water softening and a replaceable KDF media that lasts for two hundred to three hundred baths. Place the ball in the tub for a minute or two before you get in. These are available online from a variety of sources.

POOLS AND HOT TUBS

The number of pool chemicals is overwhelming: disinfectants, algaecides, clarifiers, surface cleaners, scale inhibitors, shock treatments, defoamers, and so on. No wonder many children are allergic to swimming pools! There are other options in pool cleaning.

Ozone is a much more powerful oxidant than chlorine, and it leaves no harmful by-products. Ozone does not leave swimmers with red eyes, rashes, itching, or other skin irritations. Over thirty thousand pools are ozonated in Europe. Germany has used the technology for more than thirty years. All their Olympic pools are ozonated. Perhaps this is one reason some Olympic swimmers have refused to swim in chlorinated, U.S. pools.

Chemicals Negate Water's Positive Effects

Water can be a powerful tool for healing and for exercise. Yet the chemicals we use for disinfection can often interfere with its positive effects. It is well-known that chlorine absorption by swimmers is a health hazard. For those who regularly use chlorinated or brominated hot tubs and Jacuzzis, the health effects may be even more critical.

One of the main reasons for the resistance to ozonation in the United States is that there is a higher initial cost. However, over the life of the pool, ozone reduces the ongoing operating and maintenance costs. Chlorine is famous for destroying pool infrastructures, for rusting out ventilation systems, and for destroying pool liners. Ozone poses no such problems. With the current level of knowledge, many pool owners feel that failure to use ozone in an indoor pool constitutes professional negligence. If you own a hot tub or a personal spa, perhaps it is time to make the switch. (See sources for information on the installation of ozone technology.)

MINERALS

There has been significant debate over the health benefits of minerals from drinking water; the bioavailability of minerals from the water source has been questioned for many years. Although drinking water is not the *major* source of minerals for the human body, drinking mineralized water has been shown to make a contribution to the mineral balance in the body. Nowhere in nature is water without minerals. The bioavailability of minerals from water is dependant on several factors: the presence of flora and other conditions within the intestines, the presence of food at the time of consumption, age-related metabolic efficiency, and mineral deficiencies.[49] Each of these factors can affect the degree to which minerals are absorbed from water.

Demineralized/distilled water has several negative health effects. It causes increased urination and the excessive elimination of minerals and electrolytes. It also causes a build-up of extra-cellular fluid (edema or puffiness), fewer red blood cells, and other changes in the blood.[50] According to the World Health Organization's *Guidelines for Drinking-Water Quality*, the following essential minerals have a high bioavailability from water: sodium, phosphorous, potassium, selenium, molybdenum, fluorine, boron, and iodine. Those with a moderate bioavailability from water include calcium, magnesium, copper, zinc, and manganese.[51] A review of four calcium bioavailability studies found that calcium was at least as bioavailable from water as it is from dairy products (though this isn't as high as calcium absorption from raw fruits and vegetables). Magnesium absorption from water is also very good—between 45 and 50 percent. These studies indicate that minerals in water are as available as minerals from food—sometimes to an even greater extent. However, the *form* of the minerals is also important. Calcium carbonate (not a well-absorbed form of calcium) can be difficult to break apart in the stomach, and it may be taken up as a whole molecule that is then deposited in joints and arteries. Underground sources of water often have high concentrations of calcium carbonate and magnesium oxide which should be avoided by those with arthritis or atherosclerosis. Minerals in ionic form are generally more easily absorbed. This is the way minerals are found in spring water.

> **Many of the best water treatment systems today provide remineralization chambers, where beneficial minerals are put back into purified water (see sources). Another way to add minerals back to distilled or RO water is by adding ¼ tsp. of a natural, unprocessed salt to every quart of water.**
>
> 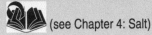 (see Chapter 4: Salt)

ALKALINE WATER

Drinking "alkaline" water has gained popularity over the last decade. Alkaline water is produced either by using a device called an ionizer or by adding pH drops to water. Either way, the pH level of the water is raised well above neutral—sometimes as high as 9 or 10. Drinking this water adds imbalanced alkaline ions to the body and neutralizes acids in the stomach that are necessary for proper digestion.

Ionizing machines called water ionizers make alkaline water by placing the water in an electric field—separating the positively charged (alkaline) ions from the negatively charged (acidic) ions in water. This produces two streams of water: alkaline water and acidic water. The alkaline water has been advocated for drinking whereas the acidic water has disinfecting qualities and can be used topically. Ionizers, because they place water within an electric field, have a negative effect on the electromagnetic field of water molecules. They produce aggressive water, which is potentially imbalancing for the body.[52] Drinking ionized water or water with a pH higher than 8.5 for long periods of time can be detrimental.[53]

Gabriel Cousens, MD, explains that the water inside the cell (intracellular water) is slightly acidic and that the water outside the cell (extracellular water) is slightly alkaline. This creates an osmotic potential and an electrical gradient that draws water into the cells.[54] When wastes build up in the body because of poor diet, stress, and disease, the extracellular water becomes acidic. This condition, referred to as acidosis, reverses the osmotic potential and the electrical gradient at the cell membrane and makes hydration difficult. The addition of alkaline minerals without their acidic counterpart also robs hydrogen from the body. Active hydrogen is required to acidify the water inside the cell. It is also often the limiting factor in the production of adinosine triphosphate (ATP)—the cell's source of energy. Providing alkaline minerals without their acidic counterpart causes numerous imbalances. The best way to maintain a balanced pH is to eat raw foods. Raw foods contain an abundance of organic acids (a source of active hydrogen) as well as a plethora of alkaline minerals, which are electrically balanced and available for absorption.

WATER STRUCTURE

The emerging science of quantum physics describes the human body as a living crystal—an organized matrix of crystal-like fluids that are capable of supporting almost instantaneous communication.[55] Water is the key. Under certain circumstances, water molecules organize to form a liquid crystal with properties that are different from normal water. This is what is referred to as "structured" water. The difference between normal water and its liquid crystalline form (structured water) has been described as similar to the difference between a piece of quartz and a quartz crystal. A crystal has different properties because of the way the molecules are organized.

In the 1960s, it was discovered that crystalline water immediately surrounded the collagen molecule that makes up the connective tissues of the body. This crystalline water-connective tissue system has recently been implicated as one of the major communication systems within the body.[56]

Structured water has been described as *more efficient* water, with the potential to hydrate more effectively and therefore to enhance energy, soften skin, improve bowel regularity, and enhance mental clarity.[57] Structured water can be purchased as a concentrate (intended to be mixed with distilled water), or it can be made at home using a variety of devices. Some water treatment systems now have structuring components at the end of the purification process (see sources).

WATER CONTAINERS

The vast majority of bottled waters come packaged in plastic, even though there is increasing concern that plastic leaches a variety of chemicals into water. Plastic is made by combining a number of synthetic chemicals in a process called polymerization. The plastics industry tells us that the process binds toxic chemicals so tightly that they are not able to escape. However, the polymerization process is never 100 percent complete. It always leaves some toxic chemicals available to migrate out of the plastic and into whatever contacts it—that's why for years the EPA referred to plastic as an "indirect food additive." Today, plastic is called a "food contact substance."

 (see Chapter 5: Plastic)

Many of the chemicals used to make plastic are toxic. Some are known to cause cancer; others are endocrine disruptors because they disrupt the normal functioning of hormones. Hormones are active in tiny concentrations (parts/per/trillion) and have an effect on virtually every bodily function. The effects of disrupting the normal activities of hormones can be devastating—even permanent. There are two types of plastic that are predominantly used to package water—both should be avoided. In fact, all plastic should be avoided whenever possible.

PET or PETE

PET or PETE stands for polyethylene terephthalate. This type of plastic is characterized by a clear, glasslike transparency. It is used almost exclusively for bottled water and juice drinks. PET plastic is thought to be the safest plastic for water. However, evidence indicates that PET leaches a class of chemicals known as phthalates when temperatures rise above room temperature. The longer the water is in the bottle, the more of a problem it becomes—especially if water remains in warm warehouses for extended periods of time, or if water sits in the sun.

 (see Chapter 5: Phthalates)

Research by world expert Dr. William Shotyk has found traces of antimony (used to make PET plastic) in water stored in PET bottles. A Canadian source of ground water contained 2 parts per trillion (ppt) of antimony. However, the same ground water stored in a PET plastic bottle had 630 ppt of antimony when opened six months later. Dr. Shotyk's experiments were duplicated in Germany, where forty-eight brands of water in PET bottles were studied. The water had an average of 4 ppt antimony before being bottled; the contents of a newly filled bottle had 360 ppt. When bottles were opened three months later, 700 ppt were measured.[58]

Even though health authorities maintained that the higher levels of antimony were far below official safety guidelines, the study illustrates an interesting point—that chemicals do leach from PET plastic bottles.

Polycarbonate

Polycarbonate plastic is another plastic that is widely used for bottling water. It is characterized by the number 7 within the triangle on the bottom of a container.

 (see Chapter 5: Classifications of plastic)

Polycarbonate bottles are hard—used as five-gallon water containers and for reusable drinking bottles. Polycarbonate, or Lexan, is used because it is durable. It neither holds flavors nor does it deliver them to the fluid it holds. However, in 1998, Dr. Patricia Hunt of Case Western University in Ohio accidentally discovered that polycarbonate plastic leaches bisphenol A (BPA), a potent hormone disruptor. During research, she discovered that all of her laboratory mice, including those not treated in any way, began exhibiting chromosomal abnormalities. Her investigation revealed that BPA was leaching from the animals' polycarbonate cages, and that it was the cause of the chromosomal changes.[59] Another researcher, Ana Soto, noticed that her lab mice treated with BPA were a lot fatter than her other mice. More alarming still was the work of later scientists who found that cancer cells placed in test tubes containing BPA grew rapidly—even at doses lower than what people are normally exposd to.

> **BPA may impair reproductive organs and may have adverse effects on breast tissue development and prostate development by reducing sperm count. The widespread use of plastic is now being blamed, at least in part, for early breast development in young girls and for reduced sperm counts in men.**

BPA can be leached into the water through normal wear and tear, as well as exposure to heat and cleaning agents. A 2003 study conducted at the University of Missouri confirmed Dr. Hunt's conclusions but also found that detectable levels of BPA leached into liquids at room temperature. This means that water in a plastic water bottle at room temperature can be potentially harmful. (Note: Baby bottles made from polycarbonate plastics are quietly disappearing from the market despite industry assurances that polycarbonate plastics are safe.)

 (see chapter 5: Bisphenol A)

Epoxy

There are numerous water bottles that contain *supposedly inert* epoxy liners. Yet even epoxy can contain BPA. SIGG reusable water bottles have long been perceived as the eco-friendly alternative to plastic water bottles. For years they marketed a light-weight, extruded aluminum bottle with an epoxy lining, claiming that it did not *leach* BPA. Yet in 2009 they came out with a new "EcoCare" BPA-free formula admitting that all of their bottles manufactured before August of 2008 contained BPA. Even though their new formula is BPA-free, many users feel betrayed by the company's earlier lack of disclosure.

Stainless steel

Stainless steel water bottles are light, durable, and hold both hot and cold liquids. They do not leach contaminants into the water. Klean Kanteen makes a complete line of stainless steel water bottles (see sources).

BOTTLED WATER

Bottled water is a four-billion-dollar-a-year business in the United States. It has also become a serious health and environmental issue. The National Resources Defense Council conducted a four-year study of the bottled water industry and concluded that bottled water is not always better or safer than tap water.[60] According to industry and government estimates, about 25 percent of bottled water is actually bottled tap water. This may be due to the fact that a large portion of the bottled water that is sold is Aquafina (owned by Pepsi) and Dasani (owned by Coca-Cola); both are processed tap water. Even when bottled water complies with the EPA's bottled water standards, those rules are weaker in many ways than EPA rules for city tap water. Fluoride is even added to some bottled water. Dannon's bottled water has added fluoride.

Comprehensive testing released in an October 2008 report by the Environmental Working Group (EWG) revealed an array of chemical contaminants in each of the ten bottled water brands analyzed. Contaminants included toxic by-products of chlorination at levels no different than routinely found in tap water. In fact, further investigation showed that the contaminants were often the same—and at similar levels to those found in the local water supply where products were bottled. This would indicate that many store brands are simply bottling the local tap water. Some store brands exceeded legal limits for water contaminants; four brands contained bacteria, some contained pain medication.[61]

The other issue with bottled water is the plastic that creates health and environmental concerns. The 2008 EWG study included assays for breast cancer cell proliferation. One bottled water brand caused a 78 percent increase in the growth of breast cancer cells compared to a control sample. When estrogen-blocking chemicals were added, the effect was inhibited, showing that the cancer-producing chemicals mimicked estrogen. The ingestion of endocrine-disrupting chemicals from plastics is an important health concern for those who exclusively drink bottled water.

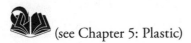 (see Chapter 5: Plastic)

One-and-a-half million tons of plastic are used to bottle water every year. Even though the plastic is recyclable, most of it ends up in landfills, slowly leaching its harmful components into the soil—a good reason to purchase bottled water from a source that bottles in glass. As much as possible, use and buy water in glass containers. If you choose to buy bottled water, look for brands that are sold in glass bottles or for brands that are more than just purified tap water (see sources).

WATER AND CONSCIOUSNESS

Dr. Masaru Emoto, author of the best-selling *Messages from Water* books, has gained worldwide acclaim through his research and his belief that water is deeply connected to our individual and collective consciousness. His work gained worldwide renown when it was featured in the film *What the Bleep Do We Know*.

Dr. Emoto postulated his theory of "Hado," which states that since everything is energy, by changing the vibration, we change the substance. Conventional science still does not support this idea, yet quantum physics clearly suggests we do alter our environment. By producing different energetic vibrations through words or music, the same water sample appears to "change its expression." Photographic documentation is found in several of his books. Dr. Emoto found that some of the most beautiful water crystals were formed in conjunction with the energy of love and gratitude.

We have the same ability to "change our expression" or to literally change who we are by changing our vibration and by resonating with thoughts and emotions based on love and gratitude. When we resonate at a higher level, we can have an influence on others around us—perhaps through the water. Just as a vibrating violin string can cause another string of the same frequency to vibrate, we may be able to awaken the vibrations of love and harmony in our fellow beings by holding these same frequencies ourselves. In turn, this will positively influence the water on the entire planet so that it can hold the frequencies that will connect us with the divine. Drinking water with the highest vibration can make a huge difference—not only in your physical health, but in your level of consciousness.

SOURCES (In the order they appear in the chapter):

Water filters:
http://www.berkeyfilters.com/
Radiant Life: http://www.radiantlifecatalog.com/sec.cfm/ct/7

Shower filters:
Wellness shower filter: www.wellnessfilter.com
Radiant Life shower filter: http://www.radiantlifecatalog.com/prod.cfm/ct/7
VitaCshower: http://vitacshower.com/FAQ.html

Vitamin C tablets for dechlorination of bathwater:
http://vitacshower.com/FAQ.html

Ozonation for pools:
www.Airwaterbestprices.com
www.intec-america.com/intec/

Water bottles:
Klean Kanteen: http://www.kleankanteen.com/

Bottled water:
Mountain Valley Spring Water (glass bottle) originates at a protected natural spring in Hot Springs, Arkansas: www.mountainvalleyspring.com

VOSS Artesian Water (glass bottle) from a virgin aquifer in central Norway: www.vosswater.com

Evian Water (glass and plastic bottles); a French mineral water from several sources near Évian-les-Bains, on the south shore of Lake Geneva: www.evian.com

Fiji water (plastic bottle); drawn from an artesian aquifer located at the edge of a primitive rainforest in Fiji: www.fijiwater.com

Volvic water (plastic bottle) from deep inside the ancient volcanoes of the Auvergne in France: www.volvic-na.com

Structured water:
Vitalizer Plus: www.wyntersway.com

Chapter 3

ELECTROMAGNETIC SMOG

✦

Another form of pollution

Dr. Neil Cherry, one of the first scientists to document the negative health effects of electromagnetic fields, declared, "No level of exposure to artificial fields is safe ... The safe level of exposure to 50/60 Hz fields is zero."[62] Since his early work, many more scientists have begun to document the link between artificial electromagnetic fields and a variety of cancers, diseases, and other health concerns.

Electromagnetic smog is a *major* cause of health problems in our modern world. It is invisible, silent, odorless, and tasteless; and unless we have become sensitized to it—often to the point of becoming sick—we are unaware of its presence. We are surrounded by a sea of electromagnetic frequencies unprecedented in the history of the human race. Consider how many devices and silent sources of electromagnetic interference have entered our modern world: high-voltage power lines; cell phones; computers; video display units; microwave ovens; electronic games; radio, television, and cell phone towers; satellites; police and military radar; and countless others. This form of invisible pollution permeates our homes, our work places, and the outdoors, and it creates a tremendous stress on all living systems.

Immediate symptoms of electromagnetic (EM) pollution include headaches, fatigue, dizziness, nausea, dehydration, lethargy, spaciness, depression, insomnia, irritability, anger, rage, and violence. Long-term effects include cancer, birth defects, blood sugar imbalances, multiple sclerosis, chronic fatigue, asthma, decreased immunity, and cognitive and other neurological disorders.[63]

The human body is an electrical system. Nearly every biological function depends on electrical signals. EM pollution disrupts the body's electromagnetic field and creates chaos and confusion to the point where cellular communication is impaired. Shielding has been placed into newer heart pacemakers so that interference does not cause misfiring and incorrect signaling to be sent to the heart. Organs also become strained in the presence of unnatural EM fields; the bloodstream holds more toxins, glands emit fewer hormones, and cells mutate.

At some level, governments, manufacturers, and medical groups acknowledge the potentially harmful effects of EM pollution. That's why EM shields are used in *every* industry. So, why have we not protected ourselves? The answer to this question is because we have been led to believe that the EM frequencies we are exposed to are safe. Nothing could be further from the truth! In 1984, the U.S. Navy conducted well-funded studies demonstrating that exposure to EM radiation resulted in altered cellular behavior, altered hormone levels, altered cell chemistry, altered immune function, modified human brain waves, and sterility in male animals. Their results have been reproduced in laboratory tests. However, these studies have been repressed and are not well known.[64]

Two organizations were charged by Congress to review the scientific literature and to assess the biological effects of exposure to low-frequency EM fields (the type generated by wiring and power lines). In 1997 and 1998, these reviews were released, downplaying the effects and concluding that there was no cause for alarm. But an in-depth review of these and other documents reveals bias and inconsistency.[65] Studies continue to document the effects of EM exposure on the nervous system, the blood, and on growth and development.

OUR ELECTRICAL CONNECTION WITH THE EARTH

Every minute, thousands of lightning strikes occur on the surface of the earth. These maintain the earth's direct current (DC) electrical field. Lightning has a high-frequency component followed by a low-frequency component. This produces electromagnetic waves and harmonics that characterize what is known as the Schumann Resonance—the frequency of the earth. Although the existence of the Schumann Resonance is an established scientific fact, there are very few who are aware of the importance of this frequency as a tuning fork for life.

All life on earth has evolved within the gentle DC electrical field of the earth. Without our connection to this field, we suffer. This has been documented in a study conducted at the Max Planck Institute for Behavioral Physiology. In an underground bunker that completely screened out the natural electromagnetic field of the earth, student volunteers lived for thirty days. These healthy students suffered emotional distress and migraine headaches, and it was noted that their normal circadian rhythms lost synchronicity.

However, after a brief exposure to 7.8 Hertz (the Schumann Resonance), the volunteers' state of health returned.[66] Similar symptoms were reported by the first astronauts and cosmonauts who were no longer exposed to the natural frequencies of the earth. Modern spacecraft are said to contain devices that simulate the earth's Schumann Resonance.

Our delicate electrical systems are finely tuned to the DC currents of the earth. Beyond synchronizing the biological rhythms that influence emotional and psychological balance, our connection with the earth has been shown to balance brain waves,[67] to reduce stress,[68] to improve sleep,[69] to relax muscles,[70] and to reduce inflammation.[71] Our electrical systems are disrupted when they are exposed to alternating current (AC), microwaves, and other unnatural EM fields that make up the electrical milieu of our modern world. Simple, direct connection with the earth (grounding) is often enough to relieve the symptoms of EM pollution.

EM smog, like other forms of pollution, has created an environment that is literally *out of tune* with nature. The consequences, although they are being covered up by utility companies and by the wireless technology industry, will add to our demise unless we protect ourselves and unless we demand the truth. Fortunately, necessity has guided the development of methods to shield and protect us from the damaging effects of EM pollution. The law of resonance is the key to the concept of EM protective devices, which can *re-tune* us to the frequencies of the earth and protect us from EM interference. This chapter discusses the major forms of EM pollution and some of the available technology that can protect you and your family.

SOURCES OF ELECTROMAGNETIC POLLUTION

There are three main ways we are exposed to electromagnetic radiation:

1. Through the air via wireless technologies (cell phones and Wi-Fi networks), high-frequency power lines, and satellite transmissions.
2. Via close proximity to electrical wiring in our homes and offices.
3. Through the ground via geomagnetic currents or if we live in the pathway of returning electrical currents to utility distribution hubs.

We can be affected by EM fields anywhere, any time. This is because a large portion of the problem comes through the air. Cell phone technology is now some of the most pervasive. Every year, more and more cell phone towers are erected to provide signals to cell phone users across the globe. Anyone who carries a cell phone is exposed. Wireless computer technology, otherwise known as Wi-Fi, connects people to the Internet in schools, coffee shops, and hotels. Every year, more Wi-Fi networks are established—often in homes with multiple computers. Laptop computers also use Wi-Fi technology. Other sources of EM pollution through the air include high-frequency power lines and satellite transmissions.

Cell phones and cordless phones

In 1993, the cell phone industry set up the Wireless Technology Research program and provided twenty-seven million dollars for research to prove that cell phone usage was safe. They hired George Carlo, MD, to head the program because of his long-time support for the use of cell phones. After six years, he was fired. Dr. Carlo then decided to publish his findings. His book *Cell Phones: Invisible Hazards in the Wireless Age* uncovers how the cell phone industry has distorted science and blatantly ignored evidence that suggests numerous potential health hazards.[72,73]

Since 1993, further evidence has accumulated showing that cell phones are dangerous. At least six studies have shown that cell phone radiation damages DNA—the first step to cancer. More studies have determined that sperm-making cells are particularly vulnerable to low-level radiation from cell phones.[74] This may account for the gradual reduction in sperm count in many men who carry cell phones in their pockets. Cell phones may also affect fertility in women. Since the hip produces 80 percent of the body's red blood cells, carrying a cell phone in your pocket may have a long-term effect on red blood cell supply and therefore on oxygen levels in your body.

Cell phone use has also been shown to cause damage to the blood vessels in the brain—even over short periods of time. Cell phone use opens the blood-brain barrier and allows the flow of proteins and sugar into the brain.[75] Each of these is major cause for alarm.

Thermal imaging (the ability to detect tiny temperature changes with a heat-sensitive camera) shows that within twenty minutes of cell phone use, the temperature of the head increases—up to 4° F. This is evidence that the use of cell phones can have adverse effects on the brain and other tissues.

> According to Professor Leif Salford, head of research at Lund University, Sweden,
> "The voluntary exposure of the brain to microwaves from hand-held mobile phones ... [is] the largest human biological experiment ever."

In 2008, Dr. G. Khurana, a top neurosurgeon, reviewed more than one hundred studies on the effects of mobile phones. He concluded that there is statistically significant evidence for a relationship between the long-term use of mobile phones and a delayed occurrence of brain tumors on the same side of the head. Brain tumors take several years to develop, but the odds for developing a brain tumor appear to be two to four times greater for cell phone users.[76] According to Dr. Khurana, Swedish researchers were the first to report a positive association between cell phone use and brain tumor risk. This is no surprise, since the Swedish were among the first to use cell phones.

In July of 2008, Dr. Ronald B. Herberman, director of the University of Pittsburgh Cancer Institute, issued an unprecedented warning to his faculty and staff. Based on early unpublished data, his advice was to limit cell phone use because of the possible risk of cancer.[77] The University of Pittsburgh Cancer Institute Web site contains a list of ten precautions for cell phone users.

Ten Precautions for Cell Phone Users

(From the University of Pittsburgh Cancer Institute Web site)
http://www.environmentaloncology.org/node/201

1. Do not allow children to use a cell phone except for emergencies. The developing organs of a fetus or child are the most likely to be sensitive to any possible effects of exposure to electromagnetic fields.

2. While communicating using your cell phone, try to keep the cell phone away from the body as much as possible. The amplitude of the electromagnetic field is one fourth the strength at a distance of two inches and fifty times lower at three feet. Whenever possible, use the speaker-phone mode or a wireless Bluetooth headset, which has less than 1/100th of the electromagnetic emission of a normal cell phone.

3. Avoid using your cell phone in places, like a bus, where you can passively expose others to your phone's electromagnetic fields.

4. Avoid carrying your cell phone on your body at all times. Do not keep it near your body at night such as under the pillow or on a bedside table, particularly if pregnant. You can also put it on "flight" or "off-line" mode, which stops electromagnetic emissions.

5. If you must carry your cell phone on you, make sure that the keypad is positioned toward your body and the back is positioned toward the outside so that the transmitted electromagnetic fields move away from your rather than through you.

6. Only use your cell phone to establish contact or for conversations lasting a few minutes as the biological effects are directly related to the duration of exposure. For longer conversations, use a land line with a corded phone, not a cordless phone, which uses electromagnetic emitting technology similar to that of cell phones.

7. Switch sides regularly while communicating on your cell phone to spread out your exposure. Before putting your cell phone to the ear, wait until your correspondent has picked up. This limits the power of the electromagnetic field emitted near your ear.

8. Avoid using your cell phone when the signal is weak or when moving at high speed, such as in a car or train, as this automatically increases power to a maximum as the phone repeatedly attempts to connect to a new relay antenna.

9. When possible, communicate via text messaging rather than making a call, limiting the duration of exposure and the proximity to the body.

10. Choose a device with the lowest SAR possible (SAR = Specific Absorption Rate, which is a measure of the strength of the magnetic field absorbed by the body). SAR ratings of contemporary phones by different manufacturers are available by searching for "sar ratings cell phones" on the internet.

Interesting research completed in 2008 revealed that EM frequencies from cell phones cause a significant increase in the release of mercury from dental amalgam (mercury) fillings.[78] Mercury is a neurotoxin. Increased release of mercury following cell phone use compounds the problem with EM radiation from cell phones. Researchers who conducted the study also documented increased mercury release following MRI (magnetic resonance imaging), and they suggested further work to determine the probable accelerated release of mercury in conjunction with other forms of EM pollution.

 (see Chapter 12: Mercury amalgam fillings)

Many cell phone users believe that if they use the hands-free earpiece provided with their phone, they are protecting themselves against microwave radiation directly to the head. In 2000, the British government reversed their endorsement of the hands-free earpiece when they discovered that cell phone–wired headsets can channel more than three times the amount of radiation into the head when compared to holding a phone against the ear. The headset wire connecting a cell phone and earpiece serves as an antenna that absorbs radiation. When a headset is used with a cell phone, the radiation generated by the phone *and* the airborne radiation are transferred through the wire and penetrate the head directly through the ear canal.

Air tube headsets have been designed to overcome the problem of radiation directly to the ear. The main advantage of using an air tube headset with your cell phone is that you eliminate the wire. Sound is delivered through an air-filled wireless tube. Testing shows that an air tube can reduce the amount of radiation to the head by up to 98 percent. Air tube earpieces are available for cell phones as well as for cordless phones (see sources).

> **Wireless headsets (the kind that are intended to stay in your ear for extended periods of time) represent an even greater risk because the wire is replaced with a transmitter *and* a receiver operating directly in your ear.**

Most cell phones now have the capacity to "ramp up" the signal when it is weak. This happens routinely in the car because of the blocking effect of the metal in the vehicle. This results in a greater exposure for you and others when a cell phone is used in a vehicle. It is important *not* to use your cell phone when it is roaming. This is when it is sending out the highest levels of radiation as it searches for a nearby antenna.

Children are especially susceptible to cell/cordless phone emissions for several reasons. A child's cranial bones are thinner than adult bones. Their cells are dividing much more rapidly, and their immune systems are not yet fully developed. In addition, children are likely to be exposed to many more times the radiation during their lifetime than adults who were raised before the advent of cell phones. In your home, a corded (landline) should be used whenever possible. If you use a cordless phone, use the speaker mode whenever possible.

No product can completely eliminate cell/cordless phone radiation, but it is possible to decrease emissions significantly with the use of EM shielding devices. If you use a cell or cordless phone, purchase a protective device (see sources). Remember to turn off your cell phone when it is not in use—especially while you sleep. A functioning cell phone on your night stand can be responsible for sleep disturbances and radiation damage while you sleep.

Wireless computer networks

Wireless networks (Wi-Fi) allow you to easily connect multiple computers and to move them from place to place without disconnecting and reconnecting wires. These networks are used for laptops and for other wireless devices and to connect to the Internet in public places. Like cell phones, wireless computer modems use EM radiation in the microwave frequency range. Wireless modems deliberately generate microwave radiation *all the time*.

The term *hotspot* is used to designate an area where a computer network exists—a place where a laptop or other wireless device can pick up the internet signal. This term is *literal*. If you have a computer network set up in your home, your whole home becomes a hotspot—a virtual antenna for the microwave frequencies that can heat up your body and cause numerous harmful effects. If you have a wireless modem in your home or if you use a laptop computer, it is important to install protection (see sources). Some individuals choose to wear personal protection as well.

Power lines

Another source of EM pollution is high-voltage electrical power lines which are constantly emitting both electric and magnetic fields. Even though distance reduces the danger, long-term exposure is hazardous. Secondary distribution lines, the kind you see in streets, may pose a larger problem than high-voltage transmission lines simply because they are often located so close to homes and places of business. Because the human body is mostly water and minerals, it is a *living antenna* and can absorb strong fields like those from power lines. The presence of power lines has been associated with the risk of childhood cancer in numerous epidemiological studies. If you live or work near power lines, consider the use of a protective device. Products are available that will significantly reduce EM exposure for the whole home (see sources).

Satellite dishes

If satellite dishes are even partially directed toward a power transmission line, they will absorb and focus its frequency. Main or secondary power lines in the vicinity of a satellite dish may actually be *amplified* by the satellite dish. Satellite dishes have been known to pick up and augment space satellite radiation and microwave communications between buildings. All this can create intensified hot spots in and around your home.

Electrical wiring

Being in close proximity to electrical wiring for extended periods of time exposes you to the effects of sixty-cycle (60 Hertz) alternating current (AC). The sixty-cycle AC used in American homes literally makes the electrons in your body vibrate back and forth sixty times every second. Imagine the stress this can cause to a living electrical system.

There are two components of the EM field that are produced by electrical wiring and electrical appliances. The magnetic component is only generated when an appliance is turned *on* but the electrical component exists as soon as an appliance is plugged in—even if it is turned *off*. EM fields radiate out in all directions from wiring and appliances. This includes the electrical wiring behind the walls of your home. In other words, if circuit breakers are on, there are EM fields continually radiating throughout your home, and you do not have to touch an appliance or its wiring to conduct the current running through it. All you have to do is be within several feet of it to have *induced* current running through your body as though you were part of the wiring. Because the frequency of the human nervous system is so close to the frequency of man-made electrical systems, resonance can be established. This resonance between electrical wiring and the nervous system allows for the transference of energy that can have many detrimental biological effects. One of the best studied of these effects is the body's stress response outlined in the book *Electromagnetic Fields* by Blake Levitt. Another effect is the destabilization of the body's calcium, lithium, potassium, and magnesium, which govern calmness, mood, and memory.

> **Pay particular attention to the electrical equipment in your sleeping environment. Move alarm clocks and lamps away from your bed. Avoid electric blankets and heating pads.**

The environment where you sleep is critical. Most people have bedside lamps or clock radios nearby. Heated water beds and electric blankets also produce EM fields that are right up against your body. If you have even *one* electrical device near your bed, or if your head is near to wiring within the wall (typically wiring runs about two feet above the baseboard), then your chances of insomnia and other stress-related sleep disorders is many times greater.

There are several ways to dispel the induced current we pick up from wiring and electrical appliances in our homes and offices. One way is to place shielding devices on each appliance. Another method is to use filters at each electrical outlet to reduce EM fields. In some instances, it may be wise to use several methods (see sources). Some electro-sensitive individuals turn the circuit breakers to their bedroom off during the night. Other individuals use conductive sheets that plug into the grounding system of their home and connect them to the earth during sleep. These methods reduce or eliminate many sleep disturbances, as long as there are no ground currents present carrying what has been termed "dirty electricity."

> **One of the best things you can do is to walk barefoot on the earth whenever possible. Just 30 minutes of direct earth contact every day is said to work wonders for those who are electro-sensitive.**

Dirty electricity

Electric power is intended to power our homes and buildings at a frequency of 60 Hertz. Today, the current is contaminated with micro-surges of radio frequency radiation and other EM contaminants referred to by some as "dirty electricity." Dirty electricity has increased with our use of fluorescent, energy-efficient lighting and electronic devices such as dimmer switches and video display terminals. Modern electrical appliances induce high levels of transient current (high-frequency spikes) and harmonics (multiples of the fundamental 60 Hertz frequency) back into a building's electrical system. These EM contaminants ride along on the electrical system and can contaminate nearby buildings and homes.

The National Electrical Safety Code specifically mandates that current which leaves the utility's substation over the utility's wires must return to the substation over the utility's own neutral wires. However, often the neutral wire is not adequate to carry all of the returning current. In 1992, many utility companies began installing ground rods on utility poles to eliminate overloaded neutral wires. This sends the return current into the ground rather than through the neutral wire on its way back to the substation. Some believe that if you are unfortunate enough to be in the pathway of an overloaded neutral current returning to a substation, the very ground you walk on could carry hazardous currents that enter your home via metal objects and plumbing. If your home lies in this return pathway, your whole home could be exposed to *dirty electricity*.

Ground current can carry unpredicted high frequencies and in some cases dangerous voltages into a home or building. Radio frequency waves from nearby broadcast transmitters can also enter a home through the air and be picked up and re-radiated by a building's electrical system, thus adding to a person's daily, ongoing exposure to EM energy.

Dave Stetzer has done extensive research and has designed filters that have been used with tremendous success in schools and other public buildings. Within weeks after the installation of these filters, the symptoms of chronic fatigue, multiple sclerosis, asthma, fibromyalgia, tinnitus, and diabetes have been ameliorated for both teachers and students (see sources).

Microwave ovens

Over 90 percent of American homes have microwave ovens used for meal preparation. Because microwave ovens are so convenient and so energy efficient, very few homes or restaurants are without them. Manufacturers and government agencies have told us for a long time that microwave ovens do not leak harmful radiation, and that they do not alter food. Both claims are false. Microwave oven enclosures may reduce the amount of radiation emitted, but they are not leak proof.

> ## Does your microwave oven leak? Try this simple experiment:
>
> Place your cell phone inside a microwave oven and close the door. Using another telephone, dial your cell phone number. If it rings, you know that microwave radiation penetrated the oven—and that it is able to leak into your living environment.

A large amount of literature has been published on the biological effects of microwave radiation. Exposure can result in significant amounts of energy being absorbed by the body. Just as with food, this energy is transformed into heat in the body. Sensitive body parts, such as the eyes, testes, and brain, are not able to flush the extra heat that may build up. People working in microwave fields have reported headaches, eyestrain, fatigue, and sleep disturbance. These effects have been associated with the interaction of the microwave fields with the central nervous system of the body. Those who understand the effects of microwave radiation refuse to have microwave ovens in their homes. There are other reasons not to use microwave ovens. What they do to food is equally (if not more) disturbing.

 (see Chapter 5: Microwave cooking)

Video display terminals

In 1988, researchers at the Northern California Kaiser Permanente Medical Care Program in Oakland, California, reported a statistically significant association between video display terminals and miscarriage. In a survey of 1,583 women, those using video display terminals for more than twenty hours a week during the first three months of pregnancy had nearly twice as many miscarriages as women in similar jobs who were not using video display terminals.[79] Other studies with mice support these findings.

Changes in brain wave patterns are also induced by the kind of radiation coming from video display terminals. The result is behavioral symptoms such as sluggishness, depression, and the inability to concentrate. Many computer operators experience these symptoms. Beyond these difficulties, eye strain has been a problem with those who work at video terminals, caused by the ultraviolet (UV) emissions.

Older cathode ray terminals (CRTs) are known to emit many more times the radiation—especially from the back and sides of the terminal—than the newer, liquid crystal, flat screen monitors. However, both are cause for caution. Those who work in rooms with rows and rows of computers get the most exposure and should be cautioned and protected.

Baby monitors

Baby monitors operate at a wide variety of frequencies with corresponding differences in transmitting power and range. Most baby monitors are not permitted to transmit continuously, and signals are only transmitted from a given sound level. Since little is known about the possible long-term effects of the weak, high-frequency EM fields used in baby monitors, precautionary measures should be taken. Many have noticed improvements in their baby's sleep when monitors are moved just six feet away.

- Place the monitor at least six feet away from your baby.
- Do not use systems that transmit continuously.
- Set the baby unit to "voice activation mode" rather than to a continuous transmission mode.

Hair dryers

The Department of Energy has conducted extensive research on household appliances and determined that hair dryers are responsible for emitting excessive EM fields. Because hair dryers are placed so close to the head during operation, they can cause many times the exposure as other appliances.

The link between childhood leukemia and exposure to hair dryer emissions was reported in a 1998 U.S. government report prepared under a 65 million dollar allocation under the EMF RAPID Program.[80] The University of Southern California and the National Cancer Institute have also linked children's leukemia to hair dryer usage. To date, few hair dryers have been developed and tested to limit EM exposure.

Geopathic fields

In addition to the artificially produced EM fields, we are also influenced by variations in magnetic fields in the earth itself. These fields are called geomagnetic or geopathic fields. Many people living near power lines are adversely affected when there is a synergistic effect between geomagnetic fields and the EM fields produced by power supply—they tend to enhance each other. If a bed or a workplace is situated in an area where there are high variations in the geomagnetic field, persistent health problems may occur. When a bed is moved to a more suitable position (often only two or three feet away), the person improves. Geopathic fields can be determined by using a detection instrument called a geomagnetometer (see sources).

ELECTRO-SENSITIVITY

Electro-sensitivity is a condition characterized by sensitivity to electricity. It is unique among medical conditions in that each individual reacts to different sources of electricity with his/her own set of symptoms. This uniqueness makes it difficult for the medical profession to accept. A growing number of countries are just beginning to recognize it as a medical condition.

There is a strong link between chemical toxicity and electrical sensitivities. Many people feel that electro-sensitivity is a by-product of chemical sensitivity. The UK-based Breakspear Hospital, which specializes in the treatment of environmental illness, reports: "As the food and chemical sensitivities come under control and the body detoxifies itself, the electrical sensitivities usually go as well."[81]

The Breakspear Hospital recommends the following five-point program for the treatment of many environmental illnesses that appear to be linked to a toxic overload.

1. Neutralizing food sensitivities
2. Minimizing EM exposure
3. Minimizing exposure to toxic chemicals
4. Restoring nutritional status
5. Removing heavy metals

The Environmental Health Center in Dallas, Texas, offers treatment based on a similar theory—that those with electro-sensitivity and multiple-chemical sensitivity are overburdened with chemicals, EM pollution, bacteria, viruses, and the like, causing the body to become hypersensitive. Their program of is one of detoxification and nutritional support.[82]

EM PROTECTION DEVICES

The naturally occurring frequency that is important to all life is the Schumann Resonance (7.8 Hertz). Our body and brain are balanced at this frequency when we are connected to the earth. When we are disconnected from the earth and exposed to a variety of unnatural EM frequencies, we become out of sync in many ways.

In order to protect embassy personnel against microwave radiation at the U.S. Embassy in Moscow, personnel were provided with protective devices that produced earth's natural resonant frequency. Many EM protection devices work in a similar way. They provide the frequency of the Schumann Resonance or other balancing frequencies that support coherence.

Coherence is an inherent order within a system where individual units (organs, glands, and cells) operate as components of the whole rather than as individual parts. Coherence is a fundamental factor distinguishing life from nonlife.[83] In essence, a greater degree of coherence results in a greater ability to function and in a greater ability to withstand stress. EM frequencies disrupt the electromagnetic order in biological systems. They diminish coherence and the subsequent ability to adjust to stress. Prolonged exposure to unnatural EM frequencies wears down an organism by reducing its ability to operate as a coherent whole. Chaos cannot exist in the presence of coherence. When coherence is supported or reestablished, an organism is able to function in balance despite stress from the environment.

One type of EM protection called *earthing* connects a person directly to the earth. Earthing dissipates extraneous electric fields back to the earth. Perhaps more importantly, *earthing* also connects the human body with the Schumann Resonance and provides access to the plethora of frequencies on the earth that balance hormones and biological rhythms.[84] Free electrons provided by these products from the earth have been shown to reduce inflammation and to counter the effects of free radicals[85] (see sources).

LifeBEAT products support overall coherence by supplying the frequencies that bring the body back into homeostasis. Medical imaging shows the restoration of organ balance within a few minutes after using these products (see sources).

Some protective devices eliminate the dipolar activity in the environment. The best known application of this technology is radar absorbent material— the type of material that makes the Stealth Bomber aircraft invisible to radar. This material has no polarity and allows EM fields to pass through it in such a way that they are rendered harmless.

Most types of protection are based on filtering out the chaotic EM interference. These come in the form of bracelets, necklaces, and other items that are worn on or near the body. The Teslar device is one of the best known of this type of device. It looks like a watch (see sources).

Stetzerizers, or Stetzer filters, actually filter the transient and harmonic frequencies that ride the electrical system. They are intended to be plugged into the electrical system of the home (see sources).

DIET FOR REDUCING ELECTROMAGNETIC EFFECTS

To deal with the onslaught of EM pollution and its debilitating effects, the body must operate at maximum efficiency. Most people who become sensitive to the effects of EM fields are first weakened (overburdened) in some other way. Their bodies are already out of balance and vulnerable to the additional stress caused by EM pollution.

> **Our bodies and minds cannot function properly without good nutrition—it is the basis of health. Nutritional balance and the absence of toxins are our best safeguards against disease and against the effects of electromagnetic pollution.**

EM pollution greatly accelerates the formation of free radicals. In order to protect against EM field damage, a diet high in antioxidants, including whole, fresh fruits and vegetables that are high in antioxidants, is advisable.

The largest and most recent analysis of the antioxidant content of common fruits and vegetables revealed that many beans have a higher antioxidant content than many widely acclaimed fruits. Just a half-cup of small red beans, pinto beans, or kidney beans have as many antioxidants as a cup of blueberries or cranberries, [86] although some exotic fruits have been shown to have higher antioxidant values.

Antioxidant Values of Fruits and Vegetables from the Study[87]

Rank	Food	Serving Size	Total Antioxidant per Serving
1	Small red bean (dried)	Half-cup	13727
2	Wild blueberry	1 cup	13427
3	Red kidney bean (dried)	Half-cup	13259
4	Pinto bean	Half-cup	11864
5	Blueberry (cultivated)	1 cup	9019
6	Cranberry	1 cup (whole)	8983
7	Artichoke (cooked)	1 cup (hearts)	7904
8	Blackberry	1 cup	7701
9	Prune	Half-cup	7291
10	Raspberry	1 cup	6058
11	Strawberry	1 cup	5938
12	Red delicious apple	One whole	5900
13	Granny Smith apple	One whole	5381
14	Pecan	1 ounce	5095
15	Sweet cherry	1 cup	4873
16	Black plum	One	4844
17	Russet potato (cooked)	One	4649
18	Black bean (dried)	Half-cup	4181
19	Plum	One	4118
20	Gala apple	One	3903

If you are electro-sensitive or if you want to stabilize your health, it is advisable to maintain a diet without sugar, white flour, processed foods, alcohol, dairy products, and caffeine. Many foods and whole-food nutritional supplements will bolster the immune system and nourish the cells so that the effects of electromagnetic pollution are diminished. One of the authors advocates a nutrient-dense, whole-food program. For more information visit www.wyntersway.com

IONIZING RADIATION

Ionizing radiation is an extremely strong form of radiation with exceptionally short wavelengths that are capable of breaking atomic bonds and knocking electrons from their orbits. It can cause radiation poisoning and death in large doses. Small doses can be equally fatal—they just take a longer period of time to manifest. When our DNA is exposed to ionizing radiation, genetic mutations can occur. Some radiation-induced damage is repaired by various systems within the cell, but DNA double-strand breaks are not easily repaired and can lead to mutations, chromosomal translocations, and gene fusions. Each of these is linked with the onset of cancer.[88] There are a number of different forms of ionizing radiation that we can be exposed to including cosmic radiation, nuclear fallout, radioactive elements on the earth, and medical radiology.

Cosmic radiation

Earth is continually bombarded with ionizing radiation from outer space. As a general rule, we are protected by Earth's atmosphere and by Earth's magnetic field—both of which deflect ionizing radiation. Exposure is greatest at the poles where the magnetic field is weakest and at high altitudes where the air is thinner. Ionizing radiation is a concern for airline crews and frequent passengers who spend many hours in flight.

 (see Chapter 18: In-flight ionizing radiation)

Nuclear radiation

Frequent above-ground nuclear explosions between the 1940s and 1960s scattered a substantial amount of ionizing radiation. Some of this contamination was local, although much of it was carried longer distances as nuclear fallout. The increase in background radiation due to these tests peaked in 1963 and is gradually reducing.

Terrestrial radiation

Terrestrial sources of ionizing radiation include radioactive elements found in the soil and in the water. Unless you work with these elements or live in an area known to contain higher than normal amounts of radioactivity, this need not be a problem. Radon is the exception. Although it is uncommon, radon can be found in high concentrations in many areas of the world, where it represents a significant health hazard.

 (see Chapter 1: Radon)

Medical radiology

Ionizing radiation is also used in medical and dental diagnostic procedures. On average, about 15 percent of the ionizing radiation a person receives comes from medical radiology represented by x-rays, CT scans, and a variety of other procedures including angiographies, arteriographies, barium enemas, barium swallows, cholecystograms, hysterosalpingographies, intravenous pyelograms (IVPs), kidney-urinary-bladder (KUB) studies, mammograms, and upper and lower gastrointestinal series. These procedures all require ionizing radiation directed into your body, for which there is no safe level. Cancer, which develops years after exposure, is more common than we have been told. If you are healthy or if you do not submit to these procedures, your exposure may be minimal. If, on the other hand, you are hospitalized, or in need of regular diagnostic exams, you may succumb to many of these procedures over and over again and be at greater risk of developing cancer and other diseases. It is a serious concern for children who are many times more susceptible to damage from ionizing radiation.

From the very beginning, the public has been led to believe that ionizing radiation is less harmful than it is. Nuclear testing performed in many areas of the world in the 1900s made guinea pigs of masses of the population. Today, the medical profession uses x-ray and CT scans as though they were inert forms of diagnosis. They are not. According to recent literature, over half a million Americans die every year from diseases caused by overexposure to radiation associated with medical imaging.[89] CT scans are the biggest culprit. Compared with x-rays, CT scans involve much higher doses of radiation and represent substantial risks—especially for children.[90] Children have more years of life during which a potential cancer can be expressed. Growing children also have a larger proportion of dividing cells susceptible to genetic mutation. Children may be up to fifty times more likely to develop cancer than adults receiving the same dose.[91]

Interesting research based on the data collected from survivors of the atomic bombs in Japan indicates that low radiation doses, like those used in medical imaging, are the most likely to cause cancer years after exposure.[92] Survivors of the atomic bomb who received low doses of radiation similar to the amount from a typical CT scan had significantly increased risks of cancer.[93,94] The best explanation for this is that when low doses of radiation pass through human tissue, they cause deletions in the structure of individual chromosomes. (Damaged chromosomes instruct cells to turn cancerous.) At higher doses, the chromosomes can be entirely obliterated or they can be mutated in a way that does not form cancer-instructing deletions.[95]

John Gofman, PhD, MD, worked as a nuclear physicist on the Manhattan Project (the project that created the first atomic bomb). After receiving his medical degree in cardiology, he was selected to lead the Atomic Energy Commission's research to study the effects of radiation on human health. After seven years, he and his colleague concluded the following:

- *All* forms of cancer can be induced by radiation.
- The risk of contracting cancer—per unit of radiation exposure—is twenty times worse than the official estimates.
- Children are far more susceptible than adults.
- There is *no* safe dose of radiation.[96]

Dr. Gofman testified before Congress in 1969 and reported these and other findings. Shortly thereafter, he was dismissed from his position and his research was canceled. He dedicated the rest of his life to educating the public. One of his later books uncovered the undeniable link between the medical use of radiation and both cancer and heart disease.

Of the half a million deaths caused annually by overexposure to radiation associated with medical imaging, some are due to too many diagnostic procedures performed over the course of a lifetime. Others are due to equipment that is not properly calibrated. Most x-ray and CT scan equipment made before 2005 does not come with a gauge. Often, the dose dialed in is not accurate. A 1977 publication reported data from 1,433 clinics showing that radiation dosages for a chest x-ray varied from 3 to 2,300 miliroentgens.[97] Until recently, there has been little monitoring of this glaring problem.

In 2006, the FDA established new regulations to protect against excessive radiation and dose variability. Equipment manufactured after 2006 is required to include displays of duration, rate, and cumulative radiation. It is also required to filter increased radiation during longer procedures and to have tighter controls on the size of the x-ray field. Unfortunately, these measures do not apply to the equipment manufactured before 2006, which represents the majority of equipment in use today.

Before you submit to x-rays, CT scans, mammograms, or any of the above mentioned radiographic procedures, ask your health care provider these questions:

1. Is this procedure really necessary?
2. Are there non-radiological alternatives? (Often there are.)
3. Are you aware of the other sources of radiation to which I have been exposed in my lifetime—and the cumulative risk?
4. How much radiation will be delivered during the proposed procedure? (Most doctors do not know.)
5. When was the diagnostic equipment last calibrated by a medical physicist?

Digital x-ray technology was designed to reduce radiation exposure by giving a technician the freedom to carefully select dosage and duration. Quite the opposite is more likely to occur.[98] In several U.S. hospitals evaluated, the number of examinations per outpatient visit increased by 21 percent when digital x-ray equipment was installed.[99] Reasons for this include the fact that there is a tendency to take more images than necessary and at a higher image quality (and radiation dose) than necessary. It is also easy to delete digital images and to repeat exposures.

Alternatives to medical radiology

One of the most important questions you can ask your doctor or that you can research for yourself is, what other nonradiological alternatives are there? Infrared thermography (taking heat-sensitive photos) is a very useful, inexpensive alternative to some radiological procedures. It can detect breast cancer much earlier and more reliably than a mammogram by revealing the extra heat associated with increased blood flow to developing tumors. The technique is noncontact, it emits no radiation, and is 100 percent safe. Women are in a far better position to detect breast cancer themselves if they perform regular self-exams. An inexpensive device called the Breast Chek dramatically magnifies the sensitivity of your fingertips and increases your chances of early detection (see sources).

Ultrasound, well known for fetal imaging, is another potential alternative to radiological procedures, as is magnetic resonance imaging. If you must submit to x-rays, to a CT scan, or to another radiological procedure, increase your intake of antioxidants to reduce the free radical damage and to help your body repair tissue damage caused by ionizing radiation.

SOURCES (in the order they appear in the chapter):

EM shielding devices:
LifeBEAT Products: sprays and bio-wear to enhance coherence: www.wyntersway.com

Earthing technology: www.earthing.com/. Grounding the human body to the earth.

Teslar Technology: http://www.teslartech.com. Teslar watches and other EM field protection.

Stetzer Electric: www.stetzerelectric.com. Stetzer filters and microsurge meters for EM field detection.

BlockEMF: http://www.blockemf.com. Geo-magnetometers, personal protection, shielding devices, cell phone protection, whole-home protection.

EarthCalm: http://earthcalm.com/. Personal and whole-home protection.

Shield EMF protection: www.ShieldEMF.com. Personal and cell phone protection etc.

Energy Polarity: www.energpolarit.com. Personal protection and cell phone devices, appliance diodes and whole-home harmonizers.

Air tube headsets:
http://www.wyntersway.com/eco-friendly-headsets.html
RF-3 Air Tube headset: http://www.rfsafe.com/a_rf3headset.htm

Breast Chek Kit:
http://www.betterbreastcheck.com/

 Recommended reading:
Electromagnetic Fields: A Consumer's Guide to the Issues and How to Protect Ourselves by Blake Levitt

Cellphones: Invisible Hazards in the Wireless Age by Dr. George Carlo
X-Rays, Health Effects of Common Exams by John Gofman, MD

Chapter 4

WHAT'S WRONG WITH OUR FOOD?

Hippocrates, the father of medicine, said, "Let food be thy medicine and medicine be thy food." Today, doctors swear the Hippocratic Oath, yet they ignore the original advice. The foundation for staying healthy in a toxic world is proper nutrition—often easier said than done. Especially today, making sure that the food you eat has the greatest complement of nutrients can go a long way toward your being able to thrive in a toxic world.

Each cell in your body is a living, breathing entity receiving nourishment and getting rid of wastes through the bloodstream. Whether you eat an organic carrot or a box of chemically laden cereal, your bloodstream faithfully carries it to your cells. The question arises: What exactly *is* being carried to your cells?

Pesticides are a major factor in the demise of our food. However, they represent only a portion of the problem. Before a crop is even planted, the chances that it may have been genetically modified or genetically contaminated by nearby genetic breeding programs are increasing. Next, consider the preservatives and the food additives that are routinely added during the processing of food. Even the packaging materials may contain toxic preservatives that have now been banned in some countries. What about irradiation, the practice of bombarding food with ionizing radiation? This practice has been approved in the United States for nearly every type of food, and it is nearly impossible to tell which foods have been irradiated and which foods have not. Add to all of the above the blatant fact that our soils have been depleted and poisoned by years of intensive agriculture. Unfortunately, what's in our food, today, is no longer capable of sustaining healthy life. No wonder Americans are some of the sickest, most malnourished individuals in the world.

The food industry in the United States is purely profit motivated. What ends up in the grocery store is the result of corporate America's greed and total disregard for our health. Nutritional quality is routinely cast aside in favor of yield, cost of production, shelf life, insect resistance, and so on. On a more positive note, there are a few companies and a number of small organic growers who refuse to be controlled by corporate America. They continue to provide toxin-free food capable of nourishing our bodies, minds, and spirits. The following chapter is designed to alert you to the dangers of the toxins and chemicals in the food supply and to provide information to help you make wise choices.

ORGANIC—WHAT DOES IT MEAN?

Organic farming refers to agricultural production (food and clothing) without the use of synthetic pesticides and fertilizers. Additionally, in order to be classified as organic, foods must be minimally processed without artificial ingredients, preservatives, or irradiation. By definition, organic foods are not genetically altered. However, even this has become an issue because of cross pollination.

100 Percent Organic

According to the USDA's national organic standard, products labeled 100 percent organic can only contain organically produced ingredients. Products containing 100 percent organic ingredients can display the USDA organic logo and/or the certifying agent's logo.

Organic

To be labeled as organic, 95 percent of the ingredients must be organically grown, and the remaining 5 percent must come from approved nonorganic ingredients. These products may also display the USDA organic logo and/or the certifier's logo.

Made with Organic Ingredients

Food products labeled "made with organic ingredients" must be made with at least 70 percent organic ingredients, three of which must be listed on the back of the package, and the remaining 30 percent of the nonorganic ingredients must be from an approved list. These products may display the certifier's logo but not the USDA organic logo.

Organic certification includes inspection of fields and processing facilities; it includes periodic testing of soil and water to ensure that standards are met. This does not mean that pesticides are never used, but it does mean that when pesticides are deemed necessary, permission may be granted by the certifying organization to apply *botanical* or other *nonpersistent* pest controls under restricted conditions. Botanical pesticides are derived from plants and are broken down much more rapidly than traditional pesticides.

Unfortunately, since government regulations control the certification of organic products, even the term "organic" means less than it did years ago. Many of the largest organic brands are now owned and operated by the same big corporations that sell regular brands and junk foods. The following Web site created by Phil Howard, at Michigan State University, includes a variety of charts that identify which large corporations own which organic brands: http://www.msu.edu/~howardp/organicindustry.html.

Whenever you can find local, organic growers or participate in a co-op where you know the sources of the food you eat, you will have even greater insurance of its quality. If this is not possible, make sure the organic products you purchase have certification logos.

PESTICIDES

The damage produced by pesticides is pervasive. Researchers have discovered that often pesticides do more damage at low levels than at higher doses.[100] Of the hundreds of pesticides still in use today, many are proven to cause cancer, birth defects, neurological disorders, autoimmune syndromes, and hormone disruption. One of the most recent and critical concerns with the continued use of pesticides (as well as with plastics and other chemicals) is their estrogenic effects—the mimicking of feminizing hormones that dramatically alter sexuality and fertility. The average sperm count in men has dropped from 125 million/ml in 1932 to 50 million/ml in 1998.[101]

Facts about Pesticides in the Foods We Eat:

- It is possible for a two-year-old child to have ingested more than the lifetime tolerated amount of pesticides by eating only half of one non-organic, pesticided apple.
- The average one-year-old can eat certain fruits (such as two grapes or three bites of some apples, pears, or peaches), and that amount will exceed the EPA safe *adult* exposure level to organophosphate pesticides.
- Some winter squash, green beans, spinach, celery, and lettuce were found to contain more than the daily safe limit of pesticides for children—in one serving.
- High levels of chlordane (banned in 1983) have still been found in potatoes, carrots, beets, lettuce, and zucchini. This could be due to contaminated soil or the use of chlordane that was stockpiled years ago.
- Every day, nine of ten children aged six months to five years are exposed to combinations of thirteen different nerve-damaging insecticides in the food they eat—even after washing and processing the food.

—*Our Toxic World: A Wake-Up Call* by Doris Rapp, MD

Almost nothing is known about the long-term impact of most of the pesticides in use today. A National Research Council study found that complete information on the hazards to human health were available for only 10 percent of pesticides. In a study of Mexican/Indian children, one group was routinely exposed to pesticide sprays as well as to the regular use of pesticides in the home. The other group was exposed to a pesticide only during the annual DDT spraying for malaria. When these children were evaluated at ages four and five, it was discovered that those who were exposed to pesticides could not jump up and down as well; they could not draw a stick figure; they had poor eye/hand coordination; and they were less sociable and creative. These children also had less stamina, poor short-term memory, and more behavioral problems.

Not only are we unaware of the long-term consequences of pesticide use, but pesticides are flagrantly overused and not well regulated. What may end up in our food can be anything from currently accepted levels (which are often inappropriate) to toxic doses in one meal. Many pesticides are routinely used by gardeners and homeowners with no idea of the long-term consequences.

Organochlorides
This large category of pesticides includes DDT, 2,4-D, aldrin, dieldrin, lindane (the active ingredient in lice-control shampoos), endrin, and chlordane. Although some of these pesticides have been banned, residues continue to persist in soils everywhere. Organochloride pesticides cause damage to the skin, liver, kidneys, and to the immune system.

Organophosphates
Examples of common organophosphate pesticides are diazinon, parathion, and malathion. This category was originally designed as nerve gas; these chemicals can damage the lungs, intestines, bladder, heart, muscles, nerves, and brain. They have been associated with sociopathic disorders including rage and violent behavior. Diazinon is toxic to the nervous system. It can cause headaches, blurred vision, and memory problems. The sale of diazinon for indoor use was banned in 2002, but 70 percent of agricultural use continues. Parathion is known to disrupt fertility; it has caused more deaths than any other organophosphate.

Carbamates
Carbamates are similar to the organophosphate pesticides. Common pesticides in this classification include Sevin, Carbaryl, and Aldicarb.

Carbamate chemicals are used in clothing, medicines, and plastics. They have been known to cause blurred vision, twitches, convulsions, weakness, memory loss, behavioral problems, cancer, defective sperm, and birth defects. Like the organophosphates, carbamates have been associated with extreme, unprovoked anger and violence.

One of the biggest difficulties with pesticides is *drift*. They can be carried for miles on the wind. Scientists have tracked DDT-containing clouds that originated in Africa where the use of DDT is still in full force.[102] These DDT-laden clouds eventually rain everywhere, contaminating soils and water worldwide. Even organic crops can be contaminated if farmers spray on windy days. If you live in an agricultural area, you or your own crops may be at risk.

Organic is better

There is no longer any doubt that eating organic food has its advantages. In 2003, researchers at the University of Washington compared a group of eighteen children who ate organic food with twenty-one children who all ate conventionally produced food. The children were all roughly the same age (two to five years old), gender, and of similar family income. The children with organic diets had far lower (six to nine times) levels of pesticide metabolites in their bodies.[103] Researchers in this study concluded that eating organic fruits and vegetables could significantly reduce the pesticide burden carried by children. This information provides a level of certainty for parents who choose to feed organic food to their children.

For some, switching to organic food may not be entirely possible. In this case, knowing which crops have the highest levels of pesticides may be important. There are twelve crops that are known as the "Dirty Dozen" because they contain the highest levels of pesticides, according to the Environmental Working Group, a nonprofit research organization in Washington DC. These crops, above others, should be purchased in organic form whenever possible.

Best and Worst Crops

The Dirtiest Dozen (beginning with the worst)
- peaches
- apples
- sweet bell peppers
- celery
- nectarines
- strawberries
- cherries
- pears
- grapes
- spinach
- lettuce
- potatoes

The Cleanest Dozen (beginning with the best)
- onions
- avocados
- sweet corn (frozen)
- pineapples
- mangoes
- asparagus
- sweet peas (frozen)
- kiwi fruit
- bananas
- cabbage
- broccoli
- papaya

GENETIC MODIFICATION

Genetic modification (GM), also known as genetic engineering, gene splicing, or recombinant DNA technology, is the alteration of a living organism's genetic makeup by transferring one or more genes from another organism. GMO stands for genetically modified organism, referring to a plant or other organism that has been modified.

The most common reason for genetic modification is for resistance to herbicides, pests, diseases, drought, or temperature variations. Other reasons for GM include yield enhancement, nutritional enhancement, extension of shelf-life, improved flavor, and processing characteristics.

There are still many questions about the safety of consuming genetically modified foods. Proponents argue that GM is not fundamentally different from other breeding programs. The difference, however, is that GM creates *unnatural* genetic combinations. GM recombines the genetic material from plants, insects, or animals for which there is no (or low) probability of natural breeding. New genes or DNA sequences are introduced into chromosomal locations, which can result in unpredictable effects on the environment and on human health. Several examples of this are cited:

- Tobacco plants genetically engineered to produce gamma-linolenic acid also produced actadecatetraenic acid—a toxin.
- Yeast modified to obtain increased fermentation unexpectedly accumulated methylglyoxal in toxic and mutagenic concentrations.
- Soybeans modified with a gene from the Brazil nut also had allergenic characteristics.
- In a Philippine village located near GM corn fields, fevers, respiratory illnesses, and skin reactions became prevalent. The corn, called Bt maize, contains a pesticide in the gene. Blood tests showed that the villagers had developed antibodies to the built-in pesticide. Four families left the village and recovered—and then got sick again when they returned.

All of the European Union nations as well as Japan, China, Australia, New Zealand, and many other countries require the mandatory labeling of foods that contain GM ingredients. As a result, most food manufacturers in these countries choose to use non-GM ingredients. In the United States, unless food is labeled "organic" it may contain GMOs—you will never know. There are currently *no labeling requirements* for GM products. Because of the widespread use of GM corn and soy, it is estimated that more than 70 percent of the foods in grocery stores in the United States and Canada currently contain GM ingredients. If the product label says corn, corn flour, dextrin, starch, soy, soy sauce, margarine, or tofu there is a good chance that it has GM ingredients.

Because of something called *gene flow*, even organic growers are having difficulty maintaining non-GM status. Gene flow causes genetic contamination of non–genetically engineered crops. More organic farmers are reporting traces of GM organisms in their crops all the time. This is because all genetically engineered organisms include genes that are designed to overcome natural reproductive barriers between organisms. In a study published in *Nature* it was revealed that GM mustard plants were twenty times more likely to crossbreed than regular mustard plants growing right next to them.[104]

Another recent view theorizes that GM foods are behind the new disease called Morgellons disease, which is characterized by tiny fibers that grow from skin lesions. These fibers appear to be synthetic. They cause extreme itching and the feeling that something is crawling underneath the skin. Laboratory testing discovered agrobacterium in the mysterious fibers—the same agrobacterium inserted in the DNA during genetic manipulation of plants.[105, 106]

The only way U.S. citizens are likely to be protected from GM is if they let legislators know of their concern and if they request support for legislation that requires appropriate labeling. The following Web site tells you how you can fight back against GM foods: http://www.naturalnews.com/026908_food_GMO_Monsanto.html

To read a well-researched article by Nathan Batalion titled *50 Harmful Effects of Genetically Modified Foods,* visit this Web site: http://www.raw-wisdom.com/50harmful.

IRRADIATED FOOD

Irradiation destroys harmful bacteria and fungus on fruits and vegetables, meats, and other products. This allows meat and produce to sit on the shelf for much longer than nonirradiated food. But the practice is not without tremendous health hazards.

Irradiation uses ionizing radiation to split molecular bonds with high-energy beams. This kills pathogens, but it forms an abundance of free radicals and "radiolytic" compounds in food. The damaging effects of irradiated foods have been studied and documented since the 1960s. Doses of radiation necessary for irradiating meat (fifteen to twenty million times greater than a chest x-ray) produce elevated levels of benzene, formaldehyde, and other cancer-causing compounds in food. This is the reason that irradiation must be called a food *additive*. Irradiation also reduces vitamin content[107] and kills enzymes.

The government of India carried out studies to determine if irradiated wheat was safe for consumption. During the course of their studies, several alarming things were discovered and eventually disclosed to the U.S. congressional hearing on irradiation in 1987:[108]

1. Rats and mice fed freshly irradiated wheat showed increased levels of cells with chromosome abnormalities in their bone marrow. This was repeatedly observed in several separate experiments.
2. Normal monkeys and undernourished children fed diets containing freshly irradiated wheat showed elevated levels of white blood cells

with chromosome abnormalities. Several months after the irradiated wheat was withdrawn, levels of chromosome abnormality returned to normal.

3. Mice fed freshly irradiated wheat-based diets had increased numbers of prenatal deaths.

Unfortunately, the FDA, citing five out of thousands of studies, has continued to extend its approval for the use of irradiation on more and more food products. In 1963, irradiation was approved for wheat and flour to control insects. In 1964 it was approved as a sprout inhibitor on white potatoes. In 1983, approval was given for use on spices and herbs. In 1986 it was approved for use on fresh foods to delay maturation (in other words, to delay spoiling). It was approved for poultry in 1990, red meat in 1999, and eggs in 2001. Most recently (2008), it was approved for lettuce, spinach, and many other vegetables. Irradiation has been used for years on a variety of crops including apples, strawberries, bananas, mangoes, onions, potatoes, spices, seasonings, meat, poultry, fish, and grains.

Whether it's a fruit, a vegetable, or a meat product, all foods that are irradiated are supposed to be labeled with the symbol shown below. Often they are not. Now the FDA is proposing sweeping changes that would relax labeling requirements even further.

Changes proposed and encouraged by the irradiation industry would allow

for many irradiated foods to go unlabeled. Another change would allow companies to substitute other terms in place of the word "irradiated," such as "electronic pasteurization" or "cold pasteurization." These terms are misleading and are intended to downplay the fact that food is altered by irradiation.

Like other practices (e.g., water fluoridation) irradiation is popular because it solves waste problems from other industries. The Department of Energy's By-product Utilization Program benefits by reducing disposal costs on spent military and civilian nuclear fuel wastes.[109] Irradiation also allows products that might not be appealing to be sold to unsuspecting consumers. Irradiation is another reason to shop for organic produce, to participate in co-ops, or to grow as much of your own food as possible.

 (see Chapter 4: Irradiation of meat/poultry)

BARCODE FOODS

The term *barcode food* refers to food that is packaged so that it can remain on the shelf in a grocery store for predetermined periods of time. The creation of barcode foods requires processing (e.g., cooking, drying, refining, extracting, extruding, pasteurizing, irradiation) Processing notoriously destroys nutrients or renders nutrients unavailable at the cellular level. Processing kills enzymes; it alters amino acids, promotes rancidity, and often changes the composition of minerals so that they are no longer easily assimilated. Processing also changes living food into energetically lifeless "food forms" that are unable to fulfill the nutritional needs of our bodies.

The grocery store concept is built around *barcode* foods and extended shelf life. Whatever nutritive content these foods had to begin with is largely lost in the processing, and the only way they can stay on the shelf is if they are dead. Unfortunately, 70 percent of today's diet is composed of barcode foods.

> **Whenever possible, avoid processed foods. Not only are they devoid of nutrients and enzymes, they are also the most likely to contain genetically modified ingredients.**

There is a vast difference between living and dead (cooked and processed) food. Living food has a positive energy signature that strengthens the human body (often just by being near to it). Processed foods give off little energy. In fact, they often *require* energy from our bodies in order to be assimilated. The net gain is sometimes not a gain at all but a taxing of the organs and tissues in our bodies. Barcode foods (packaged and processed) should be avoided whenever possible.

DEPLETED SOILS

As far back as the 1930s, the U.S. government was warned by nutritional experts that American soils were so deficient in mineral content that the foods grown on them could not sustain healthy life.[110] The intention of these experts was to inspire corrective action. More than seventy years later, no action has been taken. As a result, the fruits and vegetables grown in American soil and in most other parts of the world have shown dramatically reduced nutritional content.

Depleted soils and empty food may be partly responsible for the major degenerative diseases of our time. In a recent document, the FDA admitted that by setting minimum levels of nutrients in certain foods, it was possible to reduce the incidence of deficiency diseases.[111] These factors may also be one reason Americans eat too much. *Barcode* foods and foods grown on depleted soil provide empty calories devoid of nutrition; they promote weight gain and obesity. At the same time, those who consume deficient foods are starving. Their consumption has given rise to a new kind of malnutrition referred to as *over-consumptive/under-nutrition syndrome.*

How can plants grow without minerals? Most plants require only three elements to grow: nitrogen, phosphorus, and water. In the presence of these nutrients, virtually all plants will *appear* to be healthy. However, if the complete group of more than seventy minerals is either missing or deficient, food is nutritionally empty. A secondary consequence is that these plants are less able to defend themselves against natural predators. They are susceptible to damage from insects, viruses, fungi, and bacteria. In order to control this, pesticides must be used to limit the damage. It is a vicious cycle unless the root cause is addressed. And in this case the cause is really at the roots—depleted soil.

One of the simplest (and cheapest) ways to address the problem of malnutrition is to do what was recommended in the 1930s—replenish the soil by remineralizing and incorporating organic matter. Until this is done on a massive scale, U.S. farmers will continue to need to rely on chemical fertilizers, pesticides, and genetically modified versions of plants to overcome increasing growth and yield problems.

 (see chapter 11: Soil remineralization)

PRODUCE

Most produce these days is individually marked by the grower with small stickers to distinguish varieties at the checkout stand. These stickers are also your clue to whether or not the produce is organic. Organic produce has a five-digit number that always begins with the number 9. Conventionally grown produce carries a four-digit number that always begins with a 4. Genetically modified produce carries a sticker that begins with the number 8.

> **Organic produce has a five-digit number that begins with a "9."**
>
> **Conventionally grown produce has a four-digit number that begins with a "4."**
>
> **Genetically modified produce has a sticker that begins with the number "8."**

Since *organic* is your best choice for food that is free of chemical toxins, genetic modification, and irradiation, finding a source of organic produce is important. Let your grocer know you are interested in a variety of organic products. However, keep the following in mind.

When buying at a large supermarket, only eighteen cents of every dollar goes to the grower. Eighty-two cents goes to the agribusiness conglomerate that puts money back in the pockets of pesticide manufacturers, genetic engineering research, and various unnecessary middlemen. These same conglomerates are responsible for the predicament we find ourselves in. They promote chemical fertilization, the use of pesticides, genetically modified foods, irradiation, and nutritionless food.

The best way to find your way back to real food may be to support local farmers. Buying from local growers will ultimately help preserve the environment; it will also strengthen local communities by investing food dollars close to home. The following Web site contains a huge database and lets you search your local area for growers, co-ops, farmer's markets, and restaurants that participate in community sustainable agriculture. You can also order organic products online: http://www.localharvest.org/.

MEAT AND POULTRY

Before you eat another roast beef sandwich, before you purchase another Thanksgiving turkey or bite into another pork chop, think about what that meat has been fed. Consider what antibiotics or growth hormones it may have received, the circumstances in which it lived, and the manner in which it was slaughtered and packaged.

> **Some of the most important foods to purchase organically are animal foods. This is because animals tend to concentrate pesticides.**

Most people are so confident that "somebody" in the government is watching out for their welfare that they would never consider investigating the practices of the meat and poultry industry. However, in 2007 two incidents alone attempted to recall twenty-seven million pounds of E. coli contaminated beef. The U.S. meat and poultry industry is plagued with problems from beginning to end. If you understood the smallest portion of what these products were subjected to, you would be inclined to express sentiments similar to those that Oprah Winfrey expressed when she said, "It has just stopped me, cold, from eating another burger!"[112]

Hormones

Most beef calves go from eighty pounds at birth to twelve hundred pounds or more in fourteen months. The only way that amount of growth can take place is if they are fed on grain (rather than their normal diet of grass) and if they are given a variety of growth hormones. Measurable amounts of these hormones end up in human tissue. Many scientists agree that the estrogenic hormones from hormone-fed beef are partially responsible for premature puberty in young girls and for falling sperm counts in men. The poultry industry does not use hormones. The poultry industry has its own skeletons in its closet.

Arsenic in poultry

Organic arsenic is routinely fed to poultry to prevent bacterial infections and to improve weight gain. It has been approved for decades and is given to about 70 percent of chickens grown for meat—even though arsenic is a known carcinogen. Recent research revealed that arsenic in chicken was three to four times higher than in other poultry and meat.[113] An even bigger problem may be the long-term effects on the environment. Most of the arsenic fed to chickens ends up in the litter (excrement). And more than 70 percent of the arsenic in uncovered piles of poultry litter is dissolved by rainfall and leached into lakes or streams. What we don't eat in the chicken ends up in our water.

Antibiotics

In the United States the use of antibiotics is permitted to *prevent* or to *treat* diseases in all animals. In fact, the largest use of antibiotics in this country is for animals. But antibiotics are rarely required where animals are naturally raised. It is our inhumane treatment of animals that forces the use of antibiotics. Over nine million pounds of antibiotic feed are used in the cattle industry every year. These antibiotics are given in normal feed—whether animals need them or not—as part of the dietary regimen. The routine use of antibiotics in the meat and poultry industry is a major factor in the growing problem of antibiotic resistance in humans.

The words "no antibiotics added" on meat or poultry can be misleading. That statement simply means that a product has satisfied the USDA's guidelines for animals raised without antibiotics. It does not necessarily mean that the meat follows stricter organic standards. Also misleading is the use of the word "natural" on meat and poultry labels. At the meat counter, the word "natural" is often just an assurance that no artificial colors (often added to make red meat look fresh) have been added. For meat and poultry, the standard definition of the word "natural" means that the food cannot contain artificial colors, flavors, preservatives, or other artificial ingredients.

Irradiation of meat/poultry

Irradiated meat has a lower bacteria level than regular meat. It may reduce—but not eliminate—the risk of food-borne illness if your meat is undercooked. But that's the end of any benefits to irradiating meat. Irradiation does not kill resistant strains of salmonella and E. coli, nor does it eliminate mad cow disease. In most cases, irradiation is an excuse for selling under-quality meat to the consumer. Irradiation in the meat and poultry industry creates a false sense of security and allows tainted or spoiled meat to be sold. Irradiation stops the normal decay process,[114] and there is no warning when irradiated food is eventually spoiled because the beneficial organisms that warn of spoilage are also destroyed by irradiation. According to Carol Foreman, director of the Food Policy Institute of the Consumer Federation of America:

> *It's better to take steps to avoid contaminating food to begin with than it is to try to clean it up afterwards. But I'm afraid it's human nature not to spend money to change the way animals are raised, or have a trained workforce in meatpacking plants, or upgrade facilities if they can just irradiate food at the end of the line.*

Irradiation causes the release of toxic mold by-products called aflatoxins. These cause liver damage and cancer; they produce benzene and formaldehyde in food; and they destroy many vitamins and enzymes. The long-term effects of consuming irradiated food are not known and have never been fully investigated.

What Irradiation Does to Meat

1. Produces toxic mold by-products
2. Produces benzene and formaldehyde in the meat
3. Destroys vitamins and enzymes

Although labeling is required for irradiated products, it is not required in restaurants, including school lunch programs. In 2001, the proposal to allow irradiated poultry and ground beef in federal school lunch programs rather than testing for salmonella triggered such resistance that the United States Department of Agriculture (USDA) abandoned the plan. But a provision in the Farm Security and Rural Investment Act of 2002 gave the USDA the opportunity to drop restrictions. Today, every school district has the choice to buy irradiated meat and poultry.

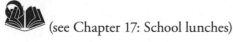 (see Chapter 17: School lunches)

> **There is nowhere on the face of the earth where there is any population that has consumed large amounts of any irradiated food over an extended period of time. I think it comes close to using the nation's schoolchildren as guinea pigs.**
>
> —Carol Foreman, director of the Food Policy
> Institute of the Consumer Federation of America

Do you know if your child's school serves irradiated meat? The following Web site provides information on how to work with your school district to stop the purchase of irradiated foods: www.safelunch.org.

Carbon monoxide

Carbon monoxide (CO), recently approved by the EPA for use in meat packaging, keeps meat red longer. The process of treating meat by removing oxygen from the package and pumping CO in, referred to as "modified atmosphere packaging," saves meat processors millions of dollars every year.

Carbon monoxide binds more effectively to hemoglobin in blood than oxygen does. That's why, in the presence of CO, a person can become oxygen starved and die. CO also competes for oxygen in muscle tissue. Myoglobin is the protein found in muscle tissue that is responsible for the same role hemoglobin fills in the bloodstream. In the presence of oxygen, myoglobin becomes oxymyoglobin and produces a red color. CO is attracted to myoglobin far more readily than oxygen, forming carboxymyoglobin, with an even more vivid and long-lasting red pigment.

Eating CO-treated meat alone may not make you sick. However, its supercharged color lasts for months—far beyond the date when it is safe to eat. The cost to shoppers is their right to know—and possibly their health. There is no requirement to let consumers know the meat was packaged using this technology.

To defend the practice, which has been banned in countries across the world, the FDA claims that consumers do not care about meat's color and that they do not consider color when making purchasing decisions. But the FDA's own Food Code warns about the dangers of a modified atmosphere packaging system.[115]

> **ROP [reduced oxygen packaging] which provides an environment that contains little or no oxygen ... raises many microbiological concerns.... the inhibition of the spoilage bacteria is significant because without these competing organisms, tell–tale signs signaling that the product is no longer fit for consumption will not occur.**
>
> FDA Food Code

During a 2007 hearing on the technology, Representative Bart Stupak (D-Mi) said: "The sole purpose of carbon monoxide packaging is to fool consumers into believing that the meat and fish they buy is fresh, no matter how old it is and no matter how decayed it might be."[116] To avoid purchasing CO-treated meat, stay away from prepackaged meat products. Make sure your meat is freshly packaged in the meat department of the store. To circumvent other problems with meat, buy only organic, grass-fed meat (see sources).

Mad cow disease

Over thirty years ago, ranchers started "factory-farming"—raising animals in penned areas, in close quarters, and feeding them hormones and other chemicals to fatten them faster for market. Huge amounts of antibiotics were necessary under these conditions because the animals became sick so easily. Ranchers also cut costs by feeding their animals alternate sources of protein (ground-up dead animals). But cows are herbivores—vegetarians. They are supposed to eat grass, not other animals. They are not intended to be confined in close quarters, nor are they meant to receive antibiotics or hormones in their feed. All of these factors have contributed to the rise of mad cow disease.

Mad cow disease is the common term for bovine spongiform encepholopathy, a progressive neurological disorder that causes a sponge-like destruction of the brain and central nervous system. The cause of mad cow disease is not virus, fungus, or bacteria. It is an abnormal protein, called a prion, that contains no DNA or RNA. Prions are transmitted from one animal to another by eating infected animal parts from the central nervous system. The disease can be transmitted to humans by eating infected meat. It is virtually 100 percent fatal.

The USDA and the beef industry continue to assure Americans that U.S. beef is safe, even though mad cow disease was documented in the United States in 2003. In fact, it has now been documented in just about every country in the world. But other countries have taken a proactive approach to the situation. Japan and European Union countries test neary *every* animal before approving meat for the market. U.S. officials still refuse to believe there is a problem, and as long as we fail to look, we will fail to know the true extent of the disease. The USDA has been unwilling to instigate any program of slaughterhouse testing. At this time, almost *no testing* is performed.

The Centers for Disease Control is equally unwilling to support any effort to document the problem. It does not require the disease to be reported. But mad cow disease is already far worse than we are being told. It has spread to many humans in this country. The human equivalent of mad cow disease is called Creutzfeldt-Jakob disease; it causes memory loss, emotional instability, an unsteady gait, rapidly progressive dementia and death, often within a year. These symptoms are surprisingly similar to Alzheimer's disease. In fact, a 1989 Yale University study reported the results of a postmortem examination of forty-six patients diagnosed with Alzheimer's disease. Six (13 percent) actually had Creutzfeldt-Jakob disease.[117] A similar postmortem study at the Pittsburgh Veteran's Hospital on demented patients reported similar findings: more than 5 percent of them had Creutzfeldt-Jakob disease.

In the United States it would appear that lobbyists for the beef industry have successfully kept regulatory agencies from taking action. In 1996, Oprah Winfrey produced a television show that uncovered the truth about mad cow disease. After the show, she found herself embroiled in a civil lawsuit brought on by the beef industry. Six years and one million dollars later, the lawsuit was finally dismissed.

How do you protect yourself and your family from mad cow (Creutzfeldt-Jakob) disease? One man, Howard F. Lyman, a fourth-generation cattle rancher, decided to become a vegetarian. Considering his knowledge of the cattle industry, vegetarianism might not be a bad idea. His book reveals the ugly facts.[118] But if you are not ready to become a vegetarian, the only way to ensure against being the next victim is to purchase organic meat from grass-fed animals. Incidentally, animals that are grass fed generally have higher levels of essential fatty acids and lean protein. Two Web sites are: http:// www.grassfedtraditions.com/grass_fed_beef.htm and www.texasgrassfedbeef .com. If you live in a rural area, seek out ranchers who may provide pasture-fed beef and other local organic products.

When it is not possible to purchase organic grass-fed beef (especially in restaurants or when you travel), consider a vegetarian meal—definitely not a burger. The kind of beef that is most likely to have mad cow disease is ground beef (because it contains meat from every part of the cow). The next most likely cuts to contain mad cow disease are those that contain bone. And don't think that just because you don't eat beef that you are protected. Pork, lamb, even wild deer and elk now have their own forms of mad cow disease.

To sign a petition for mandatory testing of all cattle brought to slaughter; to ban the feeding of blood, manure, and slaughterhouse waste to animals; and to stop the harassment of farmers and food processors who are interested

in independently testing their own beef, visit this Web site: http://www.
organicconsumers.org/madcow.cfm.

Organic meat and poultry

In order to qualify as *organic*, animals must be raised organically from the
last third of gestation (for livestock) or no later than the second day of life
(for poultry). Farmers must provide livestock and poultry food that is 100
percent organically grown. No antibiotics or hormones may be administered.
All animals must have access to pasture if they graze. They must have shade,
shelter, fresh air, direct sunlight, and room to exercise according to each
species. Organic animal products must also be kept separate from nonorganic
products during all phases of slaughter and packaging.

Meat, the Environment, and Food for Thought

It takes far more land and resources to produce red meat than it does to focus on
fruits and vegetables which should be the mainstay of the human diet. A recent
report from the Livestock, Environment, and Development Initiative identifies
the environmental cost of our addiction to red meat. Some key findings:

- Grazing lands now take up 26% (over one quarter) of the ice-free land
  on the earth.
- Seventy percent of previously forested land in the Amazon is now taken
  up by pasture.
- Livestock are responsible for 37% of all human activity-related methane
  emissions, and methane has 23 times more global warming potential
  compared to carbon dioxide.
- In the U.S., livestock are responsible for over half of the country's erosion
  issues.
- Livestock account for 20% of the earth's animal biomass.
- 30% of the earth's land surface, which was once wildlife habitat, is now
  occupied by livestock.

The Web site www.meatrix.com contains volumes of information on this subject.

FISH

According to Dr. Weston A. Price, fish is one of the best foods you can eat.
When he traveled throughout the world, studying traditional people and their
native diets, he discovered that those who ate seafood had the best health.[119]
Seafood is a source of omega-3 and other essential fatty acids found deficient in
many diets. It is also a natural source of the fat-soluble Vitamins, A and D.

> **Our soils may be depleted of certain trace minerals, but every mineral we need exists in the ocean. Seafood and sea vegetables are a sure way to get them all.**

Eating fish is healthy, but avoiding mercury and other toxins requires knowing which fish to eat. Unfortunately, we have also polluted the oceans and we have begun the practice of "farming" fish—both practices are detrimental. Many fish today contain high levels of mercury and PCBs (a family of over two hundred chemicals that end up in our air and water).

Recently, the *New York Times* had tuna tested from a number of sushi restaurants in New York City. They found so much mercury in bluefin tuna that even two or three pieces a week could be a health hazard for the average adult, based on guidelines set by the EPA.[120] These findings reinforce results in other studies showing that more expensive tuna usually contains more mercury because it comes from larger species that accumulate mercury from the smaller fish they eat. The tuna sushi in the *New York Times* tests contained far more mercury than is typically found in canned tuna. Since it is hard for anyone but experts to tell whether a piece of tuna sushi is bluefin by looking at it, it may be best to avoid tuna in sushi. When purchasing fresh tuna, buy species like yellowfin and bigeye. These smaller species generally have much less mercury.

The current FDA guidelines (released in 2004) recommend that pregnant women and young children avoid eating the kinds of fish that are likely to be high in mercury. These high-level mercury fish include shark, swordfish, king mackerel, some tuna, and tilefish. Fish known to be lower in mercury include light canned tuna, salmon, pollock, and catfish. (Light canned tuna are preferred over albacore tuna because of their size.) Most fish sandwiches and fish sticks contain pollock. The Environmental Working Group has an online calculator to calculate the amount of canned tuna that is safe to eat—based on weight and gender. Visit http://www.ewg.org/tunacalculator

 (see Chapter 19: Mercury detoxification)

Stay away from farmed fish; they are usually fed soy pellets (often genetically modified) containing pesticides. The fatty acid profile of farmed fish is greatly diminished. Coloring agents are often added (especially to salmon) to enhance color. Also avoid freshwater fish unless you know their origin—especially catfish, carp, and shoreline feeders such as sole and flounder. Shellfish and other scavengers should be eaten minimally.

EGGS

It pays to buy the best quality eggs you can find—preferably from a local grower. Eggs from free-range chickens that can eat bugs and vegetation are much better quality. Chickens fed flax meal also produce high-quality eggs. But chickens that are caged and provided with artificial lighting to encourage year-round egg production are unhealthy; they require medicated feed and they produce inferior eggs.

However, the term free range can be misleading. Although it conjures the image of open pasture, a chicken can be called *free range* if it has even limited access to the outdoors each day for an unspecified period of time—possibly only minutes. The term, *free range* does not mean that the birds actually went outdoors to roam freely, and no other criteria such as size of the area, or space per bird, are required by the term.

Paying higher prices for brown eggs or for so-called hormone-free eggs is unjustified since the color of the egg is related to the kind of chicken that laid it, not to the quality of the egg, and hormones are not used in the poultry industry. On the other hand, few chickens are antibiotic free—another reason to purchase from a local grower, where you can ask about the feeding and cultural practices.

WHAT ABOUT MILK?

Much controversy and much confusion surround the subject of milk. Today, milk is blamed for everything from chronic ear infections to cancer and diabetes—and perhaps rightfully so. However, more often than not, the milk itself is not the culprit, but rather the manner in which it has been treated.

Pasteurization

The biggest factor contributing to the degradation of today's milk is pasteurization. We have been led to believe that pasteurization protects us against bacteria in milk. The truth is that all bacterial outbreaks in recent years have occurred in pasteurized milk. Raw milk contains lactic acid–producing bacteria that protect against pathogens. Pasteurization destroys these beneficial organisms, leaving the milk without any protective mechanisms. Raw milk sours (ferments) when left at room temperature; pasteurized milk putrefies (rots).

Pasteurization (heat) also alters the amino acids in milk, making them less bioavailable; it destroys more than 50 percent of the vitamin C and over 80 percent of other water-soluble vitamins; it reduces the availability of minerals—especially calcium, magnesium phosphorus, potassium, sodium, and sulfur; and it destroys enzymes making it difficult to digest and placing unnecessary stress on the pancreas to produce digestive enzymes. This may explain why milk consumption has been linked with diabetes in industrialized nations.

Drinking pasteurized milk puts a tremendous strain on the entire digestive system. In the elderly and in those with milk intolerances or inherited weaknesses, pasteurized milk passes through the digestive system undigested. It can build up around the walls of the small intestine, preventing the absorption of nutrients. The result is allergies, chronic fatigue and a host of degenerative illnesses.[121]

Bovine growth hormone (rBGH)

The use of bovine growth hormone (rBGH) is another onslaught to milk. The *r* in rBGH refers to the term *recombinant*, because the bovine growth hormone given to cows to force the production of more milk is not a natural hormone. It is genetically engineered.

> **Since 1994, every industrialized country in the world except the United States—including Canada, Japan, and all fifteen nations of the European Union—has banned rBGH milk.**

The United Nations Food Standards Body refuses to certify that rBGH is safe. Yet, the USDA continues to endorse rBGH milk for general consumption. In the United States it is illegal to label dairy products with the phrase rBGH-free—even if it is true—because it might damage the reputation of the dairies that use the hormone. Nearly all U.S. dairies use rBGH because it increases milk production by 20 to 30 percent.

The subject of milk is voluminous and politically fraught with deception. You have two choices: avoid it or find a source of certified raw milk. In many states the sale of raw milk is illegal. For a list of raw dairies by state, visit this Web site: http://www.realmilk.com/where1.html.

Also visit: www.notmilk.com for a wealth of information on the subject.

Melamine—plastic protein

In the fall of 2008, a chemical known as melamine (used in the production of melamine/melmac dishes and other products) was found in milk powder from China. Melamine is a protein that was illegally added to show higher protein concentrations in Chinese powdered milk products. The consequences were disastrous. More than fifty thousand Chinese infants were diagnosed with kidney problems from the tiny amounts of melamine found in infant formula. Smaller amounts of melamine were found in two top U.S. infant formulas—though the FDA says these amounts are not harmful.

The U.S. FDA blocked milk-containing products from China but it has issued a growing list of products sold in the United States that may contain Chinese milk by-products. For obvious reasons, it is best to avoid all processed milk products.

SOY: PROCESSED VERSUS FERMENTED

A good portion of American consumers believe that soy milk, soy flour, and other soy products (such as soy burgers, soy ice cream, soy cheese), are heart-healthy foods. This assumption resulted from the FDA's 1999 approval of the following health claim for soy foods: *"Diets low in saturated fat and cholesterol that include twenty-five grams of soy protein a day may reduce the risk of heart disease."*

But, according to Dr. Kaayla Daniel, author of *The Whole Soy Story,* There was never a sound basis for a soy health claim and the heavy marketing of soy as a miracle food has put American men, women and children at risk. Dr. Daniel also authored a sixty-five-page petition to the FDA documenting long-standing concerns in the scientific community regarding soy's possible role in:

- Reproductive disorders
- Thyroid dysfunction
- Cognitive decline
- Immune dysfunction
- Cancer

Soy is one of the top eight foods causing allergies today, which many people experience as bloating or gas. One prominent researcher puts soy in the top six and another in the top four foods causing hypersensitivity reactions in children.[122]

One of the reasons soy is responsible for so many allergies and hypersensitivity reactions is because it contains high levels of inhibitors, which interfere with the digestion of protein and block the assimilation of minerals. These inhibitors are not neutralized by ordinary food preparation methods such as soaking, sprouting, and long, slow cooking. Also, during the high-temperature processing used to make soy protein isolate and textured vegetable protein, soy proteins are denatured, resulting in the formation of toxic lysinoalanine and highly carcinogenic nitrosamines. Another big problem with commercially available soy foods is genetic modification.

Today, more than half of the soy products available in the United States are genetically modified, unless they are organic. Genetic modification causes even more allergic reactions, and the cross-contamination of organic crops is beginning to be a big problem.

 (see Chapter 4: Genetic modification)

Approximately 25 percent of bottle-fed U.S. children receive soy-based formula. The plant-based estrogens in soy can interfere with sexual development and can influence thyroid and brain development. An infant fed exclusively on soy formula receives the estrogenic equivalent (based on body weight) of almost five birth control pills per day.[123] By contrast, almost no phytoestrogens have been detected in human milk, even when the mother consumes soy products. Anecdotal reports of other problems associated with children of both sexes who were fed soy-based formula include extreme emotional behavior, asthma, immune system problems, pituitary insufficiency, thyroid disorders, and irritable bowel syndrome.[124] Soy phytoestrogens disrupt endocrine function; they have the potential to cause infertility and to promote breast cancer in adult women.

However, Asian cultures have eaten soy for centuries without difficulty. The difference between the traditional foods eaten by Asian cultures and the processed soy products on the market today is that they are fermented. Fermentation changes this otherwise poor food choice into a healthful source of complete protein. The fermentation process neutralizes inhibitors and adds enzymes that aid in the assimilation of proteins and carbohydrates. Traditional fermented soy foods like these, listed below, are highly beneficial:

- **Natto**—-fermented soybeans with a cheeselike flavor.
- **Tempeh**—a fermented soybean cake with a firm texture and nutty, mushroom-like flavor.
- **Miso**—a fermented soybean paste with a salty, buttery texture, commonly used in miso soup.
- **Soy sauce**—traditionally, soy sauce is made by fermenting soybeans, salt, and enzymes. Many varieties on the market today are made artificially using a chemical process.

FOOD PRESERVATIVES

Unless you grow all your own food and prepare all your meals from scratch, it's almost impossible to eat food without preservatives. Manufacturers add preservatives to keep them *fresh* until they are eaten. Preservatives serve as antioxidants or antimicrobials—or both. Antioxidants suppress the reaction that occurs when foods combine with oxygen; they keep foods from becoming rancid or from discoloring. Antimicrobials are really a form of pesticide to prevent the growth of molds, yeasts, and bacteria. As with many other chemicals routinely used in food and agriculture, many of the preservatives in our food have not been thoroughly tested. Some are hormone disrupters; many have gastrointestinal side effects; and some are suspected of aggravating the symptoms of attention deficit disorder (ADD) and attention deficit hyperactivity disorder (ADHD).[125]

BHA, BHT, and TBHQ

BHA (butylated hydroxyanisole) and the related compounds BHT (butylated hydroxytoluene) and TBHQ (tertiary butyl hydroquinone) are synthetic antioxidants used to keep fats from becoming rancid. But just because they are antioxidants does not mean that they are safe to use. These compounds are among the worst of the food preservatives. Avoid them whenever possible.

BHA and BHT are found in butter, meats, cereals, chewing gum, baked goods, snack foods, and dehydrated potatoes. They are also found in animal feed and the packaging materials for many cereals and snack foods. In addition to preserving foods, BHA and BHT are used to preserve the oils in cosmetics and pharmaceuticals.

 (see Chapter 7: Cosmetics)

BHA has been identified as a carcinogen by the International Agency for Research on Cancer; both BHA and BHT have been banned in Europe and Japan. Beyond being carcinogens, these compounds are suspected hormone disrupters—thought to be partly responsible for the decrease in male fertility and the rise in testicular cancer observed since the 1950s. BHA, BHT, and TBHQ can trigger an immune system response that includes itching, burning, scaling, hives, and blistering of skin. Safer alternatives for these preservatives include the antioxidant vitamins C and E, as well as other natural antioxidants like grape seed extract.

Sulfites

Sulfites are a group of sulfur-containing preservatives that are used to protect against discoloration. They are used primarily to preserve dried fruit (to keep it from turning brown), processed potato products, and juices—including wine. Be aware that restaurant food, especially potato products, salads, and some canned foods, often contain sulfites. Lemon juice (unless it is fresh squeezed) could be a source of sulfites. The FDA prohibits the use of sulfites in foods that are important sources of thiamin (vitamin B1) because sulfites destroy this vitamin. The symptom most reported by sulfite-sensitive people is difficulty breathing. Other problems range from stomachache to hives and anaphylactic shock. Sulfites present greater problems for those who are sensitive, but sulfites should be avoided whenever possible. Currently, there are six sulfiting agents allowed in packaged foods. Watch for these forms of sulfite preservatives:

- sulfur dioxide
- sodium sulfite
- sodium bisulfite
- potassium bisulfite
- sodium metabisulfite
- potassium metabisulfite

Nitrates/Nitrites

The use of nitrates and nitrites (typically potassium nitrate and sodium nitrite) are confined to the meat industry, where they are responsible for controlling botulism bacteria in cured meats. They add a pink color and the "cured meat flavor" to products such as lunch meats, ham, and bacon. Although there is no direct evidence of carcinogenicity, nitrites are toxic. Their use is severely restricted in many countries and may provoke hyperactivity and other adverse reactions in children. The intake of cured meat should be limited.

Propionates

A group of preservatives known as propionates (propionic acid, calcium propionate, sodium propionate, and potassium propionate) are used to slow the growth of mold in the baking industry. Very few people will be affected by two slices of preserved bread, but the effects are cumulative. Like most food additives, this preservative was not tested before it was approved for use. It is a suspected gastrointestinal and liver toxicant also thought to heighten the symptoms of learning disabilities and ADD.

The use of calcium propionate is for the convenience of the manufacturer, not the consumer. Bakers who keep their work benches and slicer blades clean by wiping with vinegar every day do not need this preservative. However, bakers in large factories prefer the less time-consuming method of "fogging" their equipment with a calcium propionate spray. Perhaps more often than not, calcium propionate allows for sloppy hygiene. Preservative-free bread that is refrigerated will keep for a long time without going moldy—up to two weeks.

Benzoates

The benzoates (benzoic acid, sodium benzoate, calcium benzoate, potassium benzoate) are yeast and mold inhibitors. They are found in most soft drinks, juices, and juice drinks as well as in some salad dressings. Recently the beverage *7-Up* was reformulated in favor of more natural ingredients. Obviously, the synthetic preservatives were never really necessary. They were replaced with vitamin C and other natural antioxidants.

Sorbates

The sorbates (sorbic acid, calcium sorbate, potassium sorbate, sodium sorbate) are used in fruit drinks and vegetable products, some cheeses, and salad dressings. Also mold inhibitors, these preservatives can be replaced with vitamin C or other ascorbates.

SWEETENERS

The food-processing industry understands the addictive nature of sugars. Sugars are included in nearly everything on the grocery store shelf in order to "bring you back for more." And if you don't return for the sugar, there are other addictive ways—sugar substitutes. Some sugar substitutes are worse than the sugar itself.

Sugar (sucrose)

In 1915, the national annual average for sugar consumption was fifteen to twenty pounds per person. Today the average person consumes their weight in sugar.[126] Sugar is notoriously linked with hypoglycemia, diabetes, heart disease, and chronic tiredness. It creates a cycle of craving and bingeing and is highly addictive.

> **Sugar is a processed "food form." It contains no fiber, no minerals, no proteins, no fats, no enzymes—just empty calories. The body must draw on the vitamin, mineral, and enzyme reserves in the body to get rid of it.**

Sugar consumption itself has become a disease. In order to metabolize the huge amounts of sugar that are consumed today, the body must mobilize large amounts of adrenalin and insulin to clear the sugar from the bloodstream. Day after day, this leads to some of the problems listed below:

- Suppression of the immune system, contributing to viral and bacterial infection.

- Mineral imbalances and interference with the absorption of calcium and magnesium.
- Hyperactivity, anxiety, and difficulty concentrating.
- Overacidic condition in the body, contributing to osteoporosis, yeast infections, tooth decay, cancer, and premature aging.
- Reduction of high-density lipoproteins (HDL, good cholesterol) and elevation of low-density lipoproteins (LDL, bad cholesterol), thus increasing atherosclerosis and heart disease.
- Constipation and increased chances of irritable bowel syndrome and colon cancer.

Fructose and high fructose corn syrup

Until the 1970s, refined sugar came from beets and sugar cane. But in 1976, the sugar industry realized that it was cheaper to produce sugar from corn. Thus began the production of fructose and high fructose corn syrup. Today fructose and high fructose corn syrup have replaced sugar in many foods, especially beverages. This is a bigger problem than most people realize.

Processed white sugar (sucrose) is composed of one molecule of glucose and one molecule of fructose. When these two sugars are split apart in the intestines, the glucose is released and can be utilized by nearly every cell in the body. Fructose, however, must be sent to the liver to be broken down further. This is why fructose is often recommended for diabetics—because it does not hit the bloodstream as rapidly. However, the consumption of fructose puts a strain on the liver and on other organs of the body—beyond what regular sugar does.

As it turns out, it is the fructose in white sugar that causes the greatest number of problems. This information came as the result of a study conducted with rats. One group was fed high amounts of glucose; another group was fed high amounts of fructose. The group fed glucose was largely unaffected, but the group fed fructose showed disastrous results: Male rats were anemic; they had high cholesterol and enlarged hearts; they had delayed testicular development, and they did not reach maturity. Female rats did not give birth to live young.[127] Rats, like people, metabolize fructose via a different pathway than the pathway used in metabolizing glucose. Since the effects of fructose alone are more severe than those of normal white sugar, high fructose corn syrup and fructose should be avoided.

Aspartame

Known as Equal, NutraSweet, Spoonful, and most recently as AminoSweet, aspartame, or 1-aspartyl 1-phenylalanine methyl ester, is an engineered compound with three components: phenylalanine, aspartic acid, and methanol (wood alcohol). Phenylalanine and aspartic acid are amino acids found in many foods. However, amino acids are always consumed in combination with other amino acids. Isolated, some are able to penetrate the blood-brain barrier, causing abnormal nerve firing and cell death. A few of the side effects of aspartame are headaches, mental confusion, problems with balance, and numbness. In most instances, the effects are subtle, yet cumulative. More serious side effects of aspartame have been misdiagnosed as multiple sclerosis, Lou Gehrig's disease, and thyroid dysfunction.[128] Often, the elimination of aspartame eliminates a variety of symptoms.

The term excitotoxin has been applied to aspartame (and MSG). These chemicals cause nerve cells in the brain to fire more rapidly than normal until they become exhausted. Cell death often results. Excitotoxins have also been shown to stimulate the generation of free radicals which accelerate many degenerative illnesses.

Ten percent of aspartame is methanol—a substance with a safe limit outlined by the EPA as 7.8 milligrams per day. A one-half liter beverage sweetened with aspartame contains twenty-seven milligrams of methanol— four times the EPA limit. Of greater concern is the fact that methanol breaks down into formaldehyde. Independent studies have shown that formaldehyde from aspartame ingestion is extremely common. Each diet soda with aspartame produces six milligrams of formaldehyde—three times the daily limit established by the EPA. This amount is thirty times the established limit in New Jersey, one hundred times the limit in California, and three hundred times the limit in Maryland.[129]

 (see Chapter 1: Formaldehyde)

Despite objections from two of the original scientists who studied aspartame, it was approved by the FDA in 1980. As of 1995 more than 75 percent of the complaints received by the FDA are due to the ingestion of aspartame.[130]

Dr. Betty Martini has committed the last twenty years to uncovering the truth about aspartame and to making the world aware of its dangers. She established the worldwide volunteer force, Mission Possible World Health International (www.mpwhi.com), which is committed to removing aspartame from our food supply. If you email her, she will send you a resource guide to aspartame: bettym19@mindspring.com.

Neotame

In 2002, the FDA approved a new version of aspartame called Neotame. Neotame is chemically related to aspartame without the phenylalanine dangers. It is much sweeter than aspartame (seven thousand to thirteen thousand times sweeter than sugar). Neotame entered the market much more discreetly than the other nonnutritive sweeteners. While the Web site for Neotame claims that there are more than one hundred scientific studies to support its safety, none of these studies address the long-term health implications of using this sweetener.

Sucralose

Sucralose (otherwise known as Splenda) is produced by chlorinating sugar. This involves chemically changing the structure of the sugar molecule by substituting three chlorine atoms for three hydroxyl groups. Just like aspartame, animal studies on sucralose clearly demonstrate its toxicity. Sucralose failed in clinical trials with animals. It was found to shrink the thymus gland, to produce liver and kidney inflammation, to reduce growth, and to decrease birth weight in rats and mice.[131] Animal studies also indicate that sucralose reduces the amount of good bacteria in the intestines by 50 percent.[132]

Acesulfame-K

Acesulfame-K is an artificial sweetener that is about two hundred times sweeter than sugar. It is listed on the ingredients label as acesulfame-K, acesulfame potassium, Ace-K, or Sunett. It is used in baked goods, chewing gum, gelatin desserts, and soft drinks. The problems surrounding acesulfame-K are based on the lack of long-term studies. Acesulfame-K contains the carcinogen methylene chloride. Long-term exposure to methylene chloride can cause headaches, depression, nausea, mental confusion, liver and kidney effects, and cancer in humans.

There has been a great deal of opposition to the use of acesulfame-K without further testing, but at this time the FDA has not required that these tests be completed. Two rat studies have found that it may cause cancer. Acesulfame-K also breaks down into acetoacetamide, which has been found to adversely affect the thyroid in rats, rabbits, and dogs.

Saccharin

Saccharin was the first artificial sweetener to be discovered—in 1879. Used initially as a food preservative, saccharin wasn't sold as a sweetener until 1901, at a time when sugar was rationed during the war. In 1977, Canadian scientists found that saccharin caused cancer in laboratory animals. Canada banned it immediately. However, U.S. corporate interests won out, and for the next twenty-six years a cautionary warning label was all that was implemented on products that contained saccharin. To this day, it is classified as an *anticipated* carcinogen and is still available for use as a sweetener.

Saccharin is not metabolized in the digestive system. It is rapidly released in the urine. In fact, many individuals notice more frequent urination after the consumption of even small amounts of saccharin.[133] Perhaps this is the reason saccharin has been shown to cause bladder cancer in rats.

Sugar alcohols

Although the sugar alcohols are considered noncaloric and are much less harmful than aspartame, sucralose, saccharin, and Acesulfame-K, they are not without difficulties. The reason that sugar alcohols provide fewer calories than sugar is because they are not completely absorbed in the body. For this reason, the consumption of foods containing large amounts of sugar alcohols can lead to abdominal gas and diarrhea. Foods that contain sugar alcohols must include a warning on their label that says, "excess consumption may have a laxative effect." The class of sugar alcohols includes the following:

- Sorbitol
- Mannitol
- Isomalt
- Maltitol
- Lactitol
- Xylitol
- Erythritol
- HSH

Of the sugar alcohols, xylitol is the most widely known—for its antibacterial effects. Its use has been determined to reduce both tooth decay and ear infections because it keeps bacteria from adhering to the walls of the mucus membranes in the digestive tract. As long as they are used in small quantities, xylitol and the other sugar alcohols are good alternative sweeteners.

SWEET ALTERNATIVES

Interestingly, the "good" sweeteners that are available are all-natural, whole foods. These include raw honey, maple syrup, date sugar, brown rice syrup, agave, and an herb known as stevia. Of these, stevia is the only sweetener that does not have a glycemic impact—it is perfectly suited for almost everyone.

Raw honey

Raw honey (not heated over 115 degrees) is highly nutritious. It contains enzymes, vitamins, minerals, and numerous antimicrobial and anti-inflammatory compounds. When used in moderation, it is a good sweetener.

CAUTION: Do not give raw honey to infants. They do not have the stomach acids to inactivate naturally occurring bacteria in raw honey.

Maple syrup

Pure maple syrup, like honey, is a nutritious sweetener containing a variety of minerals and vitamins. Contrary to popular opinion, grade B does not have a greater amount of minerals, nor has it been processed differently than grade A. Grading in maple syrup is simply a matter of color and flavor—grade B has a darker color and a richer flavor. As with other foods, organic is better.

Date sugar

Date sugar is made from dehydrated dates. Although it is made from a whole food, it is highly concentrated and its use should be limited.

Brown rice syrup

Brown rice syrup is made by culturing brown rice with enzymes. It digests slowly, making it a good alternative for diabetics.

Agave

Agave nectar is a newcomer to the sweetener industry. It is a liquid, similar to honey (a bit thinner), and it contains a variety of minerals and vitamins. The one drawback to agave nectar is that it has a high fructose content—above 90 percent. Its use should be limited.

Stevia

Stevia is an herb harvested in Paraguay. Not only is this herb sweet (extracts are hundreds of times sweeter than sugar), but it has no calories, no glycemic impact, and it actually helps to balance blood sugar levels. This remarkable herb has been used as a sweetener and flavor enhancer for more than four hundred years with no adverse effects.[134] In Japan it comprises more than 40 percent of the total sweetener market. Yet this little herb has had a rough time being introduced in the United States. The sugar and artificial sweetener industries have repeatedly thwarted attempts to have stevia approved by the FDA. In 1995, the FDA lifted the import alert on stevia. This paved the way for the use of stevia as a *dietary supplement*, although it is still not approved in the United States for use as a food *additive*.

Some people have been slow to accept stevia because it has a slightly bitter aftertaste. Many companies have attempted to extract the *sweet* component (rebaudiocide, also called rebiana) from stevia to eliminate the bitter aftertaste. Some of these methods use solvents that may leave residues in the product. If you use stevia extracts, make sure the extraction process does not use harsh chemicals or bleaches. One of the authors recommends a stevia product made from the whole stevia leaf—yet it carries no bitter aftertaste. For information visit: www.wyntersway.com.

Truvia

In 2008, Coca-Cola and Cargill petitioned the FDA for approval of a new sweetener called Truvia—made from the stevia extract, rebaudiocide, and the sugar alcohol erythritol. Cargill and Coca-Cola (joint owners of the Truvia product) plan for its wide use in many foods and in diet beverages.

In studies submitted to the FDA, Truvia did not affect blood pressure in healthy individuals or blood sugar in those with type 2 diabetes. Further tests in rats showed no effects on reproduction or fertility. Because the process is proprietary, it is unknown what solvents are being used to extract the rebaudiocide from the stevia. It should also be noted that Truvia contains erythritol. Individuals consuming large amounts should be aware of the possible side effects of sugar alcohols. Pepsi is also working on its own stevia product, so stevia may finally move into the mainstream in the United States.

Just Like Sugar

Another alternative sweetener being marketed in health food stores is called Just Like Sugar. It is made of chicory root fiber (otherwise known as inulin or FOS). FOS is the acronym for fructo-oligosaccharide, which is a complex sugar derived from plants. Other ingredients in Just Like Sugar are calcium, vitamin C, and flavinoids from orange peels.

FOS is considered unique among the sugars because it has no caloric impact on the body. About 90 percent of the undigested FOS passes unchanged into the colon, where it is fermented by microflora into gases and short-chain carboxylic acids. FOS has been marketed as a "prebiotic" because it tends to encourage the growth of beneficial flora in the intestinal tract.

According to the *Physicians Desk Reference,* FOS is a source of dietary fiber that is used to improve bowel and liver function. It is also used to reduce blood cholesterol and blood pressure, but it can have side effects: increased gas (flatulence), stomach discomfort, bloating (swelling), and diarrhea.[135,136]

A more recent study confirmed these effects when twenty grams of FOS were used to sweeten lemonade on a daily basis for two weeks. Consumption of FOS increased flatulence, intestinal bloating, and mucosal irritation in healthy men.[137] Although Just Like Sugar may be an appropriate sugar substitute for some, excessive use is not recommended.

FOOD FLAVORINGS

Hundreds of chemicals are used to mimic natural flavors; many may be used in a single flavoring, such as in cherry-flavored soft drinks. The majority of flavorings are used in *junk* foods. Their use indicates that the real thing (often fruit) has been left out.

Monosodium glutamate (MSG)

Monosodium glutamate (MSG), also known as Accent, was introduced into the United States after World War II as a flavoring agent. MSG boosts the sensation of *savory* flavors in food. It has been around for a long time, even though it is a powerful neurotoxin, causing a number of toxic and allergic reactions. Symptoms can impact every part of the body including the skin, muscles, cardiovascular system, gastrointestinal system, and the brain. The recent book *The Slow Poisoning of America* by John Erb exposes the link between MSG and diabetes, migraines, autism, ADHD, and even Alzheimer's disease.[138]

> **MSG is considered an excitotoxin. It causes nerve cells in the brain to fire rapidly and erratically until they become completely exhausted. Hours later, many of these nerve cells suddenly die—as if the cells were excited to death.**

Experiments involving the feeding of MSG to infant rats and mice were done by Dr. John Olney of Washington University. The rats developed brain lesions, stunted skeletal development, marked obesity, and sterility.[139] Today, MSG is routinely used in the lab to induce obesity in experimental rats.[140]

MSG is now so widespread that it is almost impossible to avoid. More than ten thousand processed foods contain MSG, and many, such as mayonnaise and salad dressing, do not have to list it. Prepared and instant foods like soups and mixes all contain MSG. Restaurant food and fast food outlets (KFC chicken skin is loaded with it) are awash in MSG. Red meats, poultry, and other off-site prepared meat products are either sprayed with MSG-containing solutions or injected with MSG-containing compounds. Prepackaged hamburger patties have MSG. Fruits and vegetables are sprayed with MSG-containing washes. Baby foods often contain MSG, although the words monosodium glutamate will never appear on the label. Even a careful reading of the label may not always uncover the MSG; it can be disguised under any of the following names:

- Autolyzed yeast
- Broth
- Flavor enhancer
- Glutamate
- Glutamic acid
- High-flavored yeast
- Hydrolyzed protein
- Hydrolyzed plant protein
- Hydrolyzed vegetable protein
- Malt extract
- Monopotassium glutamate
- Natural flavoring
- Seasoning
- Soybean extract
- Textured protein
- Textured soy protein
- Yeast extract
- Yeast food
- Yeast Nutrient

Diacetyl

Diacetyl (also called butanedione or 2,3-butanedione) gives foods a distinctive buttery flavor and aroma. Diacetyl is used in microwave popcorn, snack foods, candies, baked goods, and other products. The National Institute for Occupational Safety and Health continues to investigate the occurrence of severe lung disease in employees at microwave popcorn packaging plants and flavorings manufacturing facilities. Medical tests of employees have shown airway obstruction and asthma—likely due to the exposure to diacetyl.[141] In light of these findings, butter flavorings should be avoided. Popcorn is better if you make your own and flavor it with real butter.

FOOD COLORINGS

Food colorings are classified as natural (derived from plants, minerals, and insects) and artificial. *Natural* food colorings are exempt from FDA certification. *Artificial* colorings (generally made from coal tar and petroleum sources) must be certified. Certified colors are listed on labels as FD&C or D&C. The letters F, D, and C stand for *food, drugs,* and *cosmetics,* indicating their approved uses. None of the artificial food colors have a clean slate.

In the 1970s, when Russian studies raised questions about the safety of FD&C Red No. 2, the FDA evaluated biological data and concluded that high dosages resulted in malignant tumors in female rats. The FDA banned the coloring agent. This had a profound effect on U.S. consumer attitudes. Retailers removed red products from their shelves for fear of backlash. Then in 1990, research showed that FD&C Red No. 3 caused thyroid tumors in male rats. But this time, rather than ban the coloring, the FDA succumbed to industry pressure and outlawed only certain uses of the coloring while continuing to allow it in food. As it turns out, FD&C Blue No.1 and FD&C Yellow No.5 are as questionable as Red No.3, but because they have been available since 1969, they are hard to remove from the FDA's "safe" list. The FDA continues to allow their use in foods.

Although the FDA dismisses his work, Dr. Ben Feingold substantiated a link between food colorings and hyperactivity in children in the 1970s.[142] More recently, the *Journal of Developmental & Behavioral Pediatrics* published information regarding fifteen trials with 219 participants; all were double-blind crossover trials. Just by eliminating artificial food colorings from their diet, children's behavior improved significantly. Furthermore, the elimination of food colorings from the diet produced one-third to one-half of the improvement typically seen with ADHD medication.[143] Amazingly, food colorings are used in many hyperactivity drugs.[144] Beyond causing behavioral problems, all artificial food colorings contain heavy metals such as lead and mercury[145]—known to aggravate attention deficit and hyperactivity in children.

Many defend the use of food colorings and other questionable food additives by saying that their use is in small quantities. This logic does not stand up to scrutiny. Biological reactions are influenced by minerals, enzymes, and hormones in the range of parts per billion or parts per trillion. Food additives, even in very small amounts, represent far greater concentrations. The average child between the ages of five and twelve takes in a daily dose of 150 milligrams of food colorings every day in foods like those listed below.

Common Foods with Food Colorings	
Gatorade Fruit Punch	Red 40
Plain M&Ms	Red 40 Lake, Blue 2 Lake, Yellow 5, Yellow 6, Blue 1 Lake, Red 40, Blue 1
Bakery Mini Chocolate Muffin	FD&C Red 40
Kraft Macaroni & Cheese	Yellow 5, Yellow 6
Eggo Waffles	Yellow 5, Yellow 6
Fruit Loops	Red No. 40, Blue No. 2, Yellow No. 6, Blue No. 1
Sprinkl'ins Yogurt	Yellow 6, Yellow 5, Red 40, Blue 1, Yellow 6 Lake, Red 3, Red 40 Lake, Yellow 5 Lake, Blue 2 Lake, Blue 1, Blue 1 Lake, Blue 2
Nutri-grain Blueberry Bars	Red 40, Blue 1
Strawberry Pop Tarts	Red 40, Yellow 6, Blue 1

The certified food colorings listed below should be avoided when possible:

- FD&C Blue 1 Brilliant Blue
- FD&C Blue 2 Indigotine
- FD&C Green 3 Fast Green
- FD&C Red 40 Allura Red AC
- FD&C Red 3 Erythrosine
- FD&C Yellow 5 Tartrazine
- FD&C Yellow 6 Sunset Yellow

FOOD ADDITIVES

Technically, the term, "food additive" refers to anything added to natural food. It includes some of the categories discussed in the previous pages. Flavorings, preservatives, food colorings, and even salt can contain many harmful substances.

Aluminum

Many common food additives contain aluminum. The average person's intake of aluminum from food additives is about 20 milligrams per day. This is a growing concern because aluminum is being linked with Alzheimer's disease and other neurological problems that are more and more common. Anticaking agents in salt, baking powders, baking mixes, self-rising flour, nondairy creamers, processed cheeses, and cheese spreads all include aluminum-containing additives. Buffered aspirin and antacids can add 500 to 5,000 milligrams of aluminum per day, depending on how many you take.

Avoid products with additives such as aluminum silicate, sodium aluminum sulfate, and sodium aluminum phosphate. Also avoid many pickled products that contain the ingredient alum. (There are pickles made using traditional recipes that utilize natural lactic acid fermentation rather than alum and other pickling agents.) Avoid the use of regular baking powder; use the Rumford brand instead—it is aluminum-free. Bake your own cakes from scratch rather than purchasing mixes, and never use self-rising flour. Purchase natural, unprocessed salt without anticaking agents. Above all, avoid the use of antacids and buffered aspirin.

Salt

Our bodies require salt in order to function. In fact, the basic makeup of our bodies is very similar to the concentration of the salts and minerals in the ocean. The fluids in our bodies—blood, lymph, bile, sweat, tears—all include salt.

The medical profession often recommends the restriction of salt because early research uncovered a correlation between salt intake and high blood pressure. However, subsequent studies indicated that salt *restriction* did more harm than good. A large study conducted in 1983 found that dietary salt did not have any significant effect on blood pressure.[146] Another study found that salt deficiency led to the loss of taste, cramps, weakness, lassitude, and severe cardiorespiratory distress on exertion.[147] Avoiding salt is a mistake. Avoiding *refined* salt is the key.

Few people realize that the majority of the salt available today—like sugar and flour—is highly refined. Unprocessed natural salt contains between seventy and eighty trace minerals. Refined salt is the product of high-temperature processing that removes all the valuable, naturally occurring minerals. Natural salt also contains traces of marine life that provide organic forms of iodine. This is the reason iodine needs to be added back to salt after the refining process. It is similar to fortifying flour after it has been processed.

Salt refiners also add other chemicals during the refining process. In order to keep salt from caking, aluminum compounds are added. To replace natural iodine, potassium iodide is added; to stabilize the volatile iodide compound, dextrose is added. This requires the addition of a bleaching agent to restore whiteness. The finished product is a far cry from natural salt. *Refined* salt *can* have a detrimental influence on the human body. Research conducted by

Henry Bieler found evidence of sodium starvation in the tissues of those who consumed refined salt.[148]

Natural salt has a crystalline structure; it contains the energy of the sun, which is stored in the bonds that make up the crystalline grid.[149] This structure is broken by high-temperature processing, and the energy is lost. On the other hand, when natural sea salt is consumed, it penetrates the cells, releasing life-giving energy. Even most sea salts on the market today are highly refined. Choose a natural, unrefined sea salt (see sources).

Oils and Fats

Oils and fats provide a valuable source of energy in the diet. They also provide the building blocks for cell membranes and a variety of hormones, and they carry the fat-soluble vitamins A, D, E, and K. Unfortunately, most commercial vegetable oils are extracted at high temperatures, causing the destruction of vitamins and the release of free radicals. Processing renders good fats indigestible or harmful to the body. Many oils are hydrogenated or partially hydrogenated, causing the formation of trans fats.

Hydrogenation and trans fats

To help foods stay fresh on the shelf or to make a solid fat from a liquid, food manufacturers "hydrogenate" unsaturated oils. Hydrogenation means to add hydrogen. During hydrogenation, oils are exposed to hydrogen at a high temperature and in the presence of a catalyst. Two things result: some double bonds are converted into single bonds and other double bonds are converted from *cis* to *trans* configuration. Both of these effects straighten out the molecules so they can lie closer together and become solid rather than liquid. Partially hydrogenated oils spoil and break down less easily under conditions of high temperature.

In nature, most unsaturated fatty acids are called cis fatty acids. This means that the hydrogen atoms are on the same side of the double carbon bond. In trans fatty acids hydrogen atoms are on the opposite side of the double bond—like having a left-handed version of the original. The problem with trans fatty acids is that they are toxic to the body. They are incorporated into cell membranes as if they were cis fats—and your cells actually become partially hydrogenated (stiff and more solid). These foreign membrane components wreak havoc with metabolic processes. Trans fats have been correlated with heart disease, diabetes, cancer, low birth weight, obesity, and impaired immune system function. This is why new labeling requirements that went into effect in 2006 require trans fat to be listed on nutrition labels.

Most of the trans fat in the American diet comes from commercially baked and fried foods that require high temperatures. French fries, donuts, pastries, muffins, croissants, cookies, crackers, chips, and other snack foods are high in trans fatty acids. There are trans, fat-free cooking oils that can easily be substituted. Tropical oils (coconut and palm oil) are naturally saturated oils—they are solid or semisolid at room temperature and are capable of being stored for long periods of time without becoming rancid. Coconut and palm oils can withstand the high temperatures of cooking without degradation. They are excellent alternatives to hydrogenated oils.

Butter versus margarine

Partially hydrogenated margarines and shortenings are even worse than the highly refined vegetable oils from which they are made. To produce them, manufacturers begin with the cheapest oils—corn, soy, cottonseed, or canola—many times already rancid from the extraction process. The oil is mixed with metal particles—usually nickel oxide—then placed with hydrogen gas in a high-pressure, high-temperature reactor. Emulsifiers and starch are forced into the mixture to give it a better consistency. Then it is steam-cleaned for the removal of its unpleasant odor. Margarine's natural color, gray, is then eliminated by bleaching. Dyes and flavors must be added to make it palatable. Does this sound like the health food it is often claimed to be?

> **Butter is an important food to purchase organic. Non-organic butter can have up to 20 times as much pesticide as non-organic vegetables.**

Butter is the best and most easily absorbed source of vitamin A. It contains lecithin, a substance that assists in the proper assimilation and metabolism of cholesterol and other fat constituents. Butter is a rich source of selenium and the antioxidant vitamin E. A Medical Research Council survey showed that men who ate butter ran half the risk of developing heart disease as those using margarine.[150]

Choose fats and oils carefully, avoiding hydrogenated and partially hydrogenated varieties. Use coconut, palm, and extra virgin olive oil rather than hydrogenated soybean, corn, canola, and cottonseed oils for cooking. Use real, organic butter rather than margarine or other artificial spreads.

Olestra

Olestra (trade named Olean) is a zero-calorie fat replacement intended to be used in the preparation of savory foods and snacks. It was approved by the FDA in 1996 for use as a fat substitute in snack foods such as potato chips. Olestra's effectiveness is due to the fact that it is not digested or absorbed into the body. Its harmful side effects are many—as indicated by the warning that was originally required to accompany products containing it:

> *Olestra may cause abdominal cramping and loose stools. Olestra inhibits the absorption of some vitamins and other nutrients. Vitamins A, D, E, and K have been added.*

The FDA lifted the requirement for the warning label in 2003 but still requires manufacturers to add vitamins A, D, E, and K to compensate for the fact that olestra inhibits the absorption of fat-soluble vitamins.

The manufacturer of olestra has flooded the scientific community with studies claiming it to be safe. The majority of these studies were conducted by the manufacturer. Independent evaluation of olestra has shown a significant number of short-term side effects, but the long-term effects could be even more serious. Since there have been absolutely no long-term research studies on olestra, especially independent research, the commonsense approach is to avoid it completely.

Industry-funded and industry-conducted research almost never finds difficulty with its own products.

RAW FOOD

The original human diet consisted primarily of raw vegetables, fruits, seeds, sprouts, and nuts. Raw, plant-based foods have been the staple throughout the vast majority of human history. One of the best virtues of raw food, sometimes referred to as "live" food, is that it contains enzymes, which are destroyed by cooking. Enzymes are considered the life force of food because they assist in digestion and absorption. When you eat food without enzymes, your body has to produce the enzymes necessary to breakdown and absorb food. This depletes the available enzymes in your body and reduces the nutritional value you receive from the food you eat. Incompletely digested food causes numerous problems and food allergies. Cooking also destroys the active forms of many vitamins. It renders many minerals unavailable. Cooking breaks down pesticides and produces toxic residues. It also coagulates about 50 percent of the protein in foods.[151]

Those who eat a raw food diet generally feel an increase in energy and in emotional balance. In time, they are more in-tune with their bodies.

Though it takes discipline to change your habits, a diet that is at least 75 percent raw food is highly beneficial and highly recommended. For ideas on how to incorporate more raw food in your diet, and for recipes specific to your body type, visit www.ahrawveda.com.

Five Element Theory and raw food

The Chinese Five Element Theory is more than five thousand years old. According to Traditional Chinese Medicine, the Five Element Theory is the key to staying healthy by keeping the five elements in balance. The five elements are Fire, Earth, Metal, Water, and Wood. These are the basic forms of energy, which are continually being transformed into one another in the natural world. The Five Element Theory classifies everything (foods, emotions, organs, seasons, planets, numbers, animals, smells) into one of the five categories. For example: Earth involves the aspects of growth, nourishment, and change. Water is associated with cold, moisture, and flowing movement. Metal is associated with clean-up, with strength, and with firmness. The theory of the five elements is the basis for a unique bond between man and nature.

Element	Taste	Color	Corresponding System
Fire	Bitter	Red	Endocrine system
Earth	Sweet	Yellow	Digestive system
Metal	Pungent	White	Respiratory system
Water	Salty	Blue or black	Circulatory system
Wood	Sour	Green	Immune system

Few people realize that balancing the foods they eat according to the five elements is one of the easiest ways to stay in balance. By balancing your diet in this way, you also help to balance your biological systems, your energy, and your emotions. Cravings are often eliminated because the five tastes are provided with each meal—or at least on a regular basis. In the creation of a balanced meal or dish, the five elements should be represented in color as well as in taste. A sampling of foods that fit each category is listed below:

Fire—(Bitter taste and/or red color)
hops, radish, romaine lettuce, alfalfa, dandelion, unsweetened chocolate, and many herbs
The large, leafy plants of summer (often bitter) belong to the Fire element.

Earth—(Sweet taste and/or yellow color)
honey, apple, cherry, banana, corn, carrot, sesame oil, yam, and millet
The late summer fruits belong to the Earth element.

Metal—(Pungent taste and/or white color)
onion, chive, coriander, parsley, radish garlic, ginger, cayenne, peppermint, clove, and white rice
The small contracted plants belong to the Metal element.

Water—(Salty taste and/or blue-black color)
salt, kelp, seaweed, Nama Shoyu, salty pickles, olives, celery, and beans
The roots of plants belong to the Water element.

Wood—(Sour taste and/or green color)
lemon, pear, plum, mango, sauerkraut, barley, and sprouts
The young plants of spring belong to the Wood element.

Living/raw foods have a higher nutrient value than foods that have been cooked or processed. They are referred to as nutrient-dense foods, and they carry a higher vibratory signature than cooked or processed food. One of the key components of the regenerative program developed by one of the authors is nutrient-dense food eaten according to the Five Element Theory. With a little practice, it is easy to create appetizing raw food, five-element meals. Several ideas are included below.

Smoothie—Banana (sweet-yellow), avocado (sweet-green), small amount of lemon (sour- yellow), raw chocolate (bitter-black), celery (salty-green), and a pinch of cayenne (pungent- red).

Salad—Romaine lettuce (bitter-green), olives (salty-black), grated carrot (sweet-yellow), red onion (pungent-red), sesame oil (sweet-yellow), lemon (sour-yellow).

Juice—Apple (sweet-red), lemon (sour-yellow), celery (salty-green), romaine lettuce (bitter-green), and ginger (pungent-white)

Flaxseed cracker—Flaxseed (sweet-yellow), tomato (sweet & sour-red), Nama Shoyu (salty-black), chive (pungent-green), and white pepper (bitter & pungent-white).

FOOD SUPPLEMENTATION

Proper diet is a cornerstone of physical health. Unfortunately, food has become increasingly devoid of essential nutrients. Poor food quality begins with the agricultural practices that have depleted soils of their minerals. Add to this the reliance on synthetic fertilizers, pesticides, antibiotics, and hormones, and the quality of our food has dropped even further. Next, food processing takes its toll with additives, preservatives, and treatments that reduce any remaining nutritive value. The result is food that can no longer sustain healthy life.

The elimination of processed, commercially grown food from your diet is important. In its place, emphasize organic fruits and vegetables, whole grains, seeds, nuts, and organically raised meat, poultry, and fish. But in today's world, even this is no longer enough. The burden placed on our bodies by chemicals, pollutants, and electromagnetic radiation is so great that without a supplementation program, few will thrive.

High-density, whole-food concentrates provide real nutrition—not isolated vitamins and minerals. In fact, many vitamin supplements may themselves be toxic to the body when they are provided *out of context*. Isolated vitamins eventually lead to imbalances and nutritional deficiencies because the body is forced to surrender its nutrient reserves to make isolated vitamins work. Many nutritionists have noted that without the whole-food complex, the body can never achieve complete nutrition because vitamin supplements lack "the rest of the story." Supplement your diet with organic, whole-food supplements—those that provide the whole complex of vitamins, minerals, antioxidants, essential fatty acids, and protein.

Bamboo

An emerging food supplement with the capacity to bridge the gap between even the best food and what is necessary to thrive is known as moso bamboo. Leaves from this bamboo have been used in Aryuvedic and Chinese medicine for centuries. It is not coincidental that the oldest living peoples in the world, including the Miao of China and the Hunzas of Tibet and Pakistan as well as the Vilcabamba of Ecuador, live into their hundreds consuming bamboo leaves from the moso bamboo family. Neither is it a coincidence that the strongest animal on earth for its size (the silverback gorilla) eats only fruit and bamboo leaves.

Moso bamboo leaves contain a balance of complementary and synergistic vitamins, minerals, amino acids, fiber, flavonoids, lactones, phenolic acids, phystosterols, antioxidants, prebiotics, carotenoids, and more. The plant's leaves are a complete, nutrient-dense food that can fill in many nutritional gaps in today's modern diet. Bamboo is also rich in organic silica. Its silica content is often more than ten times the level found in other plants used to supplement silica. Silica is essential for maintaining healthy bone and connective tissue. It is a common deficiency found with osteoporosis, arteriosclersis, and connective tissue problems.

Western medical institutions have built upon the extensive research from prestigious Chinese, Korean, and Japanese universities revealing the nutritional and health supportive qualities of moso bamboo.[152,153] The University of Hawaii John A. Burns School of Medicine even filed a provisional patent asserting that moso bamboo leaf extract inhibits breast cancer. The same researchers assert that it relieves lipotoxicity—a precursor to diabetes.[154]

Moso bamboo leaf concentrate is heralded for its ability to support all the systems of the body that are involved in any form of internal transportation. As the fastest growing plant in the world (it grows three feet per day), it is a master at moving fluids and nutrients. It has the same capacity when used as a food supplement, optimizing the transport of blood, lymph, oxygen, and bioelectric signals. Not only is moso bamboo an excellent source of complete nutrition, but it is the model of ecology and sustainability. It can be harvested again and again without damage to the plant or to the ecosystem. It yields the highest levels of oxygen (35 percent more than any other plant form) into the environment. It is self-fertilizing, and it purifies and filters the water before returning it to the soil.

Moso bamboo is available from a company known as Golden Basin International (a joint U.S./Chinese enterprise that commits profits to impoverished Chinese children and their families). The nonprofit company gathers wild bamboo from a virgin highland forest and produces the concentrate in a quality-controlled facility. Moso bamboo is available as a liquid leaf concentrate and as a powder. It is easily mixed in drinking water. It can also be infused into rice, noodles, sea salt, and other foods. For more information visit: www.wyntersway.com.

FOOD LABELS—WHAT DO THEY MEAN?
Label claims

While consumers rely on labels to make wise nutritional choices, food processors use labels to sell their product. Knowing what the words on the label really mean is important in making nutritious choices. Be wary of ambiguous terms.

The word *natural* is probably the least meaningful of all label terms. Consumers believe that natural means that the food is just as Mother Nature made it, but that really says little about the nutritional quality of the food—

or even about its safety. With the exception of the meat and poultry industry, there is no standardized meaning for the word natural. Anyone can place it on a label. Another common label phrase is *made from natural*. This simply means that the manufacturer started with a natural source. The terms: *all natural* and *no artificial ingredient*s are also virtually meaningless.

> **Only in the meat and poultry industry does the term *natural* have a meaning. For meat and poultry, *natural* means that it cannot contain artificial colors, artificial flavors, preservatives, or other artificial ingredients.**

Made with … is a good example of a misleading label. The law does not require a label to say how much of something is in the product. This type of labeling is particularly prevalent in snacks. *Made with whole grains* or *made with real fruit* says nothing about how much real anything is in the product—often it is very little.

Enriched is a tip-off that something was taken out of the food during processing that now requires another process to put it back in. Putting back isolated vitamins does not return health to the end product.

Fruit "drink" The word *drink* on a product tells you that it is *not* juice. It may, in fact, be mostly sugar and water, with added vitamin C. This enables the manufacturer to say the product is high in vitamin C, even if it is a long way from being real fruit juice.

Organic The terms *organically grown, organic,* and *pesticide-free*, unless they are accompanied with a certifying logo, may indicate that they are not totally organic. Trust in labels that say *certified organically grown* or that contain the certifying logo. This is the only way to be certain of organic status.

Ingredient lists

The ingredient list tells you what ingredients the food contains. These are listed in order, starting with the ingredient found in the largest amount (by weight). The ingredient list may be the most important information on the box to someone with food allergies. Learn to recognize all the alternate terms used to disguise MSG. Remember that fructose does not necessarily come from fruit—more likely it's from corn. Hydrogenated and partially hydrogenated oils are found in margarine, vegetable shortening, salad dressing, most chips, popcorn, French fries, cookies, crackers, candy, and pastries. It is best to avoid all packaged foods, no matter how good a label-reader you are.

Label endorsements

Americans have grown to trust organizations such as the American Heart Association (AHA) and the American Cancer Society (ACS) as benevolent benefactors of our health—not true. The ACS has gradually lost its credibility for devoting precious little of its resources to cancer prevention and for selling their endorsement to product manufacturers for a pricey sum. The AHA is also not so pure. Products displaying the AHA logo saying *"This product meets AHA guidelines"* are sometimes the worst of foods. Label endorsements are not necessarily an indication of nutritive value.

SOURCES (in the order they appear in the chapter):

Natural salt:
Celtic Sea Salt: http://www.celticseasalt.com/
Himalayan Salt: www.americanbluegreen.com
Real Salt: www.realsalt.com

Grass fed beef:
Panorama Meats' Black Angus and Red Angus: www.panoramameats.com
Country Natural Beef: Hereford and Angus: www.countrynaturalbeef.com
Tallgrass Beef: www.tallgrassbeef.com
Niman Ranch: A network of more than six hundred independent farmers and ranchers: www.nimanranch.com

Resources for finding local co-ops and local growers:
Local Harvest: www.localharvest.org This Web site will help you find farmers' markets, family farms, and other sources of sustainably grown food in your area, where you can buy produce, grass-fed meats, and many other items.

FoodRoutes: www.foodroutes.org The FoodRoutes Find Good Food map can help you connect with local farmers. On their interactive map, you can find a listing for local farmers and markets near you.

Eat Well Guide: Wholesome Food from Healthy Animals: www.eatwellguide.org The Eat Well Guide is a free, online directory of sustainably raised meat, poultry, dairy, and eggs, and online outlets in the United States and Canada.

 Recommended Reading
Regenerative Eating: A Live, Uncooked Cookbook for Addressing the Deeper Issues of Health and Wellness by Joel Gibson, Chrissy Gala, and Sharyn Wynters, ND Available online at: www.wyntersway.com

Genetic Engineering Dream or Nightmare by Mae Wan Ho

Mad Cowboy: Plain Truth from the Cattle Rancher Who Won't Eat Meat by Howard F. Lyman and Glen Merzer

Slaughterhouse: The Shocking Story of Greed, Neglect, and Inhumane Treatment Inside the U.S. Meat Industry by Gail A. Eisnitz

Spiritual Nutrition by Gabriel Cousens, MD

Chapter 5

IN THE KITCHEN

✦

Storage/ Preparation/ Cooking of Food

Harry S. Truman was known for his no-nonsense approach to life and government. He once said, "If you can't stand the heat, get out of the kitchen." Toxins infiltrate the meal preparation process from many angles. Microwave ovens, plastic food containers, aluminum and Teflon pans, lead-containing glass and ceramics, and many other challenges complicate the process. In our modern world, the heat in the kitchen is more intense than ever.

FOOD CONTAINERS

Even if food is grown under the strictest organic conditions, there are still ways chemicals can infiltrate before you have the chance to sit down and enjoy it. Many contaminants leach from food containers and food packaging materials.

Plastic

Plastic is by far the most insidious innovation ever created. Plastic releases toxins during production, during use, and after disposal. It poses serious health risks, and it endangers the environment. Once plastic is created, it exists for centuries, leaching poisonous toxins into the air, water, and soil.

Plastic is made by combining many toxic, synthetic chemicals in a process called polymerization. According to the plastics industry, polymerization binds these toxic substances so that they are locked into the plastic forever. Unfortunately, that is not entirely the case. Tiny amounts of toxins leach from plastic into any substance that is near to it—including air, water, and especially food. Scientists have been aware of this from the very beginning, and each new plastic (there are thousands of variations) that is proposed for food use must meet certain criteria. Limits have been established for the amount of toxins that can be released into food. Unfortunately, this approach is guesswork, as many of these chemicals have not been around long enough for us to understand their long-term effects on human health.

Heat, detergents, and age affect the release of toxins from plastic. Food types also have an effect. Many of the chemicals in plastic are highly fat soluble, so oily foods placed in direct contact with plastic are like blotting paper—literally pulling the toxins from the plastic into food. Acidic foods also encourage the release of more toxins.

> **Anytime you place hot foods, foods that contain fats and oils, or acidic foods (nearly all foods fit into one of these categories) in plastic, you increase the number of toxins you will eventually eat. Avoid foods stored or wrapped in plastic. When unavoidable, remove plastic wrap immediately when you arrive at home and cut off the area next to the plastic. Place foods in lead-free glass, enamel, ceramic, or stainless steel storage containers.**

Besides containing carcinogens (cancer-causing substances), plastic also contains substances that are known as *endocrine disruptors*. These substances interfere with the normal functioning of hormones. There is growing international concern about man-made endocrine disrupting chemicals. It is feared that they may be partly responsible for the decline in sperm counts and the increased rates of hormone-related cancers, such as cancers of the breast, testes, and prostate. Endocrine disruptors are also suspected of causing birth defects and early puberty onset in girls.

The reason endocrine disruptors can be so disastrous is that they have effects at extremely small concentrations—similar to the tiny amounts released into food from plastic packaging and plastic storage containers. Endocrine disruptors act in *parts per trillion*, so it takes an infinitely small amount to have an effect.

Young and developing children are the most vulnerable to endocrine disruptors in their environment and in their food. The effects may not be evident until after puberty—manifesting as physical deformities (breast, cervix, testicles), early puberty, endometriosis, skewed sexuality, low sperm count, behavioral problems, lowered intelligence, immune deficiencies, motor skill deficits, and many other problems. Each of these consequences has been seen in animal studies; many have been noted in human studies. Another difficulty is that they are not easily removed from the body and they build up over time.

> **Recently, the EPA changed the term "food additive"
> to the term "food contact substance"
> with reference to plastic.
> This was to take attention away from the fact that
> plastic adds known toxins to food.**

Evidence of the health effects of plastic already exist in sufficient quantity to halt its use in contact with food—yet it continues to be approved and used without caution. Plastic films cover almost everything from meat to mushrooms and cheese. Plastic bottles and jugs are used to contain milk, juice, honey, water, and just about every liquid preparation imaginable. Plastic dishes and plastic utensils are used in food preparation everywhere. There is almost no way to avoid plastic. However, understanding the problem will help you to find ways to minimize its use in your own kitchen.

Phthalates

Plasticizers are used to give flexibility to plastics. They intersperse around polymer molecules and prevent them from bonding as tightly to each other. The resulting plastic is not as rigid. Plasticizers migrate much more readily into food because they are not chemically bound to the plastic. The older the plastic is and the more it has been *flexed* during its lifetime, the greater the release of plasticizers. The migration of plasticizers into food can be aggravated by heat and by the presence of foods into which the plasticizing chemical will dissolve (e.g., oil, acid, or alcohol).

The most widely known plasticizers are called phthalates. They are endocrine disruptors widely used in the plastics industry. Evidence has been building for years linking phthalates to adverse health effects such as reproductive and developmental problems, respiratory impairment, and other effects.[155, 156, 157]

> **About 800 million pounds of phthalates are
> produced each year globally, and they are used
> everywhere in a wide array of products such as
> cosmetics, perfumes, paint pigments, hair sprays,
> wood finishes, and plastic.**

In 2007, thirty-five Americans from seven states participated in a national biomonitoring project. Thirty-three participants submitted urine for analysis—phthalates were found in all of them. In several instances, phthalate levels were above the 95th percentile. This means that according to the most recent figures available from the Centers for Disease Control,

95 percent of individuals supposedly have lower levels.[158] Obviously, more phthalates than expected are being ingested.

In 1997, as a seventh grade student, Claire Nelson learned that the EPA had never tested the effect of microwave cooking on plastic-wrapped food. With encouragement from her science teacher, she set out to test what the FDA had not. The National Center for Toxicological Research agreed to help. Claire's experiments revealed that a common phthalate, known as DEHA, was migrating into food oils at between two hundred and five hundred parts per million. (The FDA standard is 0.05 parts per *billion*.) Claire's findings were eventually published, and she received the American Chemical Society's top science prize for students.[159] Based on her work and on subsequent testing, many people are now aware that plastic should *never* be used in a microwave. In fact, a microwave should never be used at all!

 (see Chapter 5: Microwave cooking)

 (see Chapter 3: Microwave ovens)

Bisphenol A (BPA)

Bisphenol A (BPA) is another chemical of concern that leaches from many plastics. It is also an endocrine disruptor. In laboratory studies, BPA alters egg development in exposed fetuses and increases the risk of genetic damage in the next generation. In the biomonitoring project mentioned above, all participants were found to have BPA in their urine, and over half had it in their blood. These levels were within the range shown to cause effects in laboratory animal studies.

More than one hundred peer-reviewed studies have found BPA to be toxic at low doses, yet not a single regulatory agency has updated safety standards to reflect this low-dose toxicity. Currently "acceptable" levels of BPA are evidently not low enough. The results of research published in Europe in 2000 drew the following conclusions:

> *The over-riding conclusion of this briefing is that current legal limits are not set at low enough levels to protect human health, and that human and wildlife exposure to BPA should be eliminated where practicable. The public should be given access to all research findings, and regulators should aim to honestly inform the public about the concerns and uncertainties with regard to the effects of BPA exposure. Furthermore, the public should be given the right to know about the constituents of products, in order to enable them to make informed choices.*[160]

In laboratory animals, exposure to BPA profoundly affects the male reproductive system, with adverse changes to the testes, testosterone, and sperm production. It increases prostate and breast cancer risk, alters brain development, and causes earlier onset puberty and obesity. Researchers have found that women with a history of recurrent miscarriage have higher blood serum levels of BPA than women with successful pregnancies.[161]

A study published in the January 2008 issue of *Toxicology Letters* revealed that heating polycarbonate plastic water bottles caused the release of fifteen to fifty-five times more BPA.[162] While the leaching of BPA from polycarbonate water bottles is a concern, the danger from canned food may be even greater. There are no standards for BPA in canned foods. In 2007, the Environmental Working Group tested canned food bought throughout America and found BPA at levels two hundred times the government's traditional safe level of exposure for industrial chemicals.[163] Just one to three servings of foods with these concentrations could expose a woman or child to BPA at levels that caused serious adverse effects in animal tests.

There is only one U.S. manufacturer of canned food that uses a non-BPA lining in most of its canned food products. Eden Foods uses a lead-free, tin-covered, steel can coated with a baked enamel lining that does not contain BPA. These cans cost 14 percent more than the industry standard cans.

About 65 percent of the BPA produced is used to make polycarbonate plastic—the kind used for many rigid, reusable water bottles; approximately 25 percent is used in epoxy resin production—the kind used to line food cans. BPA is also used in dental sealants.

 (see Chapter12: Dental sealants)

Classifications of plastic

Plastic has been classified into seven categories, often identified by the number inside the triangle on the bottom of a plastic container. The numbers were originally designated for recycling—the larger the number the less recyclable the plastic. (Regardless of what you may have been led to believe, most plastic is not recycled, and most of it cannot be recycled.) For the consumer, the recycling numbers offer clues about what's in the plastic.

> **No. 1: PET or PETE** stands for polyethylene terephthalate. This type of plastic is characterized by a clear, glasslike transparency. It is used almost exclusively for bottled water and juice drinks. PET plastic is considered to be the safest, single-use plastic for water and other liquids. However, PET

plastics are loaded with plasticizers in order to keep them flexible. They leach phthalates—especially as the temperature rises. The longer your food or drink is in contact with PET plastic, the more phthalates it picks up. If you use a PET container (a commonly recycled type), remember they are not designed for reuse. Reuse will increase the leaching of phthalates.

No. 2: HDPE stands for high-density polyethylene. Milk and water jugs are made from this type of plastic. Most often it has a cloudy appearance. HDPE is considered to be a *safer* plastic, although it does not protect foods and water from odors.

No. 3: PVC stands for vinyl or polyvinyl chloride. It is used for clear food packaging and is well known for its use as piping in the plumbing industry. PVC is also used to make shower curtains, toys like big round balls, teethers, raincoats, bibs, and other products. Phthalates are added to PVC plastics to transform a hard plastic into a soft, rubbery plastic. Heavy metals like cadmium and lead are also added to make the PVC durable. You have probably noticed the smell of a new vinyl shower curtain; that is the emission of additives, particularly phthalates. Over 90 percent of the phthalates produced are used in the manufacture of PVC. One of the biggest problems with these additives is that they are not completely bound to the polymer. Over time, the phthalates and metals leach out. Each PVC product may expose you to very small amounts of phthalates and heavy metals. PVC plastic also represents a major environmental burden. It releases carcinogenic dioxins into the environment when it is manufactured and during incineration. Dioxins accumulate in fatty tissue and

contaminate the food chain. PVC is so insidious that many major companies are voluntarily phasing out its use.

No. 4: LDPE stands for low-density polyethylene. This plastic is very flexible and is made into bags for bread and frozen food, wrapping films, and grocery bags. Currently, it is considered *fairly* food safe. Companies aren't required to list what's in their plastic wrap, though, so your best bet is to be cautious. In 2006, the industry group American Chemistry Council reported that phthalates were no longer used in any U.S. plastic wraps.

No. 5: PP stands for polypropylene. This plastic is hard but somewhat flexible. It is made into yogurt, margarine, and ice cream containers; drinking straws; and syrup bottles. PP plastic uses less toxic additives than most other plastics during manufacture. It is also considered *fairly* food safe.

No. 6: PS stands for styrene or polystyrene. Styrene or its expanded form (Styrofoam) is used to make coffee cups, take-out food containers, meat trays, plastic plates, and egg cartons. It is not considered safe, nor is it recyclable. It does not degrade. Styrene itself is a carcinogen; it is also known to outgas phthalates into foods.[164] It should *never* be used in connection with food.

No. 7: OTHER. This class of plastic encompasses all others, including the plastic known as polycarbonate. Because polycarbonate is hard and durable and it does not acquire or impart odors, it has become a favorite for reusable water bottles. Sadly, plastics made using polycarbonate can leach BPA under normal wear and at room temperature. They too should be avoided.

Even though there may be *safer* plastics, the use of plastic should be phased out in the kitchen. To minimize the extent of contamination from plastic, do not buy prewrapped foods like cheese slices, and always opt for foods stored in glass or packaged fresh at the deli. When you get home, remove foods from temporary plastic and put them in natural containers such as glass, stainless steel, paper, or enamel. The longer the food is in contact with plastic and the higher the temperature, the greater the final level of contamination.

Use wood instead of plastic cutting boards, and spray your wooden board with a mist of vinegar, then with dilute hydrogen peroxide, to control bacteria. Replace food storage plastic bags with cellophane or waxed paper bags (these are great for sandwiches).

Cellophane

Cellophane (made from wood fiber) is clear and flexible (although not as pliable as plastic). It represents an alternative to plastic for the storage of food. Unlike the man-made polymers in plastic, which are largely derived from petroleum, cellophane is a natural polymer made from cellulose—a component of plants and trees. It is easily broken down by micro-organisms in the soil and does not represent an environmental burden like plastic. The NatureFlex line of cellophane is made from non-GMO trees under sustainable conditions. It is not suitable for use with high moisture content foods (see sources).

Biodegradable plastic

The biggest environmental problem with plastic is that it can take hundreds of years to break down. Thankfully, this concern is being addressed, and though the answers may not be perfect yet, they represent movement in the right direction. There are now two kinds of biodegradable plastic. One is made from polyolefin (still a petrochemical plastic), which has been modified with an additive to accelerate its breakdown. The additive causes the modified plastic to degrade in a predictable and controllable timeframe. Landfill trials demonstrated that one brand lost more than 95 percent of its molecular weight in less than ten months. The other type of biodegradable plastic is a bioplastic made from renewable resources such as corn, potatoes, and wheat. This type of plastic degrades at least 90 percent within 180 days when composting conditions (including heat, moisture, and aeration) are present.

Bioplastics include polycaprolactone, polyvinyl alcohol, and polylactic acid. Garbage bags made of bioplastic are already available in many health food stores. Many other bioplastic products are also available including food containers, plastic wrap, and cutlery. EcoProducts carries a whole line of biodegradable plastic products (see sources).

COOKWARE
Aluminum

More than half of all cookware sold today is made of aluminum because it is lightweight and because it heats evenly. If untreated aluminum is used in the preparation of salty or acid foods, large amounts of aluminum can be released into food. This is evidenced by the pitting of aluminum foil when it is in contact with these types of foods for more than several hours. In an extreme case, 0.7 milligrams of aluminum was released into three and a half ounces of applesauce after thirty minutes of cooking in an untreated aluminum pan.[165]

However, most aluminum today is anodized (dipped in a hot acidic solution). Anodization seals aluminum making it scratch resistant and easy to clean. The process modifies the molecular structure so that aluminum is not released into food. Acidic foods cooked in anodized aluminum do not react with the cookware, and most authorities believe that anodized aluminum cookware is safe. At this time, there is no evidence to the contrary. However, just like the process of polymerization, minute amounts of aluminum are bound to be released during cooking. Use your own judgment. The use of aluminum foil is another matter; it should *never* be used to cover or contain foods where the aluminum comes in direct contact with food.

> **Replace aluminum and non-stick cookware with ceramic, enamel, stainless steel, or non-leaded glass cookware.**
> (see sources)

Aluminum is a growing concern—especially because of its link to Alzheimer's disease and to other neurological problems which are becoming more and more common. But the difficulty is likely not with aluminum cookware. Many common foods and food additives contain aluminum, including pickling agents (alum), anticaking agents (aluminum silicates), baking powders (sodium aluminum sulfate), and baking mixes (sodium aluminum phosphate). The average person's intake from food additives is about 20 milligrams per day. Nondairy creamers, self-rising flour, processed cheeses, and cheese spreads also contain aluminum. These sources can provide up to 100 milligrams of aluminum a day. The largest source of aluminum is buffered aspirin and antacids. These can add 500 to 5,000 milligrams per day. Next to these sources, the amounts that have been found to leach from aluminum cookware are trivial.

 (see Chapter 4: Food additives)

Aluminum soft drink cans have also been cited as a possible source of aluminum toxicity. However, aluminum cans are lined with a plastic resin; aluminum contamination is limited to those cans that are bent or damaged, and where the resin is compromised. The greater risk from aluminum cans is the plastic resin liner known to leach BPA.

 (see Chapter 5: Bisphenol A)

Aluminum is not easily absorbed through the digestive tract, so even the above sources of aluminum may not be the cause of aluminum toxicity. Exposure to aluminum through the skin appears to be an even greater risk. Personal care products often contain aluminum—especially antiperspirant deodorants.

 (see Chapter 7: Deodorant)

Lead in glassware

Ever heard of lead crystal—those expensive crystal glasses that literally sparkle? The reason they sparkle is because they contain lead oxide, which dramatically increases the refractive index of the glass. Lead crystal can contain up to 30 percent lead oxide. When it is in contact with food, ions of iron, calcium, and magnesium in food or beverage are exchanged for the lead in the glass. A 1996 study found that beverages stored in lead crystal accumulated extraordinary concentrations of lead, and that an average of 70 percent of the ingested lead was absorbed in the human body.[166] Lead poisoning is especially dangerous for children and pregnant women. It can cause learning difficulties, behavioral problems, and serious illness.

> **Most glassware produced after 1990 for food use is lead-free. However, if you have older lead crystal glassware or decanters, never store wine or other beverages in them.**

Lead in ceramic

Lead from pottery, ceramics, and ceramic glazes also easily enters food. This includes crock pots with ceramic glazes. Ceramic ware made outside the United States—particularly in Latin America and China—is risky. Because of the possibility of lead poisoning, the FDA advises against the use of ceramic cookware from Mexico, China, India, and Hong Kong. Products made in the United States after 1990 for food use should be safe. It is still a good idea to avoid storing acidic foods such as tomatoes and tomato sauces, orange juice, and vinegar in ceramic ware, and to not wash ceramic ware in the dishwasher. Do not store food in antiques or collectibles. If you buy ceramic mugs, make sure they are lead-free and that the glazes used are also free of lead. Look for labels that say, "Safe for food use." And never use ceramic ware that is labeled "For decorative purposes only."

A test kit similar to those used by FDA inspectors to test lead levels in ceramic ware is available from Frandon Enterprises Inc. One kit costs about $30 and can be used for more than one hundred tests (see sources).

Teflon

The coating on nonstick cookware contains chemicals called perfluorinated compounds (PFC). When heated to high temperatures (above 500°F), the coating releases small amounts of PFC creating hazardous fumes. Birds are extremely sensitive to the fumes from nonstick pans. In the past twenty-five years, nonstick cookware has been linked to the deaths of hundreds of pet birds.[167] The same circumstances can cause flu-like symptoms in humans, which have been referred to as Teflon flu.

PFC can cause cancer and birth defects in animals and may pose the same risk to humans. The Society of the Plastics Industry acknowledges that PFC is found in the blood of 95 percent of the U.S. population and that it accumulates and is persistent in the environment. A study published in 2007 revealed that 100 percent of nursing mothers in Europe had PFC in their breast milk.[168] The Environmental Working Group, a U.S. advocacy organization, says DuPont (makers of Teflon) hid internal documents that showed the exposure risk is several times higher than what was reported to the government. If you choose to use nonstick pans, make sure to use low heat (better for cooking, anyway).

One of the best options for those who like nonstick cookware is a recent innovation by Ceramcor, called Xtrema cookware. This ceramic cookware is lightweight, scratch-resistant, nonstick, and made of 100 percent organic materials (see sources).

> **In the oven, glass or ceramic pans are much better than metal—you can turn down the temperature about 25°F and cook foods just as quickly.**

Kitchen utensils

Just as you want to stay away from plastic, Teflon, and aluminum cookware, you should also eliminate these materials from the utensils you use during food preparation. Even metal (stainless steel or titanium) knives tend to lose metallic ions when they are drawn through food. This accelerates wilting and oxidation (browning) and diminishes the nutritional quality of food—especially noticeable when food is in its natural, raw state.

Ceramic knives are the latest technology to overcome this problem. Made of crystalline zirconium, they are harder than steel, and they have the potential to stay sharp ten times longer than traditional knives. Because they are completely inert and nontoxic, they will not react with food acids. Fruit browns much more slowly when sliced with a ceramic knife—almost as though the knife separates the cells in food rather than slicing through them. Once you have experienced a ceramic knife, you will never want another metal knife. There are also vegetable peelers and other utensils now available from a variety of sources.

COOKING METHODS

Many processing techniques have been used throughout the ages to improve the digestibility of food. Soaking, sprouting, fermentation, aging, and acid or alkaline treatments all have their value, depending on the food in question. Often, these are better choices than cooking. Under some circumstances, cooking is helpful—overdoing it isn't. When it comes to cooking, remember two things: the less you cook it, the better (meat being an exception); and the lower the temperature, the better.

Gas versus electricity
Using gas or electricity is usually a matter of preference. Many people find that cooking with gas offers better cooking control; however, gas introduces combustion products into the house that must be vented to the outside. Sensitive individuals should avoid gas in favor of cooking with electricity. If you cook with gas, be sure to have a range hood and a ducted passage to the outside to provide adequate ventilation.

Microwave cooking
Over 90 percent of American homes have microwave ovens for meal preparation. Because microwave ovens are so convenient and so energy efficient, very few homes or restaurants are without them. But microwave cooking is not natural; it is not healthy, and it is far more dangerous to the human body than we have been led to believe.

Most everyone is aware that mother's milk should never be microwaved. Why? If microwaved food is so safe, why the caution with regard to mother's milk? In 1992, an article, "Effects of Microwave Radiation on Anti-infective Factors in Human Milk," appeared in the journal *Pediatrics*. The study found that microwaved breast milk lost lysozyme activity, antibodies, and it fostered the growth of more bacteria.[169] What really surprised the authors of the study was that even the lowest microwave setting destroyed the anti-infective properties in the milk. Adverse changes at such low temperatures suggested that microwaving itself may cause injury to the milk.

Early Russian investigations indicated that cancer-forming compounds accumulated in virtually all microwaved foods. Their research identified the following:[170]

- Microwaving prepared meats caused formation of d-Nitrosodienthanolamines, a well-known carcinogen.
- Microwaving milk and cereal grains converted some of the amino acids into carcinogens.
- Thawing frozen fruits converted glucoside- and galactoside-containing fractions into carcinogenic substances.
- Extremely short exposure of raw, cooked, or frozen vegetables converted plant alkaloids into carcinogens.
- Carcinogenic free radicals were formed in microwaved plants—especially root vegetables.
- Microwaving caused a decrease in food value from 60 to 90 percent in all foods tested.
- Microwaving decreased the bioavailability of B vitamins, vitamin C, vitamin E, and essential minerals in all food tested.
- Microwaving caused the degradation of nucleo-proteins in meats.

No wonder Russia banned the use of microwaves in 1976. Their research showed that not only did microwaved food pose health concerns; they were also among the first to acknowledge the damaging effects of microwave radiation.

 (see Chapter 3: Microwave radiation)

In 1991, Dr. Hans Hertel and Dr. Bernard Blanc of the Swiss Federal Institute of Technology published the first in-depth, clinical study on the effects of microwaved food on the human body. Their study demonstrated that microwave cooking changed the nutrients in food causing:

- Increased cholesterol levels
- Increased levels of white blood cells
- Decreased numbers of red blood cells
- The introduction of radiolytic (cancer-causing by-products) compounds
- Decreased hemoglobin levels (the ability to carry oxygen)

As soon as their study was published, the Swiss Association of Dealers for Electro-apparatuses for Households and Industry forced a gag order against the scientists, and Dr. Hertel was convicted of interfering with commerce. That gag order was eventually rescinded and damages were paid to Dr. Hertel, but the original motive was obvious.

In America, neither universities nor the federal government have conducted any tests on the effects of eating microwaved foods. Surely the industry knows what scientists outside the United States have found. If you change nothing else in your kitchen, get rid of your microwave oven.

BBQ

Barbecuing can create dangerous by-products known as heterocyclic amines (HCAs) and polycyclic aromatic hydrocarbons (PAHs). HCAs have been shown to cause cancer in lab animals and may increase the risk of cancers of the breast, colon, stomach, and prostate in humans. They are created when meat, poultry, and fish are subjected to intense high heat. Meat that is grilled, fried, or oven-broiled also produces large quantities of HCAs. PAHs are formed when animal or fish fats drip onto hot coals. The smoke and fire flare-ups drive these residues into the food. PAHs are thought to increase the risk of stomach cancer.

The biggest difficulty with barbecuing is the heat. The longer and the hotter the cooking is, the greater the problem. HCAs need intense heat to form, the reason they are absent in boiled or baked foods. One study found a threefold increase in HCAs when cooking temperatures were raised from 392 to 482 degrees. Cooking time is also important. Meats and fish cooked longer at high temperatures dry out and split open, exposing more of the meat to HCAs. Another difficulty is proper ventilation. When barbecue vents are open, the amount of smoke and PAH levels are reduced. Cancer Project nutritionists have determined the five foods containing the highest HCA levels; see their Web site.[171] If you grill, the following ideas will limit the risk of PHAs and HCAs:

- Leave the hood open when you barbecue to improve ventilation and to reduce intense heat.
- Marinate with natural marinade sauces before grilling or broiling to reduce HCAs by up to 90 percent.
- Select smaller cuts of meat.
- Select leaner cuts, to prevent dripping fat from causing flare-ups.
- Partially precook meat before grilling, to speed up grilling time.
- Flip meat frequently, which reduces the amount of carcinogens that form.

The Five Foods Highest in Heterocyclic Amines (HCAs)

1. Chicken breast, well done
2. Steak, grilled, well done
3. Pork, barbecued
4. Salmon, grilled with skin
5. Hamburger, grilled, well done

FOOD PREPARATION

Vegetable washes

Some of the simplest advice ever given has been to wash your food. Whether you purchase organic produce or not, that advice is still good. And perhaps the best time for washing it is as soon as you get home from the market. This is the perfect time to remove all the plastic, to wash fruits and vegetables, and to place them in other containers for refrigeration.

The Department of Analytical Chemistry at the Connecticut Agricultural Experiment Station conducted a study to examine the effects of rinsing fruits and vegetables under tap water as well as with a variety of commercial vegetable washing products. Four products were compared to a 1 percent Palmolive solution and to rinsing in tap water. Their findings indicated that all products, including water, removed a significant amount of pesticide residue. There were two pesticides that were unaffected, but eleven others showed significant reduction with washing.[172] Surprisingly, the commercial fruit and vegetable washes did no better than water alone. However, the duration of the rinses was only one minute. Most vegetable washes are intended for longer soaking to break down waxes and other coatings on the surface of fruits and vegetables.

A more recent study conducted in China showed that 10 percent acetic acid (vinegar) and 10 percent salt water solutions for twenty minutes outperformed water by almost four times.[173] Remember that although simple washing will remove pesticides on the outer portions of fruits and vegetables, many pesticides are systemic, which means that they are carried deep within the tissues of the plants they are sprayed on. Washing will not significantly reduce these pesticides.

Homemade Vegetable Wash

¼ cup vinegar
2 Tbsp. salt

Add these to a sink of water and soak vegetables for 15 minutes, then rinse.

Alkaline water with an abundance of negative ions (free electrons) has been used in Japan and other Asian countries for many years to soak fruits and vegetables as well as meat and fish. Negatively charged ions are attracted to positively charged bacteria and chemical residues, effectively pulling them from within the interior of produce and meat/poultry/fish products. For those who own a water ionizer, the highly alkaline water (with a pH of 10.0+) provides an excellent soak (fifteen to twenty minutes) for produce and meat. This is a great way to remove the *fishy* taste from fish and the *gamey* flavors from other meats. It is also effective for removing contaminants from deeper within fruits and vegetables. Soaking for fifteen to twenty minutes will often turn the water cloudy as pollutants are removed.

A product called NanoClean, made of ionized sea salt and shell powder, works in a similar way to add negative ions to water for soaking produce and meat. Five or six shakes of NanoClean for every gallon of water works like the highly alkaline water produced in an ionizer to effectively pull contaminants from produce and meat. The flavors of food are greatly enhanced (see sources). One of the authors recommends a fruit and vegetable wash that she feels outperforms all others. Visit www.wyntersway.com

Nonstick cooking sprays

Most nonstick cooking sprays are made with oil, water, or emulsifiers (substances that help water and oil to mix). Typically, the cheapest and least healthy oils are used in these products (such as soybean and canola), and a variety of preservatives are added to keep these products on the shelf. But why not make your own? Using your favorite organic oil (olive oil is a good choice because it does not form trans fats when heated), mix two tablespoons oil with two tablespoons of liquid lecithin (available in many health food stores and in some food markets); then fill to one cup and put in a spray bottle. Some recipes omit the lecithin and simply use oil and water (two Tbsp/cup). Just remember to shake before each use. Most women say they can't tell the difference.

Homemade Non-stick Cooking Spray

2 Tbsp. olive oil
2 Tbsp. liquid lecithin (you may omit this)

Fill to 1 cup and put in a spray bottle.
Shake before each use.

SOURCES (in the order they appear in the chapter):

Biodegradable plastic bags and other bioplastic products:
Eco Products: http://www.ecoproducts.com/

Cookware:
Xtrema cookware: http://www.ceramcor.com/

Le Creuset cookware: www.lecreusetexport.com Also often available through Whole Foods stores. French, cast-iron cookware coated with porcelain enamel; lead-free; requires no seasoning and cleans easily.

Visions cookware: http://www.visions-cookware.com/
nonporous, no lead, glass-ceramic; won't absorb food odors or flavors or react with foods.

Flavorite cookware: made by Regal Ware Inc.; it is stainless steel, waterless cookware, available online and at many outlets.

Corning and Pyrex cookware: Made by World Kitchen, LLC; each batch is tested for lead and cadmium; also available at most outlets.

Water bottles:
Klean Kanteen: http://www.kleankanteen.com/

Canned food manufacturers that don't use BPA-lined cans:
Eden Foods: www.edenfoods.com

Cellophane bags:
www.pak-sel.com, or American Environmental Health Foundation: www.ehcd.com

Frandon Enterprises Inc., P.O. Box 300321, 511 North 48th Street, Seattle, Wash., 98103, or call 1-800-359-9000.

Alkalizing Vegetable wash:
NanoClean ionized sea salt and shell powder: www.buynanoclean.com

Chapter 6

CLEANING AGENTS

✦

"A house is a home if it is clean enough to be healthy and dirty enough to be happy."

—Anonymous

For thousands of years, mankind has lived with dirt floors, open windows, and water as the only cleaning agent. Within the last fifty years, we have come to think we need floor finishes, tub and tile cleaners, and all manner of disinfecting agents. The fact is, the same cleaning agents we are using to keep our homes clean are jeopardizing our health and the health of the planet. The author of the statement quoted above (anonymous) also said, "Housework won't kill you, but why take the risk?"

Household cleaning agents are the number one source of toxins in the home—the vast majority of them contain not one but an abundance of toxic chemicals. These products are absorbed through the skin, inhaled into the lungs, and ingested as chemical residues that remain after dishes and other household items have been washed.

Most cleaning products today contain petroleum-based surfactants and solvents. These ingredients have been linked to reproductive disorders, neurological problems, and cancer. Many of them have not been thoroughly tested for their impact on human health, nor have they been tested for their impact on the environment. Unfortunately, approximately five hundred thousand tons of liquid cleaners are washed down U.S. drains every year.[174]

SURFACTANTS

Surfactants are chemicals that help to *release* the dirt and grime that water alone will not remove. Surfactant molecules have two sides: a water-attracting side and a water-repelling side. The water-repelling side is attracted to oils and dirt and helps to dislodge them from clothes or other surfaces. The water-attracting side pulls the dirt into the water. These opposing forces loosen and break up dirt particles and suspend them in the water.

Animal fats mixed with wood ashes created the earliest soap—a surfactant. This was the only cleaning product for ages, and it still works. Soap is made from a fatty acid that is reacted with an alkali. The acid side of the fatty acid forms a water soluble salt when mixed with alkali. The fatty side is attracted to dirt and grease. Modern soaps work using the same principle. However, synthetic surfactants have replaced the original, natural ingredients. Today, most surfactants are made from petrochemicals, and there are about as many different surfactants as there are people.

Surfactants are classified as *inert* ingredients and are not required to be listed on the label. Without knowing, it is nearly impossible to tell a safe surfactant from one that is toxic. Your best bet for getting safer products is either to make your own or to purchase them from companies that specialize in safe cleaning agents.

SOLVENTS

A solvent is a liquid that dissolves another substance. The term *organic solvent* sounds friendly, but the word *organic* simply means that it contains carbon. Organic solvents include alcohols and synthetic chemicals such as benzene, tetrachloroethylene, toluene, xylene, and turpentine; they often emit volatile organic compounds (VOCs) that cause headaches; eye, nose, and throat irritation; loss of coordination; nausea; and damage to the liver, kidneys, and central nervous system. Solvents are usually flammable and toxic, and like surfactants, they are not always required to be listed on the label—even though they may comprise more than 90 percent of the cleaner.

Unless they are labeled *green* or *eco-friendly*, which are the modern terms being used for safer personal care and cleaning products, practically all soaps, dishwashing liquids, shampoos, laundry detergents, conditioners, and other household cleaners contain petroleum-based surfactants and solvents and should be avoided.

COMMON HAZARDOUS INGREDIENTS IN CLEANING PRODUCTS

Although the chemicals in today's cleaning products would take volumes, the list below includes the most common. Knowing what they are will give you reasons to avoid them. Since the liver and kidneys are the major detoxification organs, toxins represent a severe burden to these organs. The term *sensitizer* is used in connection with many of these chemicals. This means that it is often the *trigger* that induces sensitivity to multiple chemicals. Note the number of chemicals that cause liver and kidney problems.

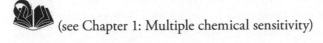 (see Chapter 1: Multiple chemical sensitivity)

Acetone—A neurotoxin, acetone may cause liver and kidney damage, and damage to the developing fetus. It is a skin and eye irritant as well as a sensitizer. Acetone is found in spot treatment cleaners; it is the main ingredient in fingernail polish remover.

Aerosol products—Products applied as aerosol sprays are broken into minute particles, which can be more deeply inhaled than larger particles. This increases their toxic effect. Aerosol propellants may contain propane; formaldehyde—a carcinogen, neurotoxin, and central nervous system depressant; methylene chloride—a carcinogen, neurotoxin; and reproductive toxin; and nitrous oxide.

Ammonia—Undiluted, ammonia is a severe eye and respiratory irritant that can cause severe burning, pain, and corrosive damage, including chemical burns, cataracts, and corneal damage. It can also cause kidney and liver damage. Repeated or prolonged exposure to vapors can result in bronchitis and pneumonia. Ammonia is a sensitizer, found in a wide range of cleaning products. It will react with bleach to form poisonous chlorine gas that can cause burning and watering of eyes as well as burning of the nose and mouth.

CAUTION: Never mix a product containing ammonia with a product containing bleach; it will form a dangerous gas.

Bleach—Bleach is the common name for the chemical sodium hypochlorite, found in a wide range of household cleaners. It is corrosive and is an eye, skin, and respiratory irritant; it is especially hazardous to people with heart conditions or asthma and can be fatal if swallowed. It may be a neurotoxin and toxic to the liver.

Diethanolamine (DEA)—Listed as a suspected carcinogen by the state of California, this chemical is a skin and respiratory toxicant and a severe eye irritant. It is used in a wide range of household cleaning products.

D-limonene—This chemical is also listed on labels as citrus oil and orange oil. D-limonene is used as a solvent in many all-purpose cleaning products especially those described as citrus and orange cleaners. Although its origin is natural—produced by cold-pressing orange peels—in its concentrated form it is a neurotoxin, a moderate eye and skin irritant, and can trigger respiratory distress when vapors are inhaled by sensitive individuals. There is limited evidence of carcinogenicity. D-limonene is not recommended for frequent use, even though it is derived from a natural source.

Ethoxylated nonyl phenol—Nonyl phenols are hormone disruptors. Some contain traces of ethylene oxide—a known human carcinogen. They are eye and skin irritants. Nonyl phenols are widely used in laundry detergents.

Formaldehyde—In lab tests, formaldehyde has caused cancer and damage to DNA. Formaldehyde is also a sensitizer, with the potential to cause asthma. It is estimated that 20 percent of people exposed to formaldehyde will experience an allergic reaction of some kind, although many may not link it to a household product. Exposure to formaldehyde may also cause joint pain, depression, headaches, chest pains, ear infections, chronic fatigue, dizziness, and loss of sleep. Several laboratory studies have shown it to be a central nervous system depressant. Formaldehyde is used in or outgassed from a wide range of other items throughout the home.

 (see Chapter 1: Volatile organic compounds)

Fragrance—The term fragrance on a label indicates the possible presence of up to five thousand different ingredients, most of which are synthetic. Many compounds included under the term fragrance are human toxins and suspected or proven carcinogens. In 1989, the U.S. National Institute for Occupational Safety and Health evaluated 2,983 fragrance chemicals for health effects. They identified 884 of them as toxic substances.[175] Symptoms reported to the FDA from fragrance exposure have included headaches, dizziness, rashes, skin discoloration, violent coughing and vomiting, and allergic skin irritation. Clinical observations have shown that exposure to fragrances can affect the central nervous system, causing depression, hyperactivity, irritability, inability to cope with stress, and other behavioral changes.

Methylene chloride—Methylene chloride is a carcinogen, a neurotoxin, and a reproductive toxin found in many stain removers. On inhalation, it can cause liver and brain damage and irregular heartbeat. It is a severe skin and moderate eye irritant.

Monoethanolamine—Found in many cleaning products, including oven cleaners, tub and tile cleaners, laundry presoaks, floor strippers, and carpet cleaners, this chemical may cause liver, kidney, and reproductive damage as well as depression of the central nervous system. Inhalation of high concentrations—when cleaning an oven—can cause dizziness or even coma. The chemical can also be absorbed through the skin. It is a moderate skin irritant and a severe eye irritant.

Morpholine—Morpholine is a moderate to severe eye, skin, and mucous membrane irritant. It is used as a solvent in a number of cleaning products, including some furniture polishes and abrasive cleansers. It is corrosive and can severely irritate and burn skin and eyes. Morpholine causes liver and kidney damage; long-term exposure can result in bronchitis. It reacts with nitrites (added as a preservative in some products) to form carcinogenic nitrosomines.

Naphthalene—This registered pesticide is listed as a suspected carcinogen in California and is most commonly found in mothballs and deodorizers. As a reproductive toxin, it is transported across the placenta and can cause blood damage. It can also cause liver and kidney damage, corneal damage, and cataracts. Skin exposure is especially dangerous to newborns.

Parabens—Parabens are hormone disruptors, widely used in cleaning products as preservatives. Paraben is usually preceded by the prefixes methyl-, ethyl-, butyl-, or propyl. Parabens may cause contact dermatitis in some individuals.

Paradichlorobenzene—This highly volatile, registered pesticide, in the same chemical class as DDT, is a suspected carcinogen and may cause lung, liver, and kidney damage. It is used in mothballs and some washroom deodorizers.

Phenol—Phenol is a highly poisonous, caustic substance derived from coal tar and used in the production of disinfectants, dyes, pharmaceuticals, plastics, germicides, and preservatives. Exposure may result in systemic poisoning, weakness, sweating, headache, shock, excitement, kidney damage, convulsions, cardiac or kidney failure, and death. Repeated exposure may also cause vomiting and mental disturbances. Phenol is considered to be corrosive to the skin and it is known to be a protoplasmic poison (toxic to all cells).

Phosphoric acid—Extremely corrosive, phosphoric acid can irritate and burn the skin and eyes. Breathing vapors can make the lungs ache, and it may be toxic to the central nervous system. Phosphoric acid is found in liquid dishwasher detergents, metal polishes, disinfectants, and bathroom cleaners—especially those that remove lime and mildew.

Sodium dichloroisocyanurate dihydrate—This corrosive chemical is a severe eye, skin, and respiratory irritant. It may cause liver and gastrointestinal damage and may be toxic to the central nervous system. It will react with bleach to form poisonous chlorine gas that can cause burning of the eyes, nose, and mouth. It is found in some toilet bowl cleaners and deodorizers.

Sodium lauryl sulfate—This chemical is a common lathering agent found in most shampoos. It is also a component of many household cleaning products. It is a known skin irritant. It also enhances the allergic response to other toxins and allergens and can react with other ingredients to form cancer-causing nitrosamines.

Toluene—Exposure to toluene may cause liver, kidney, and brain damage. It is also a reproductive toxin that can damage a developing fetus. It is found in many cleaning products as a solvent.

Turpentine—This chemical can cause allergic sensitization and kidney, bladder, and central nervous system damage. It is found in specialty solvent cleaners, furniture polish, and shoe products.

Xylene—Xylene has significant neurotoxic effects, including loss of memory. High exposure can lead to the loss of consciousness and even death. It may damage liver, kidneys, and the developing fetus. Used in some spot removers, floor polishes, ironing aids and other products, it is a severe eye and moderate skin irritant.

Cleaning Agent "Signal" Words

The three words **Caution, Warning, and Danger** are markers mandated by the EPA to appear on the label of poisonous substances. They replaced the familiar, but no longer seen, skull and crossbones symbol.

Caution: an ounce could be fatal to an adult if swallowed.
Warning: 1 teaspoon could be fatal to an adult if swallowed.
Danger: as little as five drops could be fatal to an adult if swallowed.

SAFER CLEANING AGENTS

If you have not already done so, now is a good time to phase out your old cleaning products and to replace them with safer options. Despite the continuing hype from manufacturers, cleaning rarely requires specialized or expensive ingredients. There are five basic cleaning ingredients every home should have:

1. **Baking soda** is a good scrubber. It is abrasive, soluble in water, and anti-fungal. Baking soda requires a bit more elbow grease than chlorinated powders (cleanser), but your lungs won't suffer during the job.

2. **Borax** is also an abrasive, soluble in water—with good germicidal qualities.

3. **Vinegar** is a deodorizer and sanitizer. Its mild acidity kills many bacteria and molds. The acidity will also remove mineral deposits.

4. **Castile soap** is a great natural soap. Dr. Bronners soaps include a variety of natural and castile soaps (see sources).

5. **Microfiber cloths** are a relatively new addition to the world of cleaning. These untreated, reusable cloths are made of microscopic fibers that are spun into tiny, wedge-shaped strands. They can lift off dirt and grease, reducing or eliminating the need for harsh cleaning chemicals. A good quality microfiber cloth can last for years. There are a number of different brands. The Norwegian company Norwex makes an antimicrobial microfiber cloth with silver fibers to help prevent the transfer of germs (see sources).

If you don't want to make your own, you'll find plenty of environmentally friendly products in your local health food store or online. Several good brands include Ecover, which has everything from safe laundry soap to dishwasher tablets; Heartland Natural, whose nontoxic cleaning solution is made from botanicals and amino acids and can be used for everything from dishes to laundry and carpets; and Seventh Generation, which is sold in many health food stores; Earth Friendly Products; and Nature Clean (see sources).

All-purpose cleaners

Many all-purpose cleaners contain ammonia, a strong irritant which can also cause kidney and liver damage. Many also contain DEA, which can react with nitrites (added as undisclosed preservatives) to form carcinogenic nitrosomines. Many colored products use coloring agents made from coal tar. Hormone disrupting parabens may be used as preservatives. Many cleaners also include fragrances. Even *alternative* brands may contain d-limonene, a sensitizer which can cause respiratory distress as well as liver, kidney, and nervous system damage. Here's one you can make yourself:

Homemade All-purpose Cleaner

1 tsp. borax
1/2 tsp. baking soda
2 Tbsp. vinegar
1/2 tsp. liquid castile soap
2 cups very hot water

Add the first four ingredients to a spray bottle, then slowly add the hot water and shake until dry ingredients are dissolved.

Air fresheners

Air fresheners are made from a number of chemicals, including formaldehyde, naphthalene, xylene, butane gas, cresol, ethanol, phenol, and strong fragrances. They work in one of three ways:

1. Using a nerve-deadening chemical that coats nasal passages with an oily film.
2. Masking an offending odor with a different odor.
3. Deactivating an odor.

Aerosol air fresheners release chemicals as tiny particles that can be inhaled deeply into lungs and rapidly transferred into the blood stream. Air fresheners that plug into electrical outlets break chemicals into even smaller particles and should never be used. The key to freshening air is to remove or dilute the offending odor (by cleaning, ventilation, or absorption), not to cover it with other chemicals. Baking soda in an open container will absorb many odors in an enclosed area. Zeolite, a mineral, will absorb odors as well as heavy metals (see sources). Essential oils add pleasant aromas and kill germs. Opening a window to improve ventilation will do more to freshen the air and remove odors than anything else.

Bleach

The main ingredient in chlorine bleach is sodium hypochlorite (chlorine added to lye). It is corrosive to the skin and to the eyes, nose, and throat by inhalation. Sodium hypochlorite can create poisonous chlorine gas if mixed with ammonia (which may be an unlabeled ingredient in some cleaning products) or with vinegar.

Sunshine will whiten cotton and linen clothing. Hydrogen peroxide—drug store dilution—will also whiten many fabrics without bleach (use a half-cup per wash load). Many companies now make nonbleach whiteners (see sources).

Carpet cleaner

The chemicals released from carpet cleaners and deodorizers can be considerable where there is a large carpeted area. Carpet cleaners can contain perchloroethylene, a known human carcinogen that can have immediate central nervous system consequences. Napthalene, which *is* toxic by inhalation, is another common ingredient in carpet cleaners. These cleaners may also include butyl cellosolve, a central nervous system toxin; methyl ether, which is an eye, skin, and respiratory irritant; aliphatic petroleum solvent, which is neurotoxic; isopropyl alcohol, which is carcinogenic at high concentrations; and propylene glycol.

Any less-toxic cleaning liquid will work in a carpet-cleaning machine. If using a rented machine, clean the tank first to eliminate residue from previously used products. Often, good carpet cleaning can be accomplished with hot water alone. Start off with a small amount of cleaner and adjust as necessary. Ask commercial carpet cleaning companies to clean using only water and baking soda, steam, club soda, or a less toxic cleaner like ECOgent (see sources).

Homemade Carpet Stain Remover

Mix 1/4 cup each of salt, borax, and vinegar. Rub paste into carpet and leave for a few hours. Vacuum.

Carpet deodorizer

Most carpet deodorizers contain heavy fragrances. These should be avoided. One of the easiest ways to deodorize your carpet is to sprinkle baking soda. Let it sit a few hours or overnight and then vacuum.

Dishwashing liquid (hand)

Dishwashing liquids contain detergents, coal-tar–based colors, and artificial fragrances. Most are petroleum-based. They may contain quaternium 15, an eye and skin irritant that can release formaldehyde.

 (see Chapter 7: Perfume)

Many coloring agents are known to be carcinogenic; they can penetrate the skin and be deposited on dishes. There are many alternatives (see sources).

Dishwasher detergents

Many dishwasher detergents contain dry chlorine, which is activated when dissolved in water. Chlorine fumes in the steam that leak from dishwashers may cause eye irritation and breathing difficulties. Dishwasher detergents may also contain quarternium 15. Dyes and artificial fragrances are also common ingredients. Many safe alternatives exist (see sources). Also try the following homemade version.

Homemade Dishwasher Cleaner

Mix equal parts of borax and baking soda and store in a tightly sealed container. Use 2 tablespoons per dishwasher load. If you have hard water, double the amount of baking soda in your mixture. For either mixture, use vinegar in the rinse cycle.

Disinfectants

The fad for disinfectants and antibacterial agents is based on a fear of germs perpetuated by the pharmaceutical industry. For most households, it is doubtful whether disinfectants are needed at all. Ordinary cleanliness using soap and water is the best method to prevent disease. Antibacterial agents and disinfectants should be reserved for hospitals and home care of patients with suppressed immune systems.

There are more than three hundred different active ingredients approved for use in antimicrobial products. Many of these ingredients are classified as pesticides because they kill microbes. Scientists are concerned that products containing antibacterial and antimicrobial agents kill beneficial bacteria and contribute to the creation of antibiotic-resistant bacteria. Triclosan is one of the most popular antibacterial agents. It creates dioxin, a carcinogen, as a by-product.

The following homemade solution was used at a hospital to replace other disinfectants. The bacteriologist reported that it satisfied all hospital germicidal requirements.[17]

Homemade Disinfectant

Add 1/2 cup of borax to 1 gallon of warm water.

Drain opener

Drain cleaners usually contain sodium hydroxide and sodium hypochlorite, which can cause permanent damage to skin and eyes on contact. Vapors can burn lungs. Drain cleaners may also contain dimethylbenzyl ammonium chloride, a severe eye and skin irritant, and dichlorodifluromethane, an eye irritant which is also neurotoxic. Biological products containing stabilized enzymes and bacteria are less toxic, equally effective, and more environmentally friendly (see sources). Try the following homemade version.

Homemade Drain Cleaner

1/2 cup baking soda
1/2 cup white vinegar
Boiling water

Pour baking soda down drain. Add white vinegar and cover. Let sit for 5–10 minutes. Pour boiling water down the drain. (The vinegar and baking soda break down fatty acids, allowing the clog to wash down the drain.) This method is a good preventive and can be used weekly to prevent drain clogs. If you have a difficult clog, a drain snake is recommended rather than toxic drain openers.

CAUTION: Do not use this method if you have used a commercial drain opener that may still be present in the drain.

Dusting

Dust and dust mites can be a common trigger for those with allergies. However, it is important to dust in a way that really removes dust, rather than raising it into the air where it will resettle later. Microfiber cloths are excellent for dusting. They are untreated and reusable (see sources). Dusting with a damp, lint-free cloth also works—or mix one teaspoon of olive oil with a quarter cup of vinegar on the dust cloth.

Fabric softener

Fabric softeners work by leaving a residue on the fabric which never completely washes out. It can cause allergic reactions through skin contact and inhalation. Fabric softeners may also contain coal-tar dyes, ammonia, and very strong fragrances. When fabric softeners are exposed to hot water, heat from dryers, or ironing, vapors may be emitted that can be deeply inhaled. Fabric softeners may contain quarternary ammonium compounds and imidazolidinyl, both of which are known formaldehyde releasers and are known to cause contact dermatitis. Fabric softeners are designed to reduce static in synthetic fabrics. They serve no purpose with natural fibers.

Dryerballs reduce drying time up to 25 percent while softening fabrics naturally. As dryerballs tumble with clothes in the dryer, they lift and separate clothing and allow air to flow more efficiently. Their unique design relaxes the fibers during the drying cycle, making clothes feel softer and towels more absorbent (see sources).

Homemade Anti-cling Solution

Add 1/2 cup of white vinegar, baking soda, or borax to the rinse cycle to soften water and reduce static cling.

Floor cleaners, waxes, and polishes

Conventional floor products often contain mineral spirits and petroleum solvents, both of which are neurotoxic and can cause severe eye and skin irritation. Some wax removers with ammonia contain tripropylene glycol monomethyl ether, which can cause narcosis and kidney injury with repeated and prolonged skin exposure. Alternatively, use a microfiber mop with plain water. They rinse cleaner than other mops and save on cleaning products. They are also safe for hardwood floors.

Homemade Floor Cleaner

1/4 cup baking soda
1 tablespoon liquid castille soap
1/4 cup vinegar
2 gallons hot water

Homemade Wood Floor Cleaner

1/4 cup liquid castille soap
1/2 to 1 cup vinegar
2 gallons warm water

Floor and furniture polish

Floor and furniture polishes can contain nitrobenzene, a carcinogen, reproductive toxin, and central nervous system toxicant, which can be absorbed through the skin; phenol, a carcinogen and severe skin irritant; propane; butane gas; aliphatic naptha; petroleum distillates; and turpentine—all are neurotoxins. Polishes may contain morpholine, a severe irritant which may cause kidney damage, as well as ammonia, detergents, and synthetic fragrance. Aerosol products create microscopic particles that can be inhaled deeply into the lungs and transferred to the bloodstream. Some products contain formaldehyde and nitrosamines. One of the best alternatives is unscented guitar/violin polish, available in music stores, or try the following homemade version.

Homemade Furniture Polish

1 cup olive oil, almond or walnut oil
1/2 cup vinegar or lemon juice

Shake well and apply a small amount to a soft rag. Spread evenly over furniture surface. Polish with a dry cloth.

Glass cleaner

Most glass cleaners are made of ammonia and coal-tar dyes. Some contain butyl cellosolve—a neurotoxin, alcohol, naphtha, and glycol ethers. Aerosol products create small particles that are more likely to be inhaled and to irritate eyes. Consumer Reports found plain water to be more effective than half of the glass cleaners on the market. When combined with a microfiber cloth, most people find it more than adequate. If you need to remove hard water deposits, use the homemade glass cleaner below or find another natural cleaner (see sources).

Homemade Glass Cleaner

Add equal parts of water and either vinegar or lemon juice.
Place in a non-aerosol spray bottle and mix gently.

Note: If you have a water ionizer, the acidic water easily removes water spots from glass.

Laundry detergent

Most laundry detergents are made from petrochemical ingredients. They may contain bleaches, synthetic whiteners, and chemical fragrances. Detergent residues on clothes and bed linens can be a source of skin irritation. Lingering scents from scented products can cause respiratory and other reactions for sensitive individuals. Laundry soaps, available as bar soaps or flakes, are usually made from natural minerals and fats and tend to be less toxic than conventional detergents (see sources).

Scale or mineral remover

Some lime removers contain highly caustic sodium hypochlorite and phosphoric acid, which are very irritating to lungs and dangerous for people with asthma and heart disease. Vinegar, when left to soak on hard water mineral deposits, is often effective by itself. To clean shower heads, place one-fourth of a cup of vinegar in a plastic bag and secure the bag to the shower head with a rubber band. Let it sit overnight, then rinse and buff.

Magnetic or electromagnetic treatment of the incoming water line has been discussed for many years as a way to reduce hard water deposits (and provide many other benefits). It is much less expensive than water softening and much more environmentally friendly. Some of these devices are a near miracle for eliminating scale build-up and for the prevention of future scale build-up.

 (see Chapter 2: Magnetic water conditioners)

Metal cleaner/polish

Conventional metal cleaners and polishes may contain ethylene glycol, a neurotoxin, reproductive toxin, and respiratory irritant that can cause kidney, blood, and liver damage. They may also contain ammonia and synthetic fragrances. Many tried-and-true recipes like those indicated below work just as well.

Homemade Brass/Copper/Pewter Cleaner

Lemon juice
Cream of tartar

Make a paste the consistency of toothpaste. Rub onto brass or copper with a soft cloth and leave for several minutes. Rinse with water and rub a thin layer of olive oil to prevent tarnish.

Homemade Chrome and Stainless Steel Cleaner

Undiluted, white vinegar

Rust Remover

To remove rust, rub with fine steel wool dipped in vegetable oil. The finer the steel wool, the less noticeable any scratches will be.

Homemade Silver Polish

Toothpaste can be used as a silver polish. For silverware, place silver on a piece of aluminum foil in a pot, then add 3 inches of water, 1 teaspoon baking soda, and 1 teaspoon salt. Boil for a few minutes, rinse and dry. For jewelry, fill a glass jar half full with thin strips of aluminum foil. Add 1 tablespoon salt and fill with cold water. Drop items in jar for a few minutes, rinse and dry.

Oven cleaner

Conventional oven cleaners create toxic fumes that can burn eyes, skin, and internal organs. Lye and ammonia are often the cleaning agents, and they are especially dangerous in aerosols. To avoid the need for full oven cleaning, place an aluminum foil liner in the bottom of the oven. Replace periodically. When cleaning is necessary, try a more natural cleaner (see sources) or use the cleaner below.

Homemade Oven Cleaner

Make a paste of baking soda and water and spread on oven interior. Leave overnight with oven door closed. Remove with sponge or nylon scrub pad.

Scouring powder

Most scouring powders contain bleach, crystalline silica, and oxalic acid dehydrate. All three substances are strong irritants. Bleach can also upset the balance in septic tanks by killing helpful bacteria. Alternatively, use Bon Ami scouring powder (available in many grocery stores) or the homemade version below.

Homemade Scouring Powder

1 cup baking soda
1 cup borax
1 cup regular salt

Sink, tub, and tile cleaner

Sink, tub, and tile cleaners can contain ammonia and dimethyl ethylbenzylamonium choride—both strong irritants. These cleaners may also contain ethylene glycol, a neurotoxin and reproductive toxin that may cause kidney and liver damage; sodium ortho-phenylpenol, a carcinogen and irritant; and trisodium nitrilotriacetate, a carcinogen. Some brands use highly caustic chemicals such as sodium hydroxide, sodium hypochlorite (bleach), and phosphoric acid that can burn eyes and skin. Breathing vapors can burn lungs. There are many natural alternatives (see sources).

Microfiber cloths can be used in many situations to remove grime without chemicals. They are especially good on tubs, sinks, and stoves because they won't scratch the surfaces, but the tiny, wedge-shaped fibers will cut through dirt.

Spot removers

Spot removers are often made with highly toxic petrochemical solvents, including toluene and xylene, which are neurotoxic and can cause reproductive damage; tetrachloroethylene (perchloroethylene), which is carcinogenic, neurotoxic, and an eye and skin irritant; and petroleum distillates, which can cause eye, skin, and respiratory irritation. Club soda will remove many stains. For tougher stains, mix baking soda with club soda.

Toilet bowl cleaner and deodorizer

Many toilet bowl cleaners are highly caustic and form toxic gases when mixed with water. They can contain ammonium chloride, 1,4-dichlorobenzine, hydrochloric acid, and sodium dichloroisocyanurate dehydrate. Sulfate-based products containing sodium sulfate or sodium bisulfate may cause asthmatic attacks. Try one of the following:

- Pour a can of Coke in the toilet bowl and let it sit overnight.
- To remove mineral buildup, put one or two denture cleaner tablets in the toilet bowl and let sit overnight.

Upholstery cleaner

Upholstery cleaners may contain similar products to dry-cleaning solutions. They may contain perchloroethylene, a known carcinogen and central nervous system toxicant, and naphthalene, a suspected carcinogen considered "toxic by inhalation." They may also contain ethanol, ammonia, and detergents. Aerosol products should especially be avoided. To clean upholstery, use a steam cleaner with water or a less-toxic cleaner (see sources).

DISPOSAL OF TOXIC HOUSEHOLD CLEANERS

Many communities offer options for safely disposing of toxic cleaning products, known also as household hazardous waste. Check with your local environmental, health, or solid waste agency for information. Whatever you do, don't pour unwanted household chemicals down the drain or toss them in the trash—they'll end up coming back to you one way or another.

SOURCES (in the order they appear in the chapter):

Borax: http://www.soapgoods.com/Borax-Granular-p-592.html

Microfiber cloths:
http://www.amazingcloth.com/
http://www.bluewondercloth.com/
http://www.norwex.ca/

Dr. Bronner's castile soap:
http://www.drbronner.com/

Cleaning agents:
Ecover: safe, eco-friendly cleaners available from American Environmental Health Foundation (AEHF). 1-800-428-2343 for a free catalogue.

Earth Friendly: safe, eco-friendly cleaners also available from AEHF.

Heartland Natural Cleaning Solutions: www.heartlandnatural.com

Seventh Generation: safe, eco-friendly cleaners available at many health food stores

Nature Clean: numerous safe, eco-friendly cleaners available online at: http://www.naturecleanliving.com/ and also from AEHF

Organica: Drain opener, available from AEHF

Dryerballs:
http://www.nurtured.ca/ —click the tab for diapers

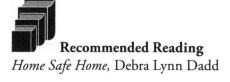 **Recommended Reading**
Home Safe Home, Debra Lynn Dadd

Chapter 7

PERSONAL CARE PRODUCTS

✦

A close-up look at cosmetics
and personal care products

Cleanliness may be next to godliness, but what if the process slowly kills you? The products we apply to our bodies on a daily basis contain hundreds of chemicals. A 2004 survey found that an average person in the United States uses nine different personal care products every day—introducing about 126 different chemicals into their body.[177] Applying products such as lotions, deodorants, moisturizers, fragrances, lipstick, and shampoos is really the same thing as ingesting these products through your skin. They are carried to your bloodstream even though they do not go through the digestive system. A certain way to expose yourself to hundreds of toxins over your lifetime is to use mainstream personal care products.

Many of the chemicals in personal care products are synthetic petrochemicals. They serve as solvents, plasticizers, preservatives, antimicrobials, dyes, and bonding agents. Because they are not natural, the body has no designated pathway for their elimination. No matter how small the amount, many of these chemicals are toxic; many mimic hormones in tiny amounts, and many accumulate with daily use. Recent efforts by consumer groups and many agencies in Europe have shed more light on what has been a hidden source of toxic exposure for many years. This research is just beginning, but the initial consensus is that the personal care and cosmetics industries are in need of a huge makeover.[178]

A study carried out in the Netherlands revealed alarming levels of chemicals commonly found in personal care products were found in baby's umbilical cords. The study discovered that a variety of chemicals used in everyday cosmetics, ranging from toothpaste to deodorants, can enter unborn babies' bodies through the umbilical cord.[179] In 2000, a group of

U.S. researchers connected with the Environmental Working Group began the quest to discover the hidden ingredients (those not required to be listed on the label) in cosmetics. The quest led them inside the offices of some of the largest U.S. cosmetics companies. Within these corporations, decisions were being made to keep the public unaware of the dangerous chemicals used in a vast array of cosmetics and personal care products. The book *Not Just a Pretty Face* chronicles the efforts of these researchers to uncover the truth. Three discoveries topped the list of their findings:

1. The cosmetics industry has known for more than twenty-five years that many of the chemicals used in personal care products cause cancer, birth defects, and reproductive damage.[180]
2. The cosmetics industry is the least regulated of all the FDA-regulated industries.
3. The cosmetics industry is allowed the freedom to make recommendations to the FDA, telling them what is safe and what is not.

As a result of their research, a huge database was compiled and cross-referenced with four similar databases. It is available at http://safecosmetics.org/ and provides information on more than fifteen thousand personal care products. The interactive Web site is capable of generating a toxic-index report on any product for which it is given the ingredients. By simply entering the ingredients, a person can get a rough idea of how their personal products rate—including which chemicals are toxic. The creators of the Web site admit it is not foolproof. However, it *does* provide the average consumer with a good idea of the safety of the products they use. It can also direct consumers to better options. The Web site includes a listing of the companies who have signed the Safe Cosmetics Compact—a commitment to work toward the use of nontoxic ingredients.

For the consumer who is attempting to decipher the myriad of chemicals on a label, the task can be indomitable. Some chemicals can have as many as five or six different chemical names. Even more problematic is the fact that many chemicals are not required to be listed on the label. The term *nontoxic* can mean that less than half of the laboratory animals died within two weeks when exposed during laboratory trials. The term *hypoallergenic* only minimizes the occurrence of well-known allergens. And especially in this industry, the word *natural* is meaningless. The term is entirely unregulated.

This chapter outlines the common toxic chemicals in personal care products and then provides guidelines for choosing safe personal care products in each major category.

COMMON TOXIC CHEMICALS IN PERSONAL CARE PRODUCTS

In 2004, the European Union implemented a ban on more than twelve hundred toxic chemicals in personal care products. A similar ban was proposed and initially defeated in the state of California. In 2005, high school students rallied, joining the Breast Cancer Fund and other activist groups against the $35 billion cosmetics industry—and this time they won. The California Safe Cosmetics Act went into effect January 1, 2007, requiring cosmetic companies to disclose chemicals containing ingredients linked to cancer or birth defects. It's the strongest law in the United States, and at the printing of this book, California is the only state with this kind of legislation protecting its consumers. Unfortunately, California's victory may be short lived. Legislature now pending, threatens to give federal law the right to overrule state mandates. It is time that more citizens got involved in campaigns to reform the laws that will protect them from toxins in personal care products.

Until further laws are passed, there are thousands of chemicals used in the personal products industry—and more are created every year. The few that are listed below represent some of the most frequently used and some of the most harmful. Being able to recognize these at a glance will enhance your ability to weed out the most suspicious products. Purchasing products from companies with a known commitment to safety will also simplify your search.

Ammonium laureth sulfate—Ammonium laureth sulfate is used as a foaming ingredient. It is less irritating than sodium lauryl sulfate (see sodium lauryl sulfate) but it is manufactured by a process known as ethoxylation, which can leave it contaminated with cancer-causing 1,4-dioxane. (Avoid ingredients that may be contaminated with 1,4-dioxane unless a process called vacuum stripping has been used. This process does not leave the end product contaminated with 1,4-dioxane.) Ammonium laureth sulfate and its chemical cousins (sodium laureth sulfate and sodium lauryl sulfate) are used in many shampoos, body washes, and toothpastes.

Benzene—Benzene (and its derivatives, naphthalene, aniline, phenol, and hydroquinone) are solvents used in nail polish remover and in the manufacture of many cosmetics, personal lubricants, dyes, and waxes. Benzene is a bone marrow poison banned in 1978 as a household solvent. It may end up in cosmetics in a number of ways. It may be used in the distillation or extraction process, or it may be contained in over-the-counter preparations labeled as drugs. As drugs, some preparations that fight such conditions as tooth decay or dandruff are not required to reveal proprietary ingredients—benzene could be one of these.

 (see Chapter 14: Gasoline pollutants)

Benzophenone family—The benzophenone family is identified by the name benzophenone followed by numbers 1 through 12. They are used as ultraviolet (UV) light absorbers in sunscreens, moisturizers, and conditioners. They can trigger itching, burning, scaling, and blistering skin.

BHA & BHT—Butylated hydroxyanisole (BHA) is used as a preservative in a variety of products. This chemical and its cousin, BHT, have been nicknamed *gender benders* because they mimic the female hormone estrogen. They are thought to be partly responsible for the decrease in male fertility and for the rise in testicular cancer observed since the 1950s. BHA can also trigger allergenic skin responses.

Centrimonium chloride—Centrimonium chloride is used as a preservative in some conditioners. It can trigger allergic skin reactions.

Ceteareth family—The ceteareth family of chemicals are identified by the name ceteareth followed by a number. There are numerous ceteareths; the most common are ceteareths 12, 20, and 30. They are used as emulsifiers and as thickening agents contained in deodorant, conditioner, lotion, cleanser, body wash, and shampoo. Ceteareth chemicals are penetration enhancers. They alter the skin's structure, allowing other chemicals to penetrate deeper into the skin. They also increase the amount of other chemicals that reach the bloodstream. Ceteareth compounds are manufactured by the ethoxylation process, which may leave them contaminated with trace amounts of 1,4-dioxane.

Cocoamidopropyl betaine—Cocoamidoproyl betaine is a foaming agent. It is a popular alternative to sodium lauryl sulfate, but it can break down when applied to the skin or react with other ingredients to form cancer-causing nitrosamine chemicals. It is found in shampoos and body wash and may cause contact dermatitis and allergies.

Cocoamide DEA & Lauramide DEA—Cocoamide and Lauramide DEA are used as foaming agents and to help keep water and oil from separating. Cocoamide DEA can break down on the skin or react with other ingredients to form cancer-causing nitrosamines. There is limited evidence suggesting that this chemical causes cancer in humans. It is found in shampoos and body wash and is manufactured by the process called ethoxylation, which may leave it contaminated with trace amounts of the cancer-causing 1,4-dioxane. Cocoamide DEA can trigger allergenic skin responses.

Colorings—Artificial colorings (made from coal tar and petroleum sources) must be certified. Certified colors are listed on labels as FD&C or D&C. The letters F, D, and C stand for food, drugs, and cosmetics, indicating their approved uses. Artificial food colorings may contain heavy metals such as lead and mercury.[181]

DEA (see triethanolamine—TEA)

Diazolidinyl and Imidazolidinyl urea—Diazolidinyl urea and imidazolidinyl urea are used as preservatives. They slowly release formaldehyde—a known carcinogen. These compounds are found in lotion, shampoo, conditioner, and body wash. They are toxic to the liver and kidneys and they can trigger an immune response that includes itching, burning, scaling, hives, or blistering skin.

Dibutyl phthalate—Dibutyl phthalate is one of the most often used phthalates. It is used in the making of plastic and is also a common ingredient in many personal care products. Dibutyl phthalate has been banned in Europe but not in the United States—though you will rarely see it listed on an ingredient label. The terms fragrance and parfum are often an indicator of the presence of dibutyl phthalate. Dibutyl phthalate is toxic to the liver and kidneys. It mimics the hormone estrogen and has been linked with reproductive and developmental problems. It can also trigger skin allergies.

 (see Chapter 5: Phthalates)

Dioxane (1,4-dioxane)—The chemical 1,4-dioxane will not appear on any label—it is not intentionally added to products. Rather, it is a by-product of a process called ethoxylation used to soften harsh detergents. Formed when foaming agents or surfactants are processed with ethylene oxide, 1,4-dioxane is classified by the EPA as a Group B2, probable human carcinogen. It is readily absorbed through the skin and lungs. Even as a trace contaminant, it is cause for concern.[182] Avoid ingredients that may be contaminated with 1,4-dioxane unless a process called vacuum stripping has been used. This process is much more effective at removing it and the end products are less likely to be contaminated.

Disodium EDTA—Disodium EDTA is used to remove cloudiness from clear liquids. It is found in shampoo and body wash. Disodium EDTA is a penetration enhancer that alters the skin's structure, allowing other chemicals to penetrate deeper into the skin and increasing the amounts of other chemicals that reach the bloodstream.

DMDM hydantoin—DMDM hydantoin is used as a preservative in lotion, shampoo, conditioner, and body wash. It can cause contact dermatitis and it may be contaminated with cancer-causing residues.

Formaldehyde—Formaldehyde is contained in many shampoos and body washes, although you will rarely see it listed on any personal care product label. Its disclosure is not required. Formaldehyde is a highly reactive chemical that combines with protein and can cause skin irritation and allergic contact dermatitis. The most widely reported symptoms from exposure to formaldehyde include headaches and irritation of the eyes. Until recently, the most serious of the diseases attributed to formaldehyde was asthma. However, recent research reports that formaldehyde is strongly suspected of causing cancer and birth defects.[183]

 (see Chapter 1: Formaldehyde)

Fragrance—The term fragrance on a label indicates the possible presence of up to five thousand different ingredients. A typical shampoo fragrance is created by mixing up to a hundred of these chemicals together. Many compounds included under the term fragrance are human toxins and are suspected or proven carcinogens. Symptoms reported to the FDA from fragrance exposure have included headaches, dizziness, rashes, skin discoloration, violent coughing and vomiting, and allergic skin irritation. Clinical observations have shown that exposure to fragrances can affect the central nervous system, causing depression, hyperactivity, irritability, inability to cope with stress, and other behavioral changes. You can avoid these chemicals by choosing products fragranced with pure essential oils.

Glycolic acid and alpha hydroxy acid (AHAs)—Glycolic acid is one of several acids known as AHAs that are used to exfoliate the skin. They are used in lotions, scrubs, and masks. As penetration enhancers, they alter the skin's structure, allowing other chemicals to penetrate deeper into the skin. AHAs are also photosensitizers, with the potential to increase the risk of sunburn and skin cancer by intensifying ultraviolet (UV) exposure. AHAs are toxic to the liver and kidneys and can trigger allergic responses: itching, burning, or blistering skin.

Hydroquinone—Hydroquinone is a skin-bleaching chemical used in many creams to reduce age spots and to lighten the color of the skin. In the United States, when used as an active ingredient, it must be listed as hydroquinone, but it may also carry these other names when it is not being used as an active ingredient: 1,4-benzenediol; 1,4-dihydroxybenzene; P-dioxybenzene; 4-hydroxyphenol; P-hydroxypnenol; or 1,4benzenediol. Hydroquinone can cause a skin disease called ochronosis, with irreversible blue-black lesions on the skin. It has also been linked to developmental and reproductive problems and is not permitted for use in cosmetics in some countries.

Imidazolidinyl urea (see Diazolidinyl urea)

Iodopropynyl butylcarbamate—Iodopropynyl butylcarbamate is used as a preservative. It is included in baby wipes, makeup, and lotion. Iodopropynyl butylcarbamate is thought to cause reproduction and developmental problems; it is linked to reduced fertility and to the reduced chance for a healthy, full-term pregnancy.

Methylchloroisothiazolinone   AND   Methylisothiazolinone—These chemicals are used as preservatives and as antimicrobial agents. They can be found in a wide range of products and can trigger allergic responses that include itching, burning, and blistering skin. They can also trigger asthma or other lung problems.

Methylene chloride—This chemical, used in nail enamel, aftershave, perfume, and cleansing cream, may cause liver and kidney damage, central nervous system disorders, headaches, and insomnia. In 1998 it was determined to be safe only for cosmetics that were intended for brief use.

Paraben family—This family of chemicals includes methyl paraben, ethyl paraben, propyl paraben, butyl paraben, and isobutyl paraben. They are used as preservatives and are included in a wide range of products. These chemicals have been included under the nickname gender benders because they mimic the female hormone estrogen and are thought to be partly responsible for the decrease in male fertility and rise in testicular cancer observed since the 1950s. Grape seed extract and rosemary extract are natural alternatives to the paraben preservatives.

Parfum (see fragrance)

Petrolatum—Petrolatum may have many names (mineral oil, petroleum jelly, paraffin oil, liquidum paraffinum, and Vaseline). Found in numerous products, it has been linked with acne and clogged pores, and reduces the ability of the skin to naturally detoxify.

PEG-family—PEG stands for polyethylene glycol. The PEG family of chemicals are identified by the name PEG followed by a number. PEGs are used to help stop water and oil from separating. They are manufactured by the process called ethoxylation which may leave them contaminated with trace amounts of 1,4-dioxane.

Phenol (carbolic acid)—Phenol is a derivative of benzene (see above), otherwise known as carbolic acid, benzophenol, and hydroxybenzene. It is found in skin creams and lotions. It is often one of the major ingredients in chemical skin peels. It penetrates the skin rapidly and has a strong corrosive effect on body tissue. Phenol can permanently lighten the skin and it can affect the skin's ability to produce pigment. It can affect the central nervous system and cause damage to the liver, kidneys, and heart. It is also a mutagen, and there is some evidence that phenol may be a reproductive hazard. Safety information for phenol advises no skin contact,[184] yet it is deliberately used to help ingredients penetrate the skin.

Polysorbate family—The polysorbate family of chemicals is identified by the name polysorbate followed by a number. These chemicals are used to help keep water and oil from separating in a wide variety of personal care products. They are manufactured by the process called ethoxylation, which may leave them contaminated with trace amounts of 1,4-dioxane. Polysorbate chemicals can trigger itching, burning, scaling, hives, and blistering skin.

Propylene glycol—Propylene glycol belongs to a family of chemicals used to help dissolve other ingredients. Lotion, shampoo, conditioner, body wash, and baby wipes may contain propylene glycol. Related chemicals include hexylene glycol and butylene glycol. These chemicals can cause contact dermatitis, irritation to eyes, skin, and mucous membranes.

Quaternium family—The quaternium family of chemicals is identified by the name quaternium followed by a number. The quaternium chemicals are used as preservatives (antimicrobials), found in lotion, shampoo, conditioner, aftershave, mouthwash, and body wash. These chemicals are potentially contaminated with cancer-causing impurities. Quaternium chemicals can trigger allergic skin responses as well as eye, nose, and throat irritations.

Benzalkonium chloride is another name for one of the most common of the quaternium compounds (quaternium 15). This compound releases formaldehyde and may cause muscular paralysis, low blood pressure, and central nervous system damage.

Sodium laureth sulfate—Sodium laureth sulfate is a foaming agent that is slightly less irritating than sodium lauryl sulfate. However, it is manufactured by the process called ethoxylation that may leave it contaminated with trace amounts of 1,4-dioxane. This chemical is found in shampoo and body washes.

Sodium lauryl sulfate—The popularity of sodium lauryl sulfate has decreased in recent years because of its harshness. It strips the skin's natural oils and can destroy eye and skin protein. It is used as a foaming ingredient and emulsifier in shampoo and body wash and is a known skin irritant. It also enhances the allergic response to other toxins and allergens and can react with other ingredients to form cancer-causing nitrosamines.

Sodium olefin sulfonate—Sodium olefin sulfonate is a foaming ingredient often used as a replacement for sodium lauryl sulfate. However, tests have shown it may be even more irritating. It is found in shampoo and body wash and can cause contact dermatitis, skin and eye irritation, and dry skin.

Styrene—Styrene is a solvent used in the manufacture of cosmetics. It is added directly to liquid eyeliners and perfumes but will rarely be disclosed on the label. It may cause eye and mucus membrane irritation, headaches, dizziness, and nerve damage.

Triclosan—Triclosan (and Triclocarban) is used as a preservative, antibiotic, and deodorizing agent. It can be found in deodorant, antibacterial soap, and toothpaste. Triclosan is a hormone disrupter in tiny amounts and has been restricted in cosmetics in Canada and Japan. It is a suspected thyroid hormone disruptor and it has also been shown to cause allergic skin responses. Triclosan is a derivative of the herbicide 2,4-D. It reacts with chlorine in tap water to form chloroform and dioxin—both suspected carcinogens.

Toluene—Toluene is a solvent used in nail polish, nail hardeners, dyes, perfumes, and other cosmetics. It will rarely be found on the ingredient label even though it may constitute over half of the volume of the product. It is a known cause of liver, kidney, and brain damage as well as damage to a developing fetus. Toluene may cause neurotoxicity and muscular incoordination, hearing loss, dizziness, and emotional instability.

Triethanolamine (TEA)—TEA (also diethanolamine, DEA and monoethanolamine, MEA) is used to control pH and to enhance foaming. It can break down when applied to the skin or react with other ingredients to form cancer-causing nitrosamine chemicals. TEA, DEA, and MEA are found in lotion, shampoo, conditioner, shaving gel, and body wash. They can cause facial dermatitis and contact dermatitis and are suspected carcinogens.

CHOOSING PERSONAL CARE PRODUCTS

Since everything you put *on* your body makes its way *into* your body, it is wise to choose products made of plant-based ingredients rather than the petroleum-based ingredients in most products. There are many companies now making good botanical products. Look for those with the most natural ingredients. Some are listed in the sources section at the end of the chapter. You will discover your own favorites.

DENTAL HYGIENE

Many of the personal care products you use on a daily basis are intended to be used directly in your mouth. The fact that they may contain poisonous and even carcinogenic ingredients is intolerable.

Toothpaste

Why would you want to brush your teeth after every meal with a product that carried the following warning?

> *If more than used for brushing is accidentally swallowed, get medical help or contact a Poison Control Center right away.*

Since 1997, the above warning has been mandatory on toothpaste containing fluoride. If fluoride is so safe—safe enough to put in our water and safe enough to use in toothpaste several times a day—why the warning? The obvious answer is that it is *not* safe!

Over forty articles can be found in the National Medical Library on the toxicity of fluoride. Half of the articles indicate that fluoride promotes cancer. A report in 2000 by the Greater Boston Physicians for Social Responsibility reviewed studies showing that fluoride interferes with brain function in young animals and children, reducing IQ with increasing exposure.[185] Fluoride is a known neurotoxin, also recognized to cause bone and teeth deformities. It can be partially responsible for weakened bones and greater numbers of bone fractures for the elderly. The toxicity of fluoride has caused many countries to rethink the use of fluoride in toothpaste; many have banned its use in water. In the United States it continues to be standard fare.

Also included on many toothpaste labels are statements of endorsement by the American Dental Association, indicating that fluoride prevents cavities. This claim has been refuted for those who are willing to push past the political hype. Not only does fluoride *not* prevent cavities, but when you get too much fluoride, your teeth can become discolored and crumble. Dental fluorosis, a mottling and deterioration of the tooth enamel, occurred in 10 percent of children's teeth in 1940. Today, it occurs at a rate as high as 55 percent.

Fluoride is most commonly listed on toothpaste labels as sodium fluoride, but it can also carry other names: phosphorofluoridic acid-sodium salt, sodium phosphorofluoridate, sodium salt phosphorofluoridic acid, and fluoride ion. Look for toothpaste without fluoride, and you will most likely find brands that are also without other harmful ingredients like Triclosan, PEG compounds, saccharin, aspartame, artificial flavors, and artificial colors (see sources).

Mouthwash

Conventional mouthwashes contain a number of ingredients that can be harmful or fatal if swallowed. They usually contain ethyl alcohol—up to 30 percent. Alcohol is used as a disinfectant, as a preservative, and as a solvent in which other additives (bactericides, colorings, flavorings) can be dissolved. Alcohol is drying; it changes the pH of the mouth and it strips away the protective mucous membrane in the mouth and throat.

> **The same germ killers used in bathroom cleaning disinfectants (phenol, cresol, and ethanol), are often used in mouthwash. Mouthwash also commonly contains formaldehyde. Many mouthwashes list a 1-800 number to a poison control facility in case of swallowing—a good clue to the toxicity of the ingredients.**

There are many other ways to combat oral bacteria and bad breath. Harsh mouthwashes represent a quick medicinal fix that cannot resolve a potentially deeper problem. Bad breath is often related to a toxic bowel, but it can also result from tooth or gum disease. Chlorophyll-rich herbs such as parsley, basil, and cilantro can be helpful to detoxify the bowel. If bad breath persists, look for the deeper cause. Make your own mouthwash with a drop of peppermint oil in a cup of water.

 (see Chapter 12: Gingivitis and periodontal disease)

Breath spray

Most breath sprays contain alcohol and isobutane (camp stove and cigarette lighter fuel) used as a propellant. As with the regular use of alcohol-containing mouthwash, the frequent use of breath spray damages the mucus membranes in the mouth and throat. As mentioned above, there are other, more effective ways to combat bad breath. Aside from making your own mouthwash, chewing fennel seeds, coriander seeds, or anise will mask odors after a meal and have a mild antimicrobial effect. Peppermint and bergamot tea may also be helpful.

HAND AND BODY PRODUCTS

The skin is the largest organ of the body. Not only is it responsible for protecting the inner organs, it is also partially responsible for detoxification. To help maintain the health of the skin, most people need extra omega-3 fatty acids from fish oil in their diet. Products for the skin should contain natural oils and plant-based ingredients rather than synthetic petrochemicals. Look for nourishing ingredients like aloe vera, coconut oil, palm oil, avocado oil, jojoba oil, and others.

The skin also needs to breathe. In order to do this, it must be kept clean without stripping the moisture-retaining oils that keep it supple. Three things to remember when caring for your skin:

1. Use warm (not hot) water and limit bath/shower time. Hot water and long showers or baths remove the natural oils from your skin.
2. Avoid strong soaps and detergents. Strong soaps are intended to remove grease and oil. They strip oil from your skin and can leave it dry and flaky. Instead, choose mild soaps with added natural oils.
3. Avoid additives and perfumes (fragrances) or dyes. These can irritate your skin and may trigger allergic responses.

Antibacterial soap

Most antibacterial soaps and hand sanitizers contain triclosan, which reacts with chlorine in tap water to form chloroform and dioxin. Because of their potential to cause antibiotic resistance, the FDA as well as the American Medical Association has expressed concern with the overuse of antibacterial soaps. Unless your profession dictates the use of antibacterial soap, avoid it. Natural soaps do a great job of cleansing the skin (see sources).

Deodorant soap

Deodorant soaps should be avoided. They work by killing the bacteria that cause body odor, but they use bactericides (antibiotics) to do the job. Triclosan and Triclocarban are typically included. The FDA warns against using deodorant soaps on infants under six months old. Better hand soaps and body lotions are listed in the sources section at the end of the chapter.

Deodorant

Deodorant has been the subject of much discussion due to the aluminum in antiperspirants and due to the preservatives, solvents, and fragrances that easily enter the body through sensitive underarm tissue. Researchers have found an association between aluminum-containing deodorant and Alzheimer's disease.

Although aluminum is poorly absorbed through the stomach, exposure to aluminum through the skin appears to be a different matter. In a 1990 study, researchers found that the overall risk of Alzheimer's disease was 60 percent greater among people using aluminum-containing antiperspirants. They also found a trend toward higher risk with increasing frequency of use.[186] Aluminum is a neurotoxin. Since exposure through the skin may be even more damaging than exposure from food, the use of aluminum-based deodorants is a significant health concern.

> **In a 1990 study, researchers found that the overall risk of Alzheimer's disease was 60 percent greater among people using aluminum-containing antiperspirants.**

The use of deodorant poses other problems. It contains preservatives known as parabens. Parabens mimic the hormone estrogen, which is known to play a role in the development of breast cancer. Scientists believe that deodorant could be responsible (at least in part) for the increase in breast cancer. This is based on the fact that women are now eight times more likely to develop breast cancer in the area of the breast closest to the underarm. Scientists in the UK analyzed twenty breast tumors and found high concentrations of para-hydroxybenzoic acids (parabens) in eighteen samples. According to researcher Phillipa Darbre, the ester-bearing form of parabens found in the tumors indicates it came from something applied to the skin, such as an underarm deodorant, cream, or body spray. Darbre said:

> *One would expect tumors to occur evenly, with 20 percent arising in each of the five areas of the breast. But these results help explain why up to 60 percent of all breast tumors are found*

in just one-fifth of the breast—the upper-outer quadrant, nearest the underarm.[187]

Since this study, many deodorants have replaced parabens with other preservatives.

 (see Chapter 7: Paraben family)

Most deodorants mask body odor with a perfumed scent; they may contain alcohol or aluminum to stop wetness. These compounds physically block or clog pores to reduce the flow of perspiration. In essence, they inhibit the body's natural release of toxins. By contrast, there are many crystal deodorants that eliminate odor-causing bacteria and therefore prevent body odor. These crystals have been used in Asia for centuries to provide protection naturally. Crystal deodorants last a long time; they don't clog pores or leave stains, and they are free from aluminum and parabens (see sources).

Exfoliants

Some of the most popular skin care products on the market today are exfoliants, commonly referred to as *skin peels*. Exfoliants are intended to remove the top layer of the skin, including dead skin and oily debris that can cause blemishes and blackheads. However, most products are acidic and can cause a variety of side effects, including increased vulnerability to the harmful effects of the sun.

In 1992, the FDA issued a consumer warning that skin peels could destroy the upper layers of the skin, causing burns, swelling, and pain. In this warning, the FDA described the effects as follows: *The skin initially reddens, as with a sunburn, then darkens and finally peels away revealing what manufacturers claim will be "new skin."* Since this initial warning, the FDA has studied the safety of alpha hydroxyl acids (AHAs) and beta hydroxy acids (BHAs). Their studies identified a doubling of UV damage to skin for people using AHA-containing products.[188] The FDA's fourteen-year review of AHAs culminated in the establishment of the need for product warnings. Unfortunately, warnings are voluntary and go unheeded by most manufacturers.

Most chemical skin peels include either alpha or beta hydroxy acid (AHA or BHA). AHA is an umbrella term for a variety of acids used in skin peels. While AHAs are water-soluble, BHAs are lipid-(oil) soluble. This allows them to penetrate the oil in the pores and exfoliate accumulated debris that can clog pores. BHAs are considered safer than AHAs but neither should be used in a concentration that exceeds 10 percent. Much higher concentrations are routinely used in salons and spas. If you choose to use these products, be aware that sun protection is important for up to a week following their use.

Another way to exfoliate the skin is referred to as microdermabrasion. This treatment typically uses tiny beads as an abrasive. Beads are often made of aluminum oxide or of plastic—neither is recommended. Aluminum is easily absorbed through the skin. The possible side-effects from the use of plastic as an abrasive are also undesirable.

Originally, natural abrasives such as apricot pits, almonds, corn cob, bamboo, and pumice were used to gently scrub the dead skin and oily build-up from the skin. More recently botanical enzymes such as pineapple enzyme and lavender enzyme have been used with success. Look for these more natural ingredients in products meant to exfoliate the skin (see sources).

An excellent exfoliant and a wonderful treatment for teenagers who struggle with oily skin and blackheads is Alexandria's Professional Body Sugaring treatment. This treatment was designed for hair removal, but it is also extremely effective as a natural, safe, painless exfoliant. It removes many blackheads and the oily build-up responsible, in part, for teenage acne. Regular professional body sugaring is one of the most effective, natural exfoliants available. It can even help with many skin conditions, including eczema and psoriasis (see sources).

Hair removal products

Hair removal includes a wide range of products and services that consist of depilatories, hair inhibitors, electrolysis, laser treatments, waxing, and the latest—sugaring. Hair removal creams (depilatories), dissolve the hair at the skin's surface. Many use harsh chemicals that are absorbed through the skin or that can cause irritation. However, there are a few more natural depilatories that use sugar or glucose and fructose, honey, and natural citrus extracts (see sources).

Hair inhibitors work by damaging the hair follicle, forcing hair to grow back thinner and lighter in color. Many of these also contain harsh chemicals and should not be used. Electrolysis uses a needle to penetrate each individual hair shaft, delivering tiny bursts of electricity to destroy hair follicles. The procedure is performed in a salon and requires multiple visits. Because the procedure uses needles, infections sometimes result. Hair removal lasers create a beam of high-intensity light that penetrates deep into skin tissue. The light delivers a controlled amount of heat which destroys the hair follicle. This procedure is also performed in a salon. The treated area may become red, lasting from a few hours to several days (an indication of skin damage), and subjects must avoid the sun for four to six weeks in preparation for the treatment.

Waxing has become very popular because it is quick and simple—although it is often painful and it can lead to infection. Waxing requires hair to be at least one-eighth of an inch long to be effective; this makes the process more of a superficial hair removal than a true hair extraction. Shorter hair and hair that is in an early stage of growth is not removed. Hair waxes are made of resins that also adhere to skin. When they are stripped away, they can cause bruising and skin damage.

Sugaring is an alternative to waxing and to other methods of hair removal. It has grown in popularity because of its ease, lack of harmful chemicals, and most importantly, because of its limited side effects. Heating sugar and water eventually forms a soft, caramel-like consistency that works similar to wax for the removal of hair, yet it is much gentler and safer. (Most people are unaware of sugar's natural antibacterial properties.) Sugaring pastes and gels are water soluble—they will not stick to anything moist like the skin, so hair can be pulled cleanly from the roots without bruising the surrounding area.

There are many sugaring products available for home and salon use, but the very best method of sugaring is performed professionally and is referred to as Alexandria's Professional Body Sugaring. This method allows a unique formula made with sugar, lemon juice, and a medley of herbs to penetrate into the skin follicle and to coat the hair on the inside of the follicle. The hair is eased out of the skin with a quick "flicking" action. Lubricating the hair eliminates relatively all discomfort. It also allows the removal of very short hairs in their earliest stages of growth. The process lasts much longer than most removal techniques, and it discourages the re-growth of hair. Cross-contamination and infection are eliminated as the paste (all natural and biodegradable) is discarded at the end of each procedure (see sources).

EYE CARE
Eye drops
Conventional eye drops that claim to whiten eyes contain chemicals that constrict blood vessels and reduce the blood supply to the eye. They may reduce redness, but they are not good for your eyes. Blood vessels bring oxygen to the optic nerve and to the rest of the eye. Restricting the blood supply restricts oxygen and nutrients. According to Marguerite McDonald, MD, clinical professor of ophthalmology at Tulane University Hospital & Clinic in New Orleans, eye drops can also be addictive. If you use them too often, you need more and more just to get the original results.[189]

Visine and Ocuclear are over-the-counter eye drops advertised to reduce redness and itching eyes. They contain an antihistamine drug called oxymetazoline ophthalmic. The warning on the package says:

Do not use oxymetazoline ophthalmic more often or continuously for longer than forty-eight to seventy-two hours without consulting a doctor. Chronic use of this medication may damage the blood vessels (veins and arteries) in the eyes.

Further warnings say:

Do not use oxymetazoline ophthalmic if you have glaucoma, except under the supervision of your doctor. Before using this medication, tell your doctor if you

- *have any type of heart condition, including high blood pressure;*
- *take any medicines to treat a heart condition;*
- *have asthma;*
- *have diabetes; or*
- *have thyroid problems.*

Murine and dozens of branded products, including Tears Plus and Eye-Sine, contain the active ingredient tetrahydrozoline hydrochloride, which is also an antihistamine that constricts blood vessels. Side effects include hypertension, heart palpitations, headache, tremors, and blurred vision. Most commercial eye drops also contain the preservative benzalkonium chloride, otherwise known as quaternium-15. Besides releasing formaldehyde, benzalkonium chloride will discolor contact lenses if they are not removed during use.

Oil is a normal part of tears. Without enough oil in your diet, tears evaporate too rapidly. Dry eye syndrome, experienced by many Americans, could be the lack of omega-3 oils in your diet. In a study of more than thirty-two thousand women, Harvard University researchers found that women eating few omega-3s were more likely to suffer from dry eye syndrome.[190] Consider taking 1000 to 3000 mg of fish oil daily. Look for brands that remove mercury and other heavy metals. If you have tired or red eyes, you might be better off using natural eye drops that combine sterile saline solutions with herbal or homeopathic remedies (see sources).

Contact lens solution

If you wear contact lenses, you are putting solutions in your eyes every day. Many of these contain preservatives and other chemicals that may not be healthy in the long run. Solutions for sensitive eyes usually have fewer chemicals and preservatives. Some individuals use commercial lens solutions for disinfection and then use a homemade solution for rinsing and placement of the lens in the eye. Debra Lynn Dadd, author of *Home Safe Home*, suggests a half teaspoon of Himalayan salt in slightly less than a cup of filtered water. (Let the undissolved minerals sink to the bottom and discard them.) Hulda Clark, author of *The Cure for All Diseases,* recommends this recipe for homemade contact lens soution:

Hulda Clark's Homemade Contact Lens Solution

A scant cup of cold water brought to a boil in a glass saucepan. After adding 1/4 tsp. aluminum-free salt and boiling again, pour into a sterile canning jar. Refrigerate or freeze.

SUN PROTECTION

Ultraviolet (UV) rays from the sun are divided into UVA, UVB, and UVC radiation. UVC radiation is filtered out by the atmosphere, leaving UVA and UVB rays that can cause skin damage by breaking chemical bonds in DNA, enzymes, and proteins. For years, the sunscreen industry has focused primarily on UVB, the light that causes the most immediate skin damage—sunburn. UVA rays, however, penetrate deeper into the skin, causing damage before any visible sunburn occurs. UVA radiation is increasingly being recognized as the *major* contributor to skin damage and aging. This shift in our understanding of UV-related skin damage brings to light the problem with many sunscreens: they shield the skin from UVB rays but leave users vulnerable to the potentially more problematic UVA damage.

The SPF (sun protection factor) test is designed to measure only the UVB protective effects of a sunscreen. In a recent survey of 878 name-brand sunscreens, a scientific review found evidence that one out of every eight high-SPF sunscreens did not protect from UVA radiation.[191] The FDA has no regulations about what degree of UVA protection a sunscreen must provide, so you may not know how much protection you are actually getting by reading the label.

Beyond being protected from the UV rays of the sun, there are other factors to consider when selecting a sunscreen—a product that may cover your entire body. Often the myriad of oils and pore-clogging ingredients can do more damage than exposure to the sun itself. Avoid products that contain the widely used ingredient called oxybenzone or benzophenone-3, which has been linked to allergies, hormone disruption, and cell damage.

In an investigation of nearly one thousand name-brand sunscreens, the Environmental Working Group found that four out of five sunscreen products either contained harmful ingredients or offered inadequate protection. Leading brands were the worst offenders. During their review of sunscreen products, the Environmental Working Group took a close look at the use of micronized minerals (especially titanium dioxide and zinc oxide), which are being incorporated in some of the newer sunscreen products. They found that these mineral powders provided excellent UVA protection. But even more importantly, repeated studies showed these products did not penetrate the skin or clog pores. [192] Micronized zinc oxide and titanium dioxide are the active ingredients in Colore Science's powder product called Sunforgettable (see sources).

It is a sad sight to see beaches and streams coated with sunscreen and tanning oil so thick that the aquatic life are literally suffocated.

Aquatic life is extremely sensitive to the synthetic petrochemicals contained in most commercial sun protection products. Micronized powders are also much friendlier to the environment.

INSECT REPELLANTS

With the concern over West Nile Virus, Lyme disease, and other insect-related illnesses, more people are using insect repellents. The most common choice is a DEET-based repellent shown to be the most effective. But DEET-based repellents aren't just hazardous to mosquitoes. DEET is short for N, N-diethyl-m-toluamide (also known as N,N-diethyl-3-methylbenzamide). It is a registered pesticide and a member of the toluene chemical family. DEET is absorbed through the skin and passes into the blood. The Medical Sciences Bulletin, published by Pharmaceutical Information Associates Ltd., reports that up to 56 percent of DEET applied topically penetrates intact human skin and 17 percent is absorbed into the bloodstream.[193] Blood concentrations of about three milligrams per liter have been reported several hours after DEET repellent was applied to skin in the prescribed fashion. DEET is also absorbed through the intestinal tract.

The most serious concerns about DEET are its effects on the central nervous system. Duke University studied muscle coordination in animals after using DEET. Those exposed to the equivalent of average human doses performed far worse than untreated animals. It was also found that combined exposure to DEET and permethrin (a pesticide routinely sprayed in mosquito abatement programs) can lead to motor deficits, learning, and memory dysfunction.[194] Products containing DEET are required to carry labels specifying the following restrictions:

- Do not apply over cuts, wounds, or irritated skin.
- Do not apply to hands or near eyes and mouth of young children.
- Do not allow young children to apply this product.

- After returning indoors, wash treated skin with soap and water.
- Do not use under clothing.
- Do not spray in enclosed areas.

Although DEET-based repellents have their place, they should only be used when the risk of insect-born infection is high. There are a number of effective, less toxic insect repellents available. They sometimes need to be applied more frequently, but they do not carry the same health risks. Citronella products provide about thirty to forty minutes of protection.[195] Bug shirts are excellent for camping and other excursions. They are made of lightweight, densely woven fabric with mesh face protection that allows air to penetrate without letting insects in. Wrist closures seal the sleeves, and a drawstring at the waist seals at the bottom edge. Many of these bug shirts fold into a zippered pocket and travel easily on a belt clip (see sources).

Many essential oils, like tea tree, geranium, citronella, cedar wood, and lemongrass, have bug-repelling properties. A product called Go Mosquito uses these and others in a spray formula to repel mosquitoes, ticks, and fleas. It can be sprayed on clothing or directly on skin. It also works for pets (see sources). BugOff also makes wristbands infused with safe insect-repelling oils. These offer good protection (see sources).

Mosquito coils for backyard protection produce smoke that contains about seventy different volatile organic compounds, including phenol, benzene, toluene, and xylene. Using yellow outdoor lightbulbs which do not attract insects can help reduce mosquito populations at night. Another option is to use a fan when there is little wind since mosquitoes are not strong flyers. Planting mosquito-repelling plants like lemon balm, catnip, basil, and lemon geraniums around outdoor sitting areas and encouraging mosquito predators like bats and dragonflies can help reduce mosquito populations as well.

Mosquitoes hate garlic. It contains natural sulfur, which repels many insects, including mosquitoes, ticks, fleas, and even black flies. One of the most effective home mosquito deterrents is liquid garlic. The odor chases them out of the area, and they stay away—for as long as they can detect the odor. Mosquito Barrier is a strong, liquid garlic made from a very powerful garlic variety, which is much more potent than the garlic found in stores. While the odor of sprayed garlic juice becomes undetectable to humans within minutes, the mosquitoes will detect it for weeks. Additionally, garlic juice, when mixed with soybean oil and water, creates a thin film that suffocates the mosquito larvae that are developing in any standing water. Garlic juice, unlike harmful chemicals, doesn't kill bees or butterflies and it is completely safe for children, fish, birds, dogs, cats, and other pets (see sources).

PERFUME

Smelling good shouldn't have to affect your health—but it often does. In 1999, the California Environmental Health Network filed a citizen petition asking for warning labels on all fragrances that are marketed without adequate safety testing. The petition was filed after two independent laboratories determined the presence of both toxic and carcinogenic ingredients in the popular perfume known as Eternity. Of the forty-one ingredients identified, toxicity data on most was either nonexistent or inadequate. Known toxins to the skin, mucous membranes, respiratory tract, reproductive system, and nervous system were identified. Two ingredients were known to cause cancer.

Eternity isn't the only offender. Most perfumes contain toxic ingredients that can cause a variety of allergic responses and respiratory troubles. Of the ingredients that have been tested, at least a quarter of the fragrance chemicals have been found to contain toxic substances. Using them day-in and day-out can have untold consequences. If you have persistent allergies; if you have a constantly stuffy nose; and if you experience regular headaches you could be suffering an allergic reaction to perfume or to the ingredients in your (or someone else's) personal care products. Essential oils and natural flower essences can be combined to make pleasant alternatives to the synthetic perfumes that dominate the market (see sources).

HAIR CARE

Hair is 90 percent protein and 10 percent water. A healthy diet rich in protein, water, and fresh fruits and vegetables will help keep hair looking healthy and shiny. With a proper diet and good care, a single hair can live four to five years. Several things to remember about caring for your hair:

1. Avoid excessive heat when blow drying and curling. Lower drying temperatures reduce hair breakage. Air dry your hair when possible.
2. Avoid harsh detergents that contain sodium lauryl sulfate, sodium laureth sulfate, ammonium laureth sulfate, and sodium olefin sulfonate.
3. Minimize the use of hairsprays and gels that contain alcohol. These products dry your hair.
4. Never brush your hair while it is wet. Wet hair breaks more easily.

Shampoo

Many shampoos contain formaldehyde, which is not required to be listed on the label. Dozens of other harsh chemicals are found in conventional shampoo and conditioner. Purchase hair care products from a growing list of manufacturers who produce safe products (see sources).

Dandruff shampoo

Dandruff shampoos are perhaps the most dangerous of all hair care products because they contain highly toxic medications to prevent the scalp from shedding skin. Antidandruff agents include recorcinol, which is rapidly absorbed by the skin and may cause inflammation, dizziness, restlessness, rapid heartbeat, and excessive sweating.

Dandruff is frequently due to digestive problems—especially yeast overgrowth. When yeast infections are cleared, dandruff often naturally resolves. If you have dandruff, you may want to try rinsing your hair in warm vinegar and wrapping your head in a towel for an hour before you wash your hair. Tea tree oil shampoo may also help (see sources). Selenium-based shampoos have also been effective because the selenium acts as an antifungal agent.[196] Sometimes dandruff is a short-term problem linked with hormone changes (especially for teenagers) and often diminishes on its own.

Hair spray and styling gels

Hair spray is essentially plastic dissolved in a solvent and put in a pressurized can or pump spray bottle. It works by gluing strands of hair together so they can form a stronger structure. And where there's plastic there are phthalates—hormone-disrupting chemicals used to keep plastics pliable.

 (see Chapter 5: Phthalates)

Breathing difficulties and contact dermatitis are common complaints from those who use hairspray. Other side effects include nail abnormalities. (When you spray and then style your hair with your fingers, the spray ends up on your fingernails. It can cause poor regrowth and infection.) Regular users of hair spray are also at risk of developing a lung disease called thesaurosis.[197] More than half the women afflicted with this disease recover within six months after discontinuing the use of hair spray. Allergic skin reactions, eye, and nasal irritation are also common reactions to exposure to hair spray and styling gel.

> **Common ingredients in hair spray and in styling gels include aerosol propellants, alcohol, carcinogenic polyvinylpyrolidone, formaldehyde, and artificial fragrances.**

As far as we are aware, there are no good hairsprays. If you must use spray, buy products with the fewest ingredients and use pump sprays rather than aerosols. As an alternative, aloe vera gel—worked into the hair while damp—may work well for some styles.

Hair dye

If you use permanent hair dye regularly, you should know about a 2001 study from the University of Southern California that analyzed the association between hair dying and bladder cancer. The concern is with a family of chemicals called arylamines—ingredients in many hair dyes that are a known risk factor for bladder cancer. What the study found:

- Women who use permanent hair dyes once a month for one year or longer have twice the risk of bladder cancer.
- Women who use permanent hair dyes for fifteen or more years at least monthly have three times the risk of bladder cancer.
- Those who have worked as hair dressers for ten years or more have five times the risk of bladder cancer.[198]

Further research showed that the use of dark colors doubled a person's risk of certain blood cancers. Women who used dark-colored permanent hair-coloring products for more than twenty-five years doubled their risk of non-Hodgkin's lymphoma. The risk was nearly the same for women who used more than two hundred applications of these products. No increased risk was seen in women who used semipermanent dyes or temporary rinses.[199] Permanent hair dyes change the natural pigment within your hair whereas semipermanent hair color has less structural impact and uses fewer, less harsh chemicals. In essence, semipermanent colors stain the hair, and they fade after six to eight shampoos. Dark colors (especially black) and some men's gray hair formulas may contain lead in the form of lead acetate.[200] These studies were enough of a concern that the European Commission changed their policy regarding ingredients in hair dyes. The United States still does not require manufacturers to file data on ingredients or report cosmetic-related injuries for these products.

Certified organic henna is a good alternative to commercial hair color. Henna utilizes a gentle and natural approach with no synthetic chemicals, no preservatives, and no harsh oxidizing chemicals. These pure vegetable products do not alter the structure or natural color of your hair and may actually condition your hair while imparting color and sheen (see sources).

If you are attempting to cover gray hair, consider that gray is caused by a lack of phenylalanine, an amino acid that, in combination with enzymes in the hair, creates the pigment called melanin, responsible for color in hair. Phenylalanine is found in nuts, meats, and eggs.

Hair regrowth formulas

There are many circumstances that can interrupt the normal hair growth rhythm. They produce a shock (stress) to the system. Common shocks include:

- Childbirth, pregnancy, and menopause (hormone imbalances)
- High fever
- Malnutrition as a result of crash dieting or long-term nutritional deficiencies
- Surgery
- Chemotherapy
- Long-term emotional stress

If shock is the reason for hair loss, it generally comes back when the stress subsides. However, if a stressful lifestyle is the cause of hair loss, hair may never return. This could also be the case when hair loss is due to nutritional deficiencies, ongoing illness, thyroid disorders, or immune dysfunction. According to the American Hair Loss Council, genetics accounts for 95 percent of all cases of hair loss in the United States.[201] This means that a person may experience hair loss beginning in their teens. When genetics are the cause, many people turn to hair regrowth formulas.

Minoxidil (Rogaine) is an over-the-counter liquid medication for the treatment of hair loss. The difficulty with formulas that contain minoxidil is that the quality of the new hair is usually poor (thin and weak) and if you stop, the hair you gained will fall out again. Once you begin, you are in it for the long term—and that may be the biggest problem. Extended use of minoxidil could cause changes in heart rate. This is not surprising since minoxidil was originally developed to treat high blood pressure. Other side effects include local itching, headaches (in 40 percent of users), dizzy spells, and lightheadedness. Unfortunately, it also takes six to eight months before you know whether minoxidil works for you. Another often recommended treatment is corticosteroid injections. Apart from the painful injections, this treatment has serious side effects.[202]

Traditional Chinese Medicine teaches that the condition of the hair is a direct reflection of the condition of the blood and the organs that are responsible for cleansing the blood (particularly the kidneys). In other words, the condition of the hair follicles may be affected by toxins in the body and blood. Some individuals have seen improvement by undergoing a detoxification program. As we have stated previously, there is no substitute for whole-food nutritional supplementation to compensate for a severe lack in most diets.

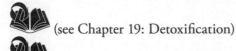 (see Chapter 19: Detoxification)

(see Chapter 4: Whole-food supplements)

Wigs

As one of the best alternatives to medications and surgery, even wigs and hair pieces can have drawbacks. When made of synthetic materials, they keep your scalp from breathing. Depending on the materials used, they may even contribute to the toxic load. This could be especially problematic for cancer patients following chemotherapy. Since the head perspires and releases wastes like the rest of the body, a good wig or hairpiece should provide adequate air circulation. Only one wig designer advertises human hair wigs made with nontoxic, breathable (see-through) materials (nylon, cotton, and silk) that allow adequate air circulation to the scalp. These hair pieces are created by a woman who lost her own hair as a young girl. After many treatments and many wigs she was guided to design her own (see sources).

Lie control

There are numerous methods recommended for lice control—everything from pesticides to mayonnaise. Manual removal of nits (eggs which are attached to the base of the hair) is crucial. Many shampoos (with and without pesticides) have been formulated to remove the nits but few are successful because they do not break down the cementlike adhesive that attaches the egg to the base of the hair. Eggs hatch about every seven to ten days.

Pesticides that are used for lice are lindane, malathion, and pyrethrin compounds. Despite the fact that the EPA says lindane products should be used as a last resort against head lice, more than one hundred sixty-six thousand prescriptions (10 percent of all prescriptions for head lice and scabies) were written from January to November 2007.[203] Lindane was banned as an agricultural insecticide in 2006. Its effects on the environment have been disastrous. The Los Angeles County Sanitation District calculated that a single head lice treatment could contaminate 6 million gallons of water—and cost an average of $4000 to remove from wastewater. Malathion is equally noxious, and pythrethrins have limited success.

A natural enzyme shampoo called Lice R Gone is being used with great success and is recommended by schools across the country. It contains no toxic ingredients, pesticides, or harmful irritants. It works by enzymatically breaking down the protein exoskeleton of the insect, killing the adult insect, and removing the nits—often in one application (see sources).

COSMETICS

The FDA does no systematic review for the safety of cosmetics before they are sold. A cosmetic manufacturer may use almost any raw material without approval from the FDA. This means that nearly 90 percent of ingredients used in cosmetic products have not been evaluated for safety. The Cosmetics Ingredients Review (CIR), the cosmetic industry's self-policing safety panel, ends up making safety recommendations to the FDA—which is like letting the fox guard the henhouse. In its thirty-year history, the CIR has reviewed the safety of 13 percent of the ten thousand five hundred ingredients used in personal care products. In 1997, Senator Edward Kennedy said this of the cosmetics industry: "The cosmetic industry has borrowed a page from the playbook of the tobacco industry by putting profits ahead of public health."[204]

Lipstick

Lead is known to brighten colors—that's why it was used in paint for many years. But while Congress still fights to stop lead paint on imported toys, many women unknowingly ingest it every day in their lipstick. Lead is not a contaminant in lipstick—it is not a by-product of other ingredients—it is purposefully added to help strengthen and brighten colors—especially the color red.

Rumors had circulated for some time that lipstick contained lead, but since lead is not required to be disclosed on the ingredient label, the only way to find out if it was there was to test. That's what the Environmental Working Group did in 2007. Thirty-three brand-name lipsticks were tested by an independent lab—twenty tested positive for lead with levels from 0.3 parts per million (ppm) to 0.65 ppm. (The safe upper limit is 0.1 ppm, established for lead in candy.)

Lead is a potent neurotoxin linked to numerous health and reproductive problems. It accumulates over time; long-term exposure can build up to toxic levels causing brain damage and learning disabilities. Because lipstick is applied to the lips and often reapplied several times during the day, the risk from lead in lipstick is more than significant.

> **Does your lipstick contain lead? Since there is no FDA requirement to report lead in lipstick, there is absolutely no way to know unless you have it tested.**

Lipsticks that also contain the following ingredients should be avoided: BHT, coal-tar dyes, colors with the word "lake" after them (they are derived from aluminum), FD&C colors, fragrances, and petroleum products. Purchase lipstick only from companies that have a strong commitment to safety (see sources).

Mascara

Mascara was created in 1913 by a chemist for his sister, Mabel. It was made from coal dust mixed with petroleum jelly. The product became a huge success and eventually a company was formed to market the product—Maybelline. The original mascara was available in cake form. Users would wet the cake with a brush, then apply. Today mascara may contain alcohol, formaldehyde, and various plastic resins. The primary danger is eye irritation, redness, burning, and swelling. There are numerous good brands (see sources),

Fingernail polish

There is no question that fingernail polish contains some of the most toxic ingredients in the cosmetics industry: phthalates, formaldehyde, toluene, acetone, resins, and methylacrylates—many are not required to be listed on the label.

A survey of nail technicians in Boston found considerable awareness that their occupation was affecting their health. Survey respondents reported work-related headaches, skin problems, and respiratory problems.[205] Occupational health studies show decreased attention and processing skills as well as increased asthma in nail salon workers. Women of childbearing age are particularly vulnerable because many of the offending chemicals in nail polish are hormone disruptors known to harm the developing fetus. If you use nail polish, apply it in a well-ventilated room. Only patronize salons that are well ventilated. Look for brands without toluene, formaldehyde, and phthalates (see sources).

FEMININE HYGIENE

Unfortunately, even feminine hygiene products can be a source of toxicity. These products are placed inside or next to some of the most delicate and absorbent tissues in the female body—they should be made of the cleanest and most sanitary ingredients, but often they are not. Both the materials and the manufacturing processes for these products are cause for concern.

Tampons and sanitary pads

Most manufacturers of tampons and sanitary pads use rayon and cotton fabric because of their absorbent properties. Both of these materials are bleached during manufacture—this is the first cause for concern. Chlorine-bleached products (including tampons, sanitary pads, cotton balls, facial wipes, paper towels, and facial tissues) contain traces of carcinogenic dioxins—some of the most dangerous chemicals in the environment. Dioxins are persistent and they accumulate. Even though a product may contain tiny amounts, they build up over time. Considering the fact that a woman may use as many as twelve thousand tampons during her forty-plus years of menstruation, tiny amounts become more than problematic. Swedish studies have shown a link between tampons containing dioxin and other chlorine by-products, and an increased risk of cancers of the female reproductive organs (especially the uterus, ovaries, and bladder). Although the FDA currently requires tampon manufacturers to monitor dioxin levels, the results are not available to the public. Tampon manufacturers are not required to disclose test results or ingredients to consumers, although many will do so voluntarily.

Rayon itself poses another risk. Unlike cotton, rayon encourages bacterial growth and causes excessive drying of vaginal tissues. The rayon used in feminine hygiene products is treated to increase absorbency. These super-absorbent fibers cause excessive drying by drawing normal secretions from vaginal tissues. Rayon fibers may also become imbedded in vaginal walls. Rayon fibers have been shown to amplify the production of the bacteria that causes toxic shock syndrome. Toxic shock syndrome is a rare bacterial illness that caused over fifty deaths between 1979 and 1980. It caused the recall of at least one brand of tampons.

Though cotton is a natural fiber, the majority of cotton crops grown today are heavily treated with pesticides. Switch to a nonchlorine-bleached, rayon-free, 100 percent–organic cotton product. Organic cotton tampons and pads are not only free of pesticides, but they are also bleached with hydrogen peroxide rather than chlorine bleach to make them safer in both ways (see sources). Many women now favor reusable natural sponges called Sea Pearls or menstrual cups (see sources).

Douches

Similar to the beneficial flora (good bacteria) in the intestinal tract, the healthy vagina also contains beneficial flora. Douching can change this delicate balance and make a woman more prone to vaginal infections. Research shows that women who douche regularly have more female health problems than those who do not. Most doctors and the American College of Obstetricians do not recommend douching. The following or similar warning must now appear on douche products:

> *An association has been reported between douching and pelvic inflammatory disease, ectopic pregnancy, tubal infertility, chlamydia, and bacterial vaginosis.*

Many douches contain the same harmful ingredients found in other personal care products. Here is the ingredient list from one widely used douche: Water (purified), Sodium Citrate, Citric Acid, SD Alcohol 40, Diazolidinyl Urea, Octoxynol 9, Fragrance, Cetyl Pyridinium Chloride, Edetate Disodium, FD&C Blue 1. Even the simplest douches (vinegar and water) will alter the natural balance in the vaginal lining and should be avoided.

> **The vagina cleans itself naturally by producing vaginal secretions. A mild odor is natural; an unusually offensive odor could be a sign of infection or of a more serious problem— douching may make the problem worse.**

Sexual lubricants

Sexual lubricants fall into one of four categories: petroleum based, oil based, water based, and silicone based. Considering what we know of petroleum products, any lubricant with mineral oil, Vaseline, petrolatum, or petroleum jelly should be avoided.

The use of water-based products or those with natural botanical oils is much safer, but watch for preservatives such as the commonly used parabens and pesticides which may be referred to as preservatives. K-Y Jelly has both (methylparaben and chlorhexidine gluconate—a bacteriocide, viricide, and fungicide).

 (see Chapter 7: Paraben family)

Also be aware of nonoxynol-9 (N-9), the active ingredient in spermacides. Studies show that N-9 may cause urinary tract infections as well as vaginal lesions that increase the risk of infections.

One of the best natural lubricants is organic virgin coconut oil. It is a gel-like semi-solid at room temperature and rapidly liquefies at body temperature. Coconut oil also has natural antiseptic properties because of the lauric acid it contains. Another excellent choice is a product called Climaxima. It is made with organic jojoba and essential oils. The product contains no synthetic or petroleum chemicals. It is tasteless, warming, stimulating, anti-infectious, and nonsticky (see sources).

WRINKLE TREATMENTS

The most obvious sign of aging is the formation of wrinkles on your skin. As you age, the collagen and elastin fibers which are intermingled with connective tissue undergo numerous changes that make your skin less resilient and more prone to wrinkles. Wrinkle treatments and antiaging creams have been around for centuries. Two of the largest factors in the aging of your skin are the sun's rays and the amount of water you drink. Hence, the simplest and most natural wrinkle treatments are hydration and moderation with regard to solar radiation. Some of the more recent wrinkle treatments may be cause for concern.

Botox

The popular antiwrinkle drug called Botox is a toxin produced by the bacteria that causes botulism—a type of food poisoning. Botulinum toxin, type A (Botox) and a similar product called Myobloc are nerve toxins. When they are injected into a muscle, they block signals that cause muscles to contract. In essence, the muscles are paralyzed. If they can't tighten, the skin flattens and appears smoother and less wrinkled. Although the treatment is very effective, the cosmetic effects of Botox are only temporary (three to six months); the process must be repeated to maintain the effects.

Studies have not been conducted to determine the long-term safety of Botox—especially when it must be used again and again. In an editorial in the *British Medical Journal,* Dr. Peter Misra, of the National Hospital for Neurology and Neurosurgery in London, said that the use of Botox was based on small-scale studies—that its very long term effects are still unknown.[206]

In February 2008, the FDA issued a warning for Botox-type drugs. In their statement, they revealed that they were investigating reports of illnesses in people of all ages who used the drugs for a variety of conditions. Their investigation included at least one hospitalization of a woman given Botox for forehead wrinkles and several deaths of children given the drug for muscle spasms. The FDA warned that the botulism toxin may spread throughout the body, resulting in respiratory paralysis. They stated that patients receiving Botox for any reason should be told to seek immediate care if they suffer symptoms of food poisoning, including difficulty swallowing or breathing, slurred speech, muscle weakness, or difficulty holding up their head.[207]

Acetyl hexapeptide-3

Acetyl hexapeptide-3, also called argireline, is another recent wrinkle treatment incorporated in a variety of antiaging creams. It is an artificially created peptide (a chain of six amino acids) that was developed by a company in Spain. It claims to be nontoxic but the mode of action is suspect. It works by reducing muscle contractions and by limiting the neurotransmitters that tell your facial muscles to move. In one trial of ten women volunteers, a 10 percent concentration for thirty days reduced the appearance of wrinkles by 30 percent. This limited testing is all that has been clinically performed to date.

Hyaluronic acid

Hyaluronic acid (HA) is a natural component of the skin that holds water and helps to prevent the cross-linking of collagen and elastin fibers as you age. HA helps keep skin smooth because of its ability to hold huge numbers of water molecules and because it has the ability to bring water into skin cells. HA levels gradually diminish over time as a part of the aging process. HA may not flatten wrinkles like the nerve toxin botulinum toxin type A, or the muscle contraction reducing ingredient acetyl hexapeptide-3, but it may reduce wrinkles without side effects. It is being used effectively in many new antiaging creams as a moisturizer. Make sure the product you choose uses other natural ingredients.

Accent XL

The Accent XL radio-frequency device is a revolutionary new method for treating loose, sagging skin and cellulite. Using Accent XL, qualified physicians and other professionals are now able to heat the underlying tissue in a controlled fashion without pain or discomfort. The procedure tightens loose, thinning skin, promotes healthy collagen production, and improves body contours. It is used for firming facial, neck, and arm skin, and on postnatal abdomens, thighs, or breasts. This form of thermotherapy causes the deep structures of the skin to tighten. New collagen develops in time, and further tightening yields more natural looking, firmer skin (see sources).

SOURCES (in the order they appear in the chapter):

Toothpaste:
Peelu Toothpaste (Peelu): www.peelu.com/

Hand soap:
Pure soap (Nature Clean): www.naturecleanliving.com/
Green Mountain Soap: www.gmsoap.com/
Pure Olive Oil Soap (Kiss My Face): www.kissmyface.com/
Glycerine Soap (Clearly Natural): www.clearlynaturalsoaps.com/

Lotion and Moisturizers:
Oil Free Moisture Lotion (Magick Botanicals): www.magickbotanicals.com/
Nature's Balance Hand and Body Lotion (Aubrey Organics): www.aubrey-organics.com/
Ultimate Moist Unscented Hand and Body Lotion (Aubrey Organics): www.aubrey-organics.com/

Deodorant
Deoderant crystal: http://thecrystal.com/

Exfoliants:
Exfoliating Enzyme Scrub (Avalon Natural Products): http://avalonorganics.com/
Apricot Sugar Scrub (Eminence Organic Skin Care): http://www.eminenceorganics.com/
Microdermabrasion Scrub (Zia Natural Skincare): http://www.zianatural.com/
Alexandria's Professional Body Sugaring: http://www.alexandriaprofessional.com/

Hair removal:
Aussie Nad's No-Heat Hair Removal Gel (Aussie): Available in many stores
Alexandria's Professional Body Sugaring: http://www.alexandriaprofessional.com/

Natural eye drops:
Homeopathic Herbal Eye drops with chamomile and eyebright (Primavu): Available in many stores
Optiquel (Bioron): Available in many stores

Sunscreen:
Sunforgettable Rock & Roller Ball, SPF 30 (ColoreScience):
http://colorescience.com

Insect repellents:
Go Mosquito (Bioexcel): www.bioexcel.com
Buzz Away (Quantum Inc.): www.quantumhealth.com/
Bug Off - repelling wrist band for kids (Kaz, Inc.): Available in many drugstores
Bug shirts - Insect barrier clothing (InsectOut):
Bug Shirt: www.bugshirt.com/
Mosquito Barrier: http://www.mosquitobarrier.com/

Botanical perfume:
Roxana Illuminated Perfume: http://www.illuminatedperfume.com/

Human hair wigs with breathable caps:
Crown and Glory: www.crownandgloryenterprises.com

Lice elimination:
Lice R Gone enzyme shampoo: http://www.safesolutionsinc.com/Lice_R_Gone.htm

Shampoo:
Herbal Shampoo (Nature Clean): www.naturecleanliving.com/
Oil Free Fragrance Free Shampoo (Magick Botanicals):
www.magickbotanicals.com/
Shampoo for Thinning Hair (Magick Botanicals):
www.magickbotanicals.com/
Solay Shine Organic Green Tea Natural Shampoo (Solay): Recommended for dandruff and itchy scalp:
http://www.natural-salt-lamps.com/natural-shampoo.html
Tea Tree Shampoo (Naturally Direct): www.naturallydirect.net
Pure Essentials Shampoo (Earth Science): Available from American Environmental Health Foundation (AEHF). 1-800-428-2343 for a free catalog.

Conditioners:
Hair Conditioner, Detangler, & Shine Spray (Magick Botanicals)
Herbal Conditioner (Nature Clean): www.naturecleanliving.com/

Heartland Natural Mint Conditioner (Heartland Products): www.heartlandnatural.com

Oil Free Fragrance Free Conditioner (Magick Botanicals)

Pure Essentials Conditioner (Earth Science): Available from AEHF (see above)

Natural Hair color:
Henna hair color (Naturally Direct): www.naturallydirect.net

Lipstick/lip liner brands:
ColoreScience: http://colorescience.com
Aubrey Organics: www.aubrey-organics.com/
Earth's Beauty: Available from many stores
Ecco Bella: Available from many stores

Mascara:
ColoreScience: http://colorescience.com
Real Purity: Available in many stores
Miessence: http://www.miessenceproducts.com/

Feminine Hygiene:
NatraCare: www.natracare.com/: Also available from AEHF (see above)
Seventh Generation: Sold in many health food stores
Organic Essentials: http://www.organicessentials.com
SeaPearls—naturalsponges:http://www.jadeandpearl.com/catalog/index.php
Mooncup—reusable feminine hygiene:
http://www.jadeandpearl.com/catalog/index.php
Diva Cup—reusable feminine hygiene: http://www.divacup.com/

Sexual lubricants:
Climaxima (Bioexcel): www.bioexcel.com

Body contouring and skin tightening:
Accent XL http://www.accentyourbody.com/index.html. In the Los Angeles area see www.bellabeverlyhills.com

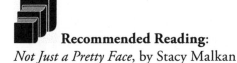 **Recommended Reading**:
Not Just a Pretty Face, by Stacy Malkan

Chapter 8

BABY PRODUCTS

Barbara Seifert is credited with having said, "A baby is a blank check made payable to the human race." Many people prepare for a new baby by painting and carpeting the baby's room. When the baby arrives, parents bathe with chemically based detergents; they apply lotions, creams, and powders filled with fragrances; they feed from plastic bottles; diaper with chemically laden disposable diapers; and clothe in fire-retardant pajamas. Although parents act out of love, their actions are often responsible for a baby's allergies, respiratory problems, skin rashes, and many more serious health problems. Each toxic exposure reduces the potential amount from the blank check written at the birth of every child.

For a number of reasons, a baby's body is more vulnerable to contaminants in air, water, food, and everyday products:

1. The potential dose of a chemical following skin exposure is likely to be about three times greater for infants than for adults. This is because infant skin is considerably thinner than adult skin. Thin skin is more permeable to chemicals. The surface area of a child's skin, relative to body weight, is also greater than adults.
2. Babies breathe more air per body weight than adults. This increases their exposure by inhalation.
3. Infants and young children are uniquely sensitive to the effects of neurotoxic agents. The blood-brain barrier, which can protect the brain from many toxic chemicals, is not fully formed until a child is six months old.
4. Children are uniquely sensitive to hormone disruptors that mimic the hormone estrogen. Hormone disruptors influence puberty for young girls and maleness for boys.
5. A baby's immune system and central nervous system are still developing—their bodies are less capable of eliminating toxins.

Scientists have developed a much greater understanding of children's vulnerability to chemicals. They have discovered links between asthma, childhood cancer, and brain damage, and such common contaminants as solvents, pesticides, and lead. Early exposure to chemicals may *prime* children for adult diseases, just as a few severe sunburns during childhood increase the likelihood of developing skin cancer later in life.[208] There is no longer any doubt that subtle damage to developing bodies may lead to disease and developmental problems later in life.

In the recently updated cancer risk guidelines, the EPA acknowledged the serious nature of childhood exposure. After reviewing twenty-three studies of early life exposures to cancer-causing chemicals, the EPA concluded that carcinogens are ten times more potent for babies than for adults, and that some chemicals are up to sixty-five times more potent.[209] Despite these concerns for children's sensitivity to harmful substances, no special protections exist regarding ingredients in personal care products for babies and children.

Amid rising concern over toxic chemicals in children's products, the Kid Safe Chemicals Act was introduced to Congress in May 2008. It is intended to amend the Toxic Substances Control Act, which has not been amended since it was passed in 1976. It would place the burden of proof on the chemical industry to show that chemicals are safe for children before they are added to consumer products. The act would also reduce childhood and consumer exposure to toxic chemical substances.

Decreasing a child's exposure to chemicals, even in the womb, could mean a lower risk of allergies and chemical sensitivities, and a lower risk of cancers and other illnesses. An early environment that is free of fabric softeners, air fresheners, commercial disinfectants, and antibacterial cleaners will decrease a child's sensitivity to many chemicals. Choosing less-toxic baby products can make a big difference. This chapter discusses the areas of concern for babies and small children.

BABY FOOD

Even though few food sources, including breast milk, are free of environmental contamination, all experts agree: breast-fed is best. Unfortunately, many toxins are transferred from mother to baby in the womb and via breast milk after birth. Breast-feeding moms should eat organic food as much as possible and avoid environmental toxins during pregnancy and nursing.

> **Nipple cracking is a common problem for women who are breastfeeding. Rather than using lotions and creams that will be ingested by baby, lactation specialists recommend spreading breast milk on the cracked area and letting it dry after each feeding. Since mother's milk contains healing ingredients, this practice helps prevent cracking and soothes/heals already cracked nipples.**

Formula

There are reasons why families need to rely on formula for some or all of a baby's diet. These babies need a safe and healthy source of food. Aside from the nutritional needs of babies, powdered formula may be the best bet. This choice reduces exposure to a chemical known as bisphenol A (BPA), which is used to line the cans of all liquid baby formulas (as well as most cans that contain food). Exposure to even tiny amounts of BPA profoundly affects the male reproductive system with adverse changes to the testes, testosterone levels, and sperm production. BPA increases prostate and breast cancer risk, it alters brain development, and it causes earlier puberty onset and obesity. BPA has been detected in sixteen of twenty liquid baby formula samples tested by the FDA and by the Environmental Working Group. Concentrations range from less than one part per billion (ppb) to seventeen ppb in these samples, with an average of five ppb.[210] For one out of three cans of infant formula tested, a single serving contained enough BPA to expose an infant to two hundred times the FDA's traditional safe level of exposure.[211] Even powdered formula is sold in cans with BPA linings, but because this formula is diluted with water, the amount of BPA that a baby consumes is reduced. Avoid ready-to-eat formula in metal cans; these have the highest BPA leaching potential.

 (see Chapter 7: Bisphenol A)

Babies can be allergic to the ingredients in some formulas. If your baby is fussy, has colic, or develops allergies, consider switching to another formula. Always use filtered water for mixing baby formula. If your water is fluoridated, use reverse osmosis to filter your water.

 (see Chapter 2: Fluoridation)

CAUTION: Never microwave mother's milk (or any baby food).

(see Chapter 5: Microwave cooking)

Baby food

Children eat more food relative to body weight than adults. Their consumption of pesticides and other toxins from food is several times that of the average adult. When you are ready to introduce other foods to your baby's diet, organic food is a worthwhile investment. The elimination of additives, preservatives, colorings, and flavorings from your child's food is also a key to keeping them healthy—and a good reason to make your own baby food.

The recent Mercer Island study funded by the EPA found that switching from conventionally grown food to organic food eliminated pesticide markers in the urine of young school children within thirty-six hours.[21]

> **During the Mercer Island study, twenty-three children aged three to eleven switched from a conventional diet to eating only organic food for five days during two test periods (summer and fall). Pesticide metabolites in the urine of these children were undetectable at the end of a five-day intervention of organic foods during both seasons. This shows the importance of eating an organic diet. It also illustrates how rapidly the body is able to clear the pesticide burden of organophosphate pesticides (the pesticides studied) when organic food is consumed.**

Baby food is easy to make. All you need is a blender or food grinder. Babies don't miss salt and sugar, so there is no need to add these seasonings. Whether you are buying baby foods or making your own, make sure they are stored in glass jars. Plastic can leach hazardous chemicals like phthalates and BPA into food.

 (see Chapter 5: Plastic)

Baby bottles

The most commonly used plastic baby bottle is made of polycarbonate. This plastic releases the hormone-disrupting chemical bisphenol A (BPA) into infant formula during heating. Because most infant formulas are already contaminated with BPA from the can lining, the issue becomes significant. Japanese scientists found that used bottles leach more than six times as much BPA as new bottles. Water heated in new polycarbonate bottles picked up between 1 and 3.5 parts per billion (ppb) BPA. Water in worn and heavily scratched bottles acquired between 10 and 28 ppb of BPA.[213]

Disposable bags for bottles may leach other hormone-disrupting chemicals known as phthalats. Hormone-disrupting chemicals affect the male reproductive system; they increase the risk of breast cancer and contribute to earlier puberty and obesity. The best option for baby bottles is glass. Glass bottles are easily cleaned and sterilized; they can be handed down from baby to baby. Evenflo makes glass bottles and Nurtured Products for Parenting in Canada stocks glass baby bottles and stainless steel sippy cups (see sources).

 (see Chapter 5: Phthalates)

Nipples and pacifiers

Nipples for bottles are usually made of latex or silicone. Latex nipples can release nitrosamines (potent carcinogens) when babies suck on the nipple. Latex is also responsible for some allergic reactions. It also breaks down faster, causing cracks where bacteria can hide. Purchase silicone nipples and pacifiers.

PERSONAL CARE PRODUCTS FOR BABY

What you put *on* your baby is just as important as what you put *in* your baby—in many cases it is the same thing. According to a new study of babies born in Los Angeles and two other U.S. cities, infants and toddlers exposed to baby lotions, shampoos, and powders had four times the concentration of phthlates in their urine.[214] The study is the first to report that skin transfer may be a main route of phthalate exposure for babies. In their report, scientists advised parents who want to reduce their baby's exposure, to stop using lotions and powders unless their doctors recommend them for medical reasons. They also suggested limiting the use of shampoos and other commercial products.

 (see Chapter 5: Phthalates)

Baby soap

Like most commercial soap, baby soap can contain numerous harmful ingredients including fragrances, petroleum products (especially mineral oil), antibacterial chemicals, ammonia, formaldehyde, glycols, phenol, and colorants. These chemicals contribute to allergies and other skin problems.

Babies' skin contains natural oils. Washing too frequently can remove these oils, causing skin to be dry and irritated. Some dermatologists suggest bathing a baby only once or twice a week—washing bums, faces, and hands as needed. Use plain warm water with a mild soap when necessary.

Natural soap is made from animal or vegetable fat and an alkali. There is a tremendous variety of good soap available (see sources). Most natural soaps are also suited for babies. Bar soaps often contain fewer chemicals than body washes and liquid hand soaps.

Antibacterial soap

Children do not have to be protected from all bacteria. In fact, some bacteria are beneficial. Scientists are concerned that antibacterial soaps kill beneficial bacteria and also contribute to the creation of antibiotic-resistant bacteria. Antibacterial soaps are usually more drying and irritating. They contain ingredients like triclosan, which is a derivative of the herbicide 2,4-D. Avoid the use of antibacterial soap.

 (see Chapter 7: Triclosan)

Bubble bath

The use of commercially available bubble bath is not recommended. Bubble bath consists mainly of detergent and artificial fragrances. The FDA receives many complaints of skin rashes, irritations, and urinary tract, bladder, and kidney infections reported by those who use bubble bath. Vaginal irritations and infections are common, especially with children who have extra-sensitive skin.

Soaking in any bath product prolongs its contact with the skin, increasing the risk that chemicals will be absorbed.

Bubble bath is likely to contain sodium laureth sulphate and cocamidopropyl betaine (the latter is a penetration enhancer, allowing other chemicals to be more easily absorbed). Both bubble bath and shower gels have the potential to penetrate the skin and lungs.

Shampoo

Shampoos cause the greatest number of adverse reactions of all hair care products. When choosing shampoo for your children, avoid sodium lauryl sulfate/sodium laureth sulfate, DEA, TEA, and MEA, which are hormone disruptors and can release carcinogenic nitrosamines. Also avoid quaternium chemicals, PEG compounds, DMDM hydantoin, polyethylene glycol, fragrances, and propylene glycol.

"Tear free" shampoos are made with a pH (acidity level) that matches baby's tears. This is why they don't sting. It doesn't necessarily mean they are safer to use. A neutral pH is less irritating to the scalp and skin. The best option is to use a less toxic shampoo with a neutral pH and to make sure to keep it out of eyes (see sources).

Lotions and diaper cream

A baby's delicate skin is easily penetrated by the chemicals in lotions and diaper creams. Safer products are free of boric acid and sodium borate—ingredients that the cosmetic industry's own safety advisory panel says are unsafe for infants. The industry's safety panel states that these chemicals are readily absorbed. Once absorbed, boron accumulates in the brain and liver and is eliminated very slowly. Despite this understanding, boric acid and sodium borate are found in many diaper rash ointments.

Other ingredients to avoid in lotions for babies are mineral oil—a petroleum product, BHA—a carcinogenic preservative banned from use in Europe and Japan, parabens—estrogen mimicking preservatives, PEG compounds, TEA, DEA, and MEA, DMDM hydantoin, quaternium compounds, sodium lauryl/laureth sulfate, and fragrances.

Another group of chemicals that will seldom be listed on the label is phthalates. These are especially harmful to children because they are suspected of altering sexual development. Phthalates, used in the manufacture of cosmetics and plastic products—including baby toys—get into the air and liquids, and they penetrate the skin. Young children have been shown to have especially high concentrations. A study published in the *Pediatrics* journal measured phthalates in the urine of 163 infants. The mothers were asked about their use of infant powders, diaper creams, wipes, shampoo, and lotion. They were also asked how many hours their infants played with items such as teething rings and pacifiers. All the infants tested had phthalates in their urine. The use of powder, lotion, and shampoo was tied to the highest concentrations, especially in younger infants.[215]

 (see Chapter 5: Phthalates)

You can reduce the need for lotions and oils if you don't remove the natural oils on a baby's skin by bathing more than necessary or by using harsh soaps. The application of single organic oils such as grape seed, wheat germ, olive, apricot kernel, almond, jojoba, or vitamin E oil will help replenish natural oils and may provide a temporary barrier on little bums.

Baby wipes

Most baby wipes on the market today contain a variety of harmful ingredients including alcohol, antibacterial compounds, fragrances, preservatives, and a chemical known as bronopol (2-Bromo-2-Nitropropane-1,3-Diol). Bronopol is an allergen and an irritant. It is a known skin, lung, and immune system toxicant. Breakdown of bronopol can lead to the formation of formaldehyde and nitrosamines which are known and suspected cancer-causing agents. Animal studies indicate very low doses of bronopol could trigger broad systemic health effects.[216]

The second problem with baby wipes is that they are made of cotton fabric that has been bleached with chlorine. This process leaves traces of dioxins—some of the most dangerous chemicals in the environment. According to the EPA, there is no safe level of dioxin. Dioxins are persistent; tiny amounts accumulate over time. Additionally, unless the cotton is organic, it has most likely been grown with genetically modified seed, pesticides (conventional cotton is one of most pesticide-poisoned crops in the United States), and synthetic fertilizers. Conventional baby wipes are not a good idea, but there are some alternatives that meet higher standards (see sources).

Powder (talc)

Talc is a naturally occurring mineral that can cause respiratory problems when inhaled. Talcum powder is reported to cause coughing, vomiting, and even pneumonia. Beyond the respiratory difficulties, baby powder may also contain fragrances (that fresh baby scent), preservaties, and sodium borate. Use any powder with caution.

DIAPERS
Disposable diapers

Disposable diapers consist of a plastic exterior, a super-absorbent layer, and a liner. The absorbent layer contains a powdery substance made of sodium polyacrylate. Sodium polyacrylate forms a gel when moistened, absorbing two to three hundred times its weight in liquid. It was developed by NASA and is used to clean up chemical spills and in potting soil as a moisture-retaining substance. Because it is a powder, it is not always contained within the diaper. Most mothers who have used disposable diapers recall the small jellylike crystals that remain on a child's genitals when the diaper is removed.

Sodium polyacrylate is a skin irritant. Though it is considered safe, there is a large data gap for toxicological information. Disposable diapers may also contain dyes, fragrances, and dioxin.

> **The average child uses over 5,000 diapers during the 30-month period before toilet training, contributing to a total of over 3 million tons of landfill refuse each year.**

Disposable diapers have been linked to respiratory problems and to increasing asthma rates in children. A study conducted by Anderson Laboratories in 1999 found that disposable diapers release volatile organic chemicals (VOCs), including toluene, ethylbenzene, xylene, and dipentene.[217] All of these VOCs have been shown to have toxic health effects with long-term or high-level exposure. Researchers also determined that mice exposed to the chemicals released by disposable diapers were more likely to experience irritated airways than mice exposed to emissions from cloth diapers. These effects were increased with repeat exposures.

 (see Chapter 1: Volatile organic compounds)

Cloth diapers
The growing concern over disposable diapers along with consideration of the ecological impact on the planet have caused many parents to reconsider cloth diapers. The options now available prove that cloth diapering doesn't have to be inconvenient. Today, cloth diapers are elasticized so that they are fitted and snug, breathable, and manageable with hook and loop closures or snaps. In the long run, cloth diapers are cheaper, they are certainly healthier, and they support a more sustainable living environment. Most babies who use cloth diapers can avoid diaper rash completely (see sources).

CLOTHING

Parents spend a lot of time baby-proofing their homes—removing breakable household items, checking toys for small parts, and making sure cabinets and cupboards are secure. But how many parents think about their baby's clothes?

Synthetic fabrics
Most synthetic fabrics, from towels to bed linens, are complex. Creating a soft pullover or a wrinkle-resistant shirt out of man-made materials takes chemical manipulation. Dozens of chemicals may be incorporated before

the finished product is ready for sale. These chemicals not only leach into the environment, but they may be absorbed through the skin or inhaled directly as clothing outgases volatile compounds. The chemicals used in synthetic clothing have been linked to respiratory ailments, asthma, immune system damage, behavioral problems, hormone disruption, and cancer. The consequences for babies, whose skin and respiratory systems are considerably more delicate, can be severe.

No-iron/wrinkle-free
Some of the worst chemicals used in fabrics are perfluorinated chemicals (PFCs). These include the nonstick additive Teflon. PFCs are increasingly being added to clothing because it makes them wrinkle-free. According to the EPA, PFCs are cancer-causing compounds.

 (see Chapter 9: Fabric treatments)

> **Anything labeled static resistant, wrinkle resistant, permanent press, no iron, stain resistant, or moth repellant contains PFCs and may outgas formaldehyde.**

Fire retardants
All children's sleepwear is required by law to meet federal flammability standards. Most fabrics treated with flame-retardant chemicals continuously emit toxic formaldehyde gas. Breathing formaldehyde gas above the levels of 0.1 parts per million for an extended period of time will cause many health problems, such as headaches, dizziness, scratchy eyes and throat, nasal congestion, coughing, and immune system abnormalities.

Fire retardant chemicals are persistent in the environment and bioaccumulative—they build up in the body over a lifetime and may cause liver toxicity, thyroid toxicity, and neurodevelopmental toxicity.[218] Brominated fire retardants (polybrominated diphenylethers, or PBDEs), impair attention, learning, memory, and behavior in laboratory animals at surprisingly low levels. The most critical time for exposure is during periods of rapid brain development.[219] The European Union has banned the most toxic forms of fire retardants; Asian countries are close behind. But the EPA has set no safety standards or other regulations. Only one state, California, has banned some chemical fire retardants. Clothes and bedding treated with fire retardant must be labeled. However, companies are not required to disclose what chemical is being used. During the 1980s and 1990s, pressure from consumer groups led to the relaxation of standards for infant sleepwear. Today, snug-fitting, untreated cotton sleepwear is a legal alternative for children's sleepwear.

Natural fabrics

Natural fabrics (cotton, linen, wool, cashmere, silk, soy, bamboo, and hemp) tend to breathe better than synthetic fibers. They naturally wick moisture away from the body. But even natural fibers can be contaminated with chemicals. Seven of the fifteen pesticides most commonly used on cotton are known human carcinogens. In fact, cotton is subjected to more chemicals than almost any other crop. Twenty-five percent of the world's pesticides and 10 percent of the world's insecticides are used on cotton annually. And the problems with natural fiber clothing production do not stop in the field. During the conversion of conventional cotton into clothing, numerous toxic chemicals are added at each stage—harsh petroleum scours, fabric softeners, brighteners, heavy metals, stain repellants, ammonia, and formaldehyde. The same is true for other natural fibers.

> **For every one pair of cotton jeans and t-shirt produced, one pound of pesticides and chemical fertilizers are used.**

There are many sources of organic clothing—this market is growing rapidly as more people become aware of the problems with synthetic fabrics and with commercially produced clothing. The environmental issues alone could fill a book since the production of synthetic fabrics uses many toxic chemicals and produces considerable toxic waste. Organic fabrics and products marketed for the chemically sensitive are less likely to have chemical finishes, dyes, and fabric softeners used during processing. Yard goods are also less likely to have chemical treatments than manufactured clothing.

> **Although natural fibers are preferable, polyester and nylon outgas the least.**

Laundering

Many chemical treatments are designed not to wash out. These include fire retardant and wrinkle-resistant chemicals. However, many other "finishing" chemicals can be reduced by washing before wearing. A general rule of thumb is to wash and dry synthetic fabrics three times before wearing. To remove excess dyes or conventional detergents and fabric finishes, wash several times or soak overnight in a tub of water with one-half to one cup of distilled vinegar. Regular washing of baby clothing with scented detergents surrounds a baby with additional harmful chemicals. Select a more natural laundry detergent.

 (see Chapter 6: Laundry detergent)

Fabric softeners

Fabric softeners work by leaving a residue on the fabric which never completely washes out. The same residue is left on washing and drying equipment. (Some dryer manufacturers will void their warranty if fabric softeners are used.) Fabric softeners can cause allergic reactions through skin contact and inhalation. They can contain many irritants and carcinogenic compounds. Two less-toxic alternatives to fabric softeners are:

1. Dryerballs. These eliminate static cling by creating space between clothes. They soften clothing, reduce drying time, and contain no chemicals or fragrances (see sources).
2. Static Eliminators. Unlike conventional dryer sheets, static eliminators are nontoxic, hypoallergenic, reusable, and they contain no chemicals or fragrances. One set of static eliminators works for five hundred wash loads and removes old detergent residues (see sources).

 (see Chapter 6: Fabric softeners)

Baby Furniture

Most wood furniture is either made or finished with toxic chemicals that can outgas volatile organic compounds (VOCs). New dressers and cribs may be made of particleboard or plywood. These are notorious sources of formaldehyde. The glues and adhesives used in furniture construction also outgas VOCs—sometimes for years.

 (see Chapter 1: Volatile organic compounds)

When purchasing new wood furniture for baby's room, choose solid wood with a nontoxic finish. Metal furniture is also a good option, but stay away from plastic. Used furniture is also a good choice because it will have less outgassing, but be sure that paint or varnish is nontoxic and not peeling or chipping. Older painted furniture (before 1960) probably has lead paint. AFM sealants can be used to seal old paint (see sources).

Bedding

Babies spend up to 70 percent of their early life sleeping and playing in a crib. Making sure they are not breathing chemicals during that time is important—especially since babies have a higher metabolic rate than adults and because they breathe more air. The most common bedding materials are polyester/cotton blends or all polyester. These synthetic and synthetic combination fabrics emit low levels of chemicals throughout their lifetime. Bedding made with 100 percent cotton, hemp, linen, or wool is least toxic. However, most conventional bedding, even of natural fibers, is subjected to chemical treatments before reaching the consumer. Avoid bedding which is advertised as wrinkle resistant or no-iron. Wrinkle-resistant fabrics are treated with chemicals containing formaldehyde, which is a carcinogen and a sensitizer. This treatment is designed to last the life of the fabric and is impossible to wash out completely. Bedding may also be treated with fire retardant chemicals; wool may be treated with mothproofing chemicals—both are designed to last a lifetime.

> **Organic fabrics are best; buying cotton flannel or unbleached cottons at a fabric store to make your own baby bedding is even better.**

Mattresses

Since 1973, the U.S. government has required that all mattresses and mattress pads meet requirements to reduce the risk of bed fires. To comply, mattresses and pads are treated with fire-retardant chemicals. The most widely used of these chemicals are the class known as polybrominated diphenyl ethers (PBDEs). PBDEs are chemical cousins to PCBs, which have been banned since the 1970s. Exposure to PBDEs may be especially harmful to infants.

 (see Chapter 9: Fire retardants)

Many mattress cores (stuffing) contain polyurethane foam. These outgas volatile organic compounds (VOCs) associated with upper-respiratory problems and skin irritation. Natural latex mattress cores or cotton batting are preferred. Foundations—the industry term for box springs—are either made of hardwood or less-expensive plywood or particleboard. Hardwood is preferred over plywood or particleboard because those are treated with formaldehyde as a preservative.

> Today, the only way to purchase a cotton mattress without fire retardants is with a doctor's prescription verifying chemical sensitivities, or to purchase a mattress wrapped in a layer of wool (wool is naturally fire-retardant).

The ideal mattress has a foundation made with natural, untreated, solid wood; a core of natural (not synthetic) latex or cotton batting; and is topped with untreated, organic cotton/wool. Organic mattresses ensure against dioxins from the bleaching of both cotton and wool and against dyes, color fixers (heavy metals such as chromium, copper, and zinc), and pesticides. There are many manufacturers that make high-quality organic mattresses (see sources).

Toys

Like other industries, the U.S. toy industry is less regulated than in many other countries. That's why consumer groups are demanding much-needed information on the safety of children's toys. In December 2007, a nonprofit organization, www.healthytoys.org, released results of the testing of over twelve hundred popular children's toys. Although these toys were only tested for a few toxic elements that could be measured by x-ray fluorescence, the results were revealing. Testing showed levels of lead, PVC, cadmium, arsenic, and mercury in excess of safe levels.[220]

Lead

When children are exposed to lead, the developmental and nervous system consequences are irreversible. The American Academy of Pediatrics recommends a maximum level of lead at 40 parts per million (ppm) in children's products. There are no federal limits set for children's toys—the only existing standard is for lead in paint. HealthyToys.org found lead in 35 percent of all the products tested. Seventeen percent had levels above the 600 ppm federal recall standard for lead in paint!

 (see Chapter 1: Lead)

Polyvinyl chloride (PVC/Vinyl)

Forty-seven percent of the toys tested by HealthyToys.org contained PVC, considered to be one of the worst plastics from an environmental as well as from a health perspective.

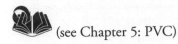 (see Chapter 5: PVC)

Even though a growing body of evidence indicates that phthalates have serious effects on sexual development, toys in the United States are still permitted to include these chemicals. Testing by Greenpeace in 1997 revealed that phthalates represented 10 to 40 percent of the weight of PVC (vinyl) toys.[221]

> In 1998 the European Chemical Bureau affirmed that phthalates easily leach from products like plastic toys; they recommended tighter standards. In 2004 Europe banned six phthalates from children's toys and teethers. Many other countries have followed, including Japan, Norway, Argentina, Mexico, and Canada. That leaves the United States as one of the few developed countries with no government limits on phthalates in toys. In the United States, if they're plastic and soft, there's a good chance they contain PVC and phthalates.

Cadmium

Cadmium is a known human carcinogen. Exposure can cause adverse effects on the kidneys, lungs, liver, and testes. Currently, there are no restrictions on cadmium in children's products in the United States. HealthyToys.org found cadmium at levels greater than one hundred ppm in 3 percent of products.

Other toxins in toys

HealthyToys.org also tested toys for arsenic, mercury, bromine, chromium, tin, and antimony—chemicals that have all been linked to health problems. The results are posted at www.healthytoys.org. Twenty-eight percent of the products tested did not contain any lead, cadmium, arsenic, mercury, or PVC. This indicates that manufacturers can make toys free of unnecessary toxic chemicals. HealthyToys.org provides specific guidelines for how to petition federal and state government agencies and toy manufacturers and to urge them to phase out toxic chemicals from toys. Visitors to the Web site can see how toys rate and can nominate others to be tested.

CAR SEATS

The same group that released the consumer guide to toxic toys also tested child car seats for dangerous chemicals. Their research, completed in May 2007 and available at www.HealthyCar.org, revealed the dangerous chemicals in a variety of car seats. Anyone shopping for a new car seat or wondering if their child's current car seat is safe can visit the Web site and search by model or compare models. Brands and models varied widely, and there was no one brand that stood out across the board for chemical safety. The full report is availableathttp://www.healthycar.org/documents/healthycarseatguide07.pdf.

Brominated fire retardants

One of the major concerns with child car seats is the outgassing of brominated fire retardants. These chemicals break down in the presence of UV light (when cars sit in the sun), leaving residue on windows and in dust particles. These residues are much higher with new child car seats. Health concerns include thyroid hormone disruption, learning and memory impairment, behavioral changes, and cancer.[222] Other safer fire retardants exist, and the fact that some child car seat manufacturers were able to meet stringent fire regulations without the use of brominated fire retardants provides ample evidence.

PVC and phthalates

Phthalates from PVC outgas during car seat use and are deposited on dust particles and on windshields as fog. These are persistent chemicals now being banned in many countries. They are suspected human carcinogens and known to cause serious effects on sexual development.

Lead

Lead is still sometimes used as an additive in plastic. Since 2000, when the European Union began restricting the use of lead in the automotive industry, many companies have reduced their usage. However, lead is still found in some car seats in the United States. According to the American Academy of Pediatrics, an estimated 3 to 4 million children in the United States under age six have blood lead levels of lead that could cause impaired development.[223] The link between lead exposure and a number of severe health effects is will established. Long-term exposure in children can affect a child's growth, damage kidneys, and cause learning and behavioral problems.[224]

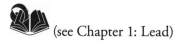 (see Chapter 1: Lead)

SOURCES (in the order they appear in the chapter):

Glass baby bottles and stainless steel sippy cups:
Nurtured Products for Parenting: www.nurtured.ca

Soap:
Natural Baby and Kids Bath Soap (Aubrey Organics): Available at many stores
Aloe Vera Baby Mild (Dr. Bronner's): Available at many stores
Calendula Baby Soap (Weleda): Available at many stores
Moonbaby Healing Soap (Moonsnail Soapworks):
www.moonsnailsoapworks.com

Shampoo:
Natural Baby and Kids Shampoo (Aubrey Organics): Available at many stores
Tribe Kids Pure Botanical Baby Shampoo and Bath Gel (Earth Tribe)
Also see sources for shampoo in the personal care chapter

Baby wipes:
Seventh Generation Unscented Baby Wipes with Aloe Vera & Vitamin E
Tushies Baby Wipes with Aloe Vera, Unscented

Cloth diapers:
Ecobaby: http://ecobaby.com
Nurtured Products for Parenting: www.nurtured.ca

Non-toxic disposable diapers:
http://www.honest.com/

Organic baby clothing:
Positively Organic: http://positively-organic.com/
Sage Creek Naturals: http://www.sagecreeknaturals.com/
Pure Beginnings: http://www.purebeginnings.com/
Mamma's Baby: http://www.mamasbaby.com/
There are many others; you will want to find your own favorites

Fabric softeners:
Dryerballs (Nurtured Products for Parenting): www.nurtured.ca
Static Eliminators: http://www.staticeliminator.ca/

Organic bedding:
Positively Organic: http://positively-organic.com/
Sage Creek Naturals: http://www.sagecreeknaturals.com/

Pure Beginnings: http://www.purebeginnings.com/
Ecobaby: http://ecobaby.com
Nature's Crib: www.naturescrib.com/
There are many others

Organic mattresses:
Simply Organic Sleep: http://simplyorganicsleep.com/
Naturepedic: http://www.naturepedic.com/
Nirvana Safe Haven: http://www.nontoxic.com/

Furniture sealants and no-VOC paint:
AFM: http://www.afmsafecoat.com/

Chapter 9

CLOTHING AND TEXTILES

✦

The toxins we wear, sit on, and sleep with

Perhaps whoever stated "Clothes make the man" knew more about the manufacture of clothing than he realized. Regardless of their source, the commercially available fabrics that are used to make dress shirts, bed linens, and couch cushions are treated with chemicals during and after their manufacture. The fabrics themselves may outgas the chemicals they are made of. These chemicals are absorbed or inhaled directly all day or all night long. Both the fabric and the process by which they are made can be cause for concern and should be considered when deciding on clothing, bedding, and home décor.

Clothing may not be the first thing that comes to mind when you think about creating a less-toxic lifestyle, but it should definitely be on your list. Your choice of clothing and other textiles not only affects your personal health, but it affects the health of the entire planet. The chemicals used in the manufacture of fabric eventually leach into the environment, leaving an impact on groundwater, wildlife, air, and soil. Just as choosing organic food and supporting sustainable agriculture sends a message to growers, choosing natural fiber clothing sends a message to textile manufacturers that will have a global impact. This chapter discusses synthetic and natural fiber fabrics. It identifies many toxic fabric treatments to be aware of—and to avoid—and it sheds light on the whole clothing industry from the perspective of fair trade and fair working conditions in the industry.

SYNTHETIC FABRICS

The invention of synthetic fibers forever changed the textile industry. Qualities like water resistance, durability, and versatility have ensured a wide range of possibilities for synthetic fabrics. But most consumers are unaware of the waste products they create, the hazards they cause, the environmental issues with disposal, or the risks they pose to those who use them.

Synthetic fabrics create huge amounts of hazardous waste during production. Chemicals that are used in the manufacture of synthetic fabrics include sodium hydroxide and carbon di-sulphide (a neurotoxin that was responsible for thousands of deaths and hospitalizations in the early days of rayon manufacture).[225] These contaminants are only two of the dozens of chemicals that leach into waterways and pollute the soil and the atmosphere. They also endanger the health of those who produce them and those who wear them. The chemicals used in the making of synthetic clothing have been linked to respiratory ailments, asthma, immune system damage, behavioral problems, hormone disruption, and cancer.[226]

The eventual disposal of synthetic fabric also creates a major environmental problem. These fabrics are not biodegradable and therefore do not break down in the soil. They are literally plastic—existing forever—leaching toxins that will have an impact for years to come.

Most synthetic fabrics are routinely treated with fire retardants, water-repellants, and permanent-press chemicals—all can outgas volatile organic compounds (VOCs) including formaldehyde. Clothing made from synthetic fibers and coated with fabric finishes will continuously outgas tiny vapors (VOCs) as the fabric is warmed against the skin, causing known and unknown side effects.

 (see Chapter 1: Volatile organic compounds)

Polyester

The basic building block of polyester is petroleum. To make polyester, crude oil is broken down into petrochemicals such as ethylene and xylene, which are then converted with heat and catalysts into polyethylene terephthalate—the same plastic that is used to make plastic water bottles. This plastic is then used to make polyester fiber for clothing.

Polyester fabric has several potential health hazards. Its production releases lung-damaging pollutants into the air. It also produces a by-product called antimony trioxide, which is toxic to the heart, lungs, liver, and skin. Long-term inhalation of antimony trioxide can cause chronic bronchitis and emphysema. Antimony trioxide also ends up in wastewater. Polyester contains chemicals called phthalates, which are used to make the fibers more flexible. These chemicals mimic the female hormone estrogen in the human body. Constant exposure to phthalates in food containers, dinnerware, polyester clothing, and other sources has been linked to a variety of developmental and reproductive problems that have increased dramatically during the last sixty years.

 (see Chapter 2: Phthalates)

Polyester also traps water vapor close to the body. It can be responsible for the perpetuation of fungal skin problems (e.g., athletes foot), night sweats (when sleeping on polyester bedding), and genital itching (when polyester is used in underwear). In spite of these health and environmental hazards, polyester outgasses the least of the synthetic fabrics.

> **Because polyester fabric is made of plastic, PET bottles may be recycled and made into clothing. Several companies now make clothing from recycled plastic. Although much credit is given to companies for discovering ways to reuse one of the worst pollutants on the planet, recycling this class of polyester only makes matters worse. The process produces more of the same pollutants. The use of natural fibers in the first place can help to eliminate a very serious pollutant.**
>
> **(see Chapter 2: Plastic)**

Acrylic

Acrylic is also a petroleum derivative. It shares many of the same problems with polyester and poses an additional hazard. Acrylic is made from acrylonitrile, a suspected carcinogen. Workers who make acrylic fiber deal daily with a probable cancer risk. Acrylic fabric typically requires gentle, cold water washing or dry cleaning, which can involve the use of the cancer-causing dry-cleaning solvent, perchloroethylene.

 (see Chapter 9: Dry cleaning)

Nylon

Nylon, too, is made from petroleum—in a process that releases many toxins into the environment. It is generally considered nontoxic for the wearer, although some people report skin reactions. Similar to polyester, nylon outgasses very little.

Polyvinyl chloride (PVC)

Polyvinyl chloride (PVC) is another plastic used for many clothing items including laminated aprons, T-shirts with plastisol prints, patent vinyl pants, and raincoats. The manufacture of vinyl (PVC) creates dioxins—potent carcinogens that accumulate in fatty tissue and contaminate the food chain. PVC also contains chemicals called phthalates, many of which affect reproduction and sexual development. PVC may also contain lead and cadmium as stabilizers. Tests by Greenpeace found lead and cadmium as well as high levels of phthalates in the plastisol ink on children's clothes sold throughout the world.[227] The major health concern about plastisol inks is not that they are PVC-based, but that they contain phthalates and lead.

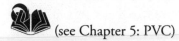 (see Chapter 5: PVC)

Spandex (Lycra)

Spandex is the generic name for Lycra—a synthetic elastic fiber made to replace rubber (latex). It is also a petroleum derivative made of polyurethane—produced by reacting polyester, polyether, polycarbonate, or polycaprolactone with diisocyanate. Spandex fibers decompose when exposed to heat and sunlight, so stabilizers must be added to protect the fibers. Phenols are used to protect spandex from heat. UV screeners such as hydroxybenzotriazoles are added to protect against light degradation. Color stabilizers are added to protect against discoloration. Since spandex is often used for swimwear, antimildew chemicals are also often added. When spandex is ready for sale to the consumer, it is loaded with chemicals and additives. This explains why some people with chemical sensitivities are unable to wear clothing containing spandex. Yet, because of the growing allergic reaction to latex, spandex is often the choice for elastic waistbands, swimwear, and other fabric that needs to stretch.

SEMINATURAL FABRICS

There are several fabrics that, although not synthetic, are not really natural either. These are made from cellulose (the basic building material of all plants). The process of turning the cellulose into fiber involves chemical reactions. The finished product is not anything like the cellulose found in nature.

Rayon

Rayon is the oldest man-made fiber. Although it is made from wood pulp, rayon is chemically and structurally engineered. It involves the use and the production of toxic chemicals. Rayon's manufacturing is a water- and chemical-intensive process that contributes to deforestation and pollution. Rayon clothes are typically dry cleaned.

 (see Chapter 9: Dry cleaning)

Tencel

Tencel (generically known as Lyocell) is a newer form of rayon that does not involve any direct chemical reaction. Tencel is considered by many to be a natural fiber, and indeed it is more natural than rayon. During the making of Tencel, wood pulp is dissolved in a nontoxic solvent. The cellulose fibers are purified and dried, and the solvent is recovered and reused. Tencel has all the advantages of rayon and in many respects is superior. It is soft, breathable, lightweight, and comfortable. It is stronger than cotton or rayon, and it stretches more than cotton. Because it is made from cellulose, it naturally wicks moisture away from the body. In addition, the closed-loop manufacturing process is much more environmentally friendly. Production emissions and wastewater are significantly lower in comparison to the processes involved in the manufacture of rayon and other textiles.

Modal

Modal is another fiber made from cellulose (in this case, beech trees). Although it, too, is a more environmentally friendly process, a small number of people experience reactions to the fiber.[228]

Acetate

Acetate (technically cellulose acetate) is also made from cellulose (wood fibers). Acetate does not absorb moisture readily but dries fast and resists wrinkling and shrinking. Fingernail polish (mostly acetate), nail polish remover, and alcohol will *melt* acetate. Triacetate is an improved acetate fabric that doesn't *melt* as easily and is easier to care for.

NATURAL FABRICS

Cotton

All natural fiber fabrics are renewable and have the potential to be sustainable.

Cotton is perhaps the universal choice in natural cloth. It is cool, soft, and comfortable. The cotton fiber is hollow in the center. This enables it to absorb up to twenty-five times its own weight in water—and it is actually stronger when wet than dry. Cotton absorbs and releases perspiration quickly, allowing the fabric to breathe. This is one of the greatest virtues of cotton. Cotton can also stand high temperatures and accepts dyes easily.

Numerous "finishing" treatments and chemicals are routinely added to give cotton wrinkle resistance, stain resistance, and other qualities. Since cotton wrinkles easily, polyester was originally added to give it wash-and-wear properties. However, consumers are beginning to realize that the addition of polyester and other synthetics takes away the breathability of cotton and adds other undesirable qualities. Discerning consumers now request 100 percent cotton. We have come full circle.

Unfortunately, cotton isn't the wholesome natural fiber it once was. Heavily laden with insecticides, herbicides, and synthetic fertilizers, cotton crops use nearly 25 percent of all the insecticides applied globally each year. The Environmental Protection Agency considers seven of the top fifteen pesticides used on cotton crops to be human carcinogens.

Organic cotton

Organic cotton is still a very small industry (only 0.03 percent of the world's cotton), but American farmers, especially in Texas, are leading the way to expand the market. The advantages of organic cotton go beyond personal health; they take into consideration the health of every living creature. Organic clothing is not only produced without pesticides, it is farmed using natural methods that include crop rotation, compost, natural fertilizers, and the use of beneficial insects. The organic clothing manufacturing process is also free of harmful chemicals and fabric finishes. Supporting this industry supports us all.

Linen

Linen and flax are interchangeable terms. Linen fibers come from the inner bark of the flax plant. Linen is resilient, durable, and is easy to produce organically. Linen also requires less water and produces fewer pollutants during the coloring process than cotton. Over the past few years, the USDA has been evaluating the economic feasibility of developing the flax plant as a U.S. commodity. However, at this time most linen comes from outside the United States.

Wool

Wool is the dense, warm coat of sheep, also called fleece. It is an amazing fabric that is naturally flame retardant and naturally soil resistant. Wool has many unique properties that make it well suited to textile production, something humans realized nearly ten thousand years ago when sheep first began to be domesticated.

Wool has excellent moisture-wicking properties, pulling moisture into the core of the fiber so that it doesn't feel wet to the wearer. Wool will absorb up to 30 percent of its weight in moisture without feeling damp. Though known for its warmth, wool is actually cooler than polyester or other synthetic fabrics because it has the ability to breathe.

Conventionally produced wool is full of pesticides and toxic chemicals incorporated during processing. With conventional wool production, sheep are given hormones and antibiotics. The sheep are often dipped in organophosphate pesticides, which create health risks for the sheep as well as the workers. Pesticides then contaminate groundwater. Wool is also traditionally processed with toxic solvents and detergents. These factors make conventionally produced wool less than desirable.

Other types of wool include:

- **Alpaca** fleece. It is very rich and silky with considerable luster.
- **Mohair** is from the Angora goat and is highly resilient and strong.
- **Angora** wool is from the Angora rabbit. This soft fiber is used in sweaters and baby clothes.
- **Camel hair** is from the extremely soft and fine fur from the undercoat of the camel.
- **Cashmere** is from Kasmir goat down.
- **Vicuna** is a member of the Llama family.

Organic wool

Like the organic cotton industry, the organic wool industry is still small—especially in the United States. Most organic wool comes from Australia. However, more wool suppliers are meeting sustainability criteria for land use, animal management, and wool processing. Supporting the organic wool industry will send out the message that will help this industry to grow.

Silk

Silk is a natural protein fiber like human hair. During their pupae stage, silkworms spin a cocoon that is collected for the making of silk thread. For hundreds of years, silk was produced without chemicals and without killing silk worms. But when it was discovered that the use of pesticides and growth regulators could prolong the life of the silk worm and increase the amount of silk in their cocoons, everything changed. Further, since the emergence of the silk worm damaged the silk, producers began to either bake or drown the silk worms to preserve the length of the fibers. As a result, silk is no longer guaranteed free of chemical additives—or cruelty, unless it is wild-crafted.

Ahimsa Peace Silk is made from the cocoons of semiwild and wild moths in India. By allowing the pupae to emerge from their cocoons on their own, this process produces silk without chemicals or cruelty. Wild-crafted silk helps maintain the forest habitat of moths by linking the livelihood of tribal spinners and weavers to the existence of these trees.

Hemp

For twelve thousand years, hemp has been cultivated to make clothing, paper, and other items—with good reason. Its bark contains some of the strongest, longest, softest fibers on the planet. Hemp clothing provides greater insulation than cotton. It is also absorbent. It wicks away moisture and has natural stain, mold, and UV light resistance. As a plant, hemp is tough enough to stand up to weeds and bugs. It requires few, if any, pesticides; it is fast growing and requires half the water of other plants; it aerates the soil, eliminating the need for crop rotation and minimizing soil erosion. So why is hemp not cultivated in the United States? Because hemp belongs to the same species as marijuana, and its cultivation has been illegal since the 1950s, despite the fact that hemp contains too little tetrahydrocannabinol (the psychotrophic ingredient in marijuana) to produce any narcotic effects. Today, hemp must be imported. It is widely grown in much of Europe and Asia, and increasingly in Canada, where hemp farming was legalized in 1998. Hemp fabric does not contain the narcotic.

Even though hemp does not typically require pesticides, this does not ensure organic status. Only a small number of companies claim to manufacture organic hemp, but there is an international certification program for organic hemp, and it is becoming more popular as a natural fabric.

Bamboo

Bamboo, the tropical grass that has come into vogue in home décor, is now making its way into retail clothing. Praised for its natural softness and sheen, bamboo has been compared to silk and cashmere. Bamboo is a prolific plant that can be harvested every three to four years. Additionally, bamboo will break down in landfills and can be grown without pesticides or chemicals. Watch for this emerging natural fabric to find its place in the textile industry.

Soy

Soybean fiber was developed in China in 1999 and is produced from the residue of soybeans after tofu manufacturing. Soy yarns are pleasantly soft like cashmere. Soy garments (socks and underwear, sheets and scarves) hit the market in 2003. Of the Earth, an Oregon-based company, introduced its line of soy yoga wear in 2005, and recently EnvironGentle started selling a line of T-shirts called Tofu T's (see sources).

FABRIC TREATMENTS

Numerous fabric finishing treatments are applied to clothes during, and at the end of the manufacturing process. These include stain resistance, wrinkle resistance, fire retardants, and petroleum-based dyes—none of which are supportive of good health.

Stain and wrinkle resistance

No-iron clothes and nonstick pans have something in common—they both contain perfluorinated chemicals (PFCs). The same characteristics that keep food from sticking to pans also keep stains and wrinkles from adhering to clothing. PFCs are increasingly being used in synthetic clothing. Anything labeled static resistant, wrinkle resistant, permanent press, no-iron, or stainresistant contains PFCs. Permanent-press treatments applied to clothing may also cause new garments to release formaldehyde gas. Formaldehyde—a probable carcinogen—can cause flulike symptoms such as headache, fatigue, runny nose, and throat irritation when inhaled for long periods of time.

In 2005, ten Washington State residents agreed to the testing of their hair, blood, and urine for the presence of six toxic chemicals. PFCs were among those chemicals tested. PFCs were found in every participant at levels that approached those causing harm to laboratory animals.[229] Recommendations at the end of the study included avoidance of the following sources of PFCs:

- Stain-resistance treatments. Choose furniture, carpets, and clothing that aren't marketed as stain resistant and don't apply finishing treatments such as Stainmaster.
- Food packaging for oily and fast foods. The packages often contain grease-repellent coatings (e.g., microwave popcorn bags and french fry boxes).
- Personal care products made with Teflon or those containing ingredients that include the words fluoro or perfluoro. PFCs can be found in a variety of cosmetics, including nail polish, facial moisturizers, and eye makeup.

- Teflon or nonstick cookware. Discard products if nonstick Teflon coatings show signs of deterioration.

Flame retardants

Synthetic materials are either considered to be inherently flame resistant or they may be treated with flame retardants at the time the clothing or furniture is made. Flame-resistant polyester textiles can be manufactured with built-in fire retardants. During manufacture, fire retardants are chemically bound to the polymer, thus making it a part of the molecular structure. The enhanced polymers are stable enough that flame resistance is maintained throughout the life of the fabric. But like other polymers, chemicals are not likely to be 100 percent bound—tiny amounts leach out—especially as the fabric is used. To be considered flame resistant, other fibers such as cotton, nylon, acetate, and triacetate must be specifically treated with fire-retardant chemicals before sale. Flame-resistant garments are usually labeled Flame Resistant.

Brominated fire retardants (Polybrominated diphenyl ethers, or PBDEs) have replaced earlier fire retardants, which were banned in 1977 when they were found to be absorbed into children's bodies and when they were discovered to be carcinogenic in animal tests. Today, children's sleepwear and the clothing mandated for occupations that require fire protection contain PBDEs. These chemicals (now banned in Europe and parts of Asia) are no less harmful than their predecessors. They are persistent in the environment and bioaccumulative—they build up in the body over a lifetime and may cause liver toxicity, thyroid toxicity, and neurodevelopmental toxicity.[230] PBDEs impair attention, learning, memory, and behavior in laboratory animals at surprisingly low levels.[231]

Even though you may not be exposed to fire-retardant chemicals in your clothing, your furniture (and other décor) is still a likely source. Today, PBDEs as well as a chemical called chlorinated Tris are used as fire retardants in furniture, in spite of the fact that chlorinated Tris was one of the fire retardants banned from children's clothing in the 1970s. It was deemed by the Consumer Product Safety Commission to be a probable human carcinogen.[232]

> **The prevalence of PBDEs in the environment is raising concern among research scientists. Studies of peregrine falcon eggs and chicks reveal that birds are ingesting high levels of PBDEs, believed to leach out of foam mattresses, synthetic fabrics, plastic casings of televisions, electronics and other products that contain fire retardants. The level of PBDEs in falcon eggs approaches the level that has caused damage to developing neurological systems.**

PBDEs have increased fortyfold in human breast milk since the 1970s. Women in North America have up to seventy-five times the levels of women in Europe or Asia, where PBDEs have been banned.[233]

Dyes

In clothing, color has become a matter of personal expression. No wonder the vibrant colors produced from petroleum-based dyes have become so popular. But many dyes are toxic and contain heavy metals, like lead, to make them colorfast. Depending on their chemical makeup, dyes can be irritants, mutagens, highly toxic—even carcinogenic. Regardless of their hazards, dyes are not required to be listed on clothing or textile labels. The clothing you purchase may contain colorants chosen from hundreds of possibilities—some toxic, some not.

Conventional dyes may cause skin irritation. Their absorption through the skin may contribute to the ever-increasing burden of toxic chemicals that wreak havoc on our immune systems, nervous systems, and detoxification systems. Very little testing has been done. Perhaps this is why many consumers are demanding natural color and choosing sustainable alternatives that don't pollute the environment during their production and disposal. Even organic cotton clothing may be dyed using toxic dyes. Look for botanical dyes or mineral-based dyes. Coloring with clay is another option.

> **Believe it or not, cotton naturally grows in a variety of colors ranging from white to green, red, pink, and various shades of brown and gray. Cultivated for thousands of years, organic "color-grown" cotton offers an eco-friendly alternative to traditional dyes and colorants.** (see sources)

Dry cleaning

Conventional dry-cleaning fluids contain highly toxic chemicals, including tetrochloroethylene (also known as perchloroethylene), a carcinogen, central nervous system toxicant, and respiratory irritant. Other chemicals typically used in the dry-cleaning process include naphthalene—a suspected carcinogen and reproductive toxin, toluene—which may cause damage to a developing fetus and is neurotoxic, xylene—a neurotoxin, benzene, formaldehyde, and trichloroethylene—all of which are carcinogenic. Many of these substances are known to cause liver and kidney damage. Fumes from dry-cleaned clothing are a common indoor air pollutant. Exposure occurs as fumes evaporate (outgas) from clothing and when contact is made with skin.

If you must use conventional dry cleaning, remove the plastic bag and hang clothes outside or in an area separate from living quarters to encourage evaporation of solvents. This could take up to a week but will be faster in warmer temperatures. Dry-cleaning fluid has a half-life of forty days.

The best option is to avoid buying clothes that need to be dry cleaned. Some clothing marked "dry clean only" does not actually need to be dry cleaned. Manufacturers simply want to avoid disgruntled customers who may wash clothes incorrectly. Generally, you can wash almost anything without harm if you know how to do it properly. Washing clothes yourself and having them pressed by a dry cleaner can provide that crisp look without the chemical exposure. Water process dry cleaning is also available with some cleaners and is an excellent alternative to traditional dry cleaning.

UNDERGARMENTS

Of all the clothing you wear, underwear fits the most snuggly and covers critical areas of your body. The last places you want exposed to toxic chemicals are your genitals and breasts. These areas are already at risk, according to the myriad of studies revealing the consequences of toxic chemicals. Many toxins are endocrine disruptors. They mimic the female hormone estrogen, and they affect fertility, sperm count, testosterone levels, onset of puberty, and the risk of prostate and breast cancer. Phthalates in polyester fabrics are endocrine disruptors. Underwear, above other articles of clothing, should be made of organic, natural fiber.

Bras with underwires

Beyond the fabric itself, there is another toxic component in bras with underwires—the wire itself. The wire that makes these bras so supportive is the very thing that can create other problems for women. It is a little known fact that metal anywhere on your body negatively affects health. The critical factor is where the metal is located and how it affects the energy flow in your body.

Acupuncture is a therapy that has been used by the Chinese for thousands of years. Metal needles are placed into different parts of the body, called acupuncture points. These points are located along energy pathways called meridians. Modern science has confirmed the existence of these pathways and the existence of the various acupuncture points along them. Wherever metal is present near a meridian, it can distort the energy flow—especially long term. A woman may never realize it. The underwires in a bra fall directly on two important neurolymphatic acupuncture points. The one under the right breast provides energy to the liver and gall bladder. The one under the left breast provides energy to the stomach. Metallic stimulation of these points initially causes an increase in associated functions. Continued stimulation causes sedation of that point and a subsequent decrease in its associated functions. If a woman wears an underwire bra for an extended period of time, it can slowly and quietly impede the functioning of her liver, gall bladder, and stomach.

Underwires can be removed and replaced by plastic knitting needles if you are willing to go to the trouble. Put plastic needles of the same diameter as the underwire in a two hundred-degree oven. Gradually turn up the temperature until the needles are bendable. Bend and hold them to the proper curve while placing them in cool water to set the new shape. Cut them to length, sandpaper the ends, and insert them into the underwire slots—then stitch closed. Nursing bras may also provide the support without wire. Be careful not to wear bras that are too tight. This compresses the lymphatic tissue around breasts and impedes the normal lymphatic flow.

FAIR TRADE

The textile industry has notoriously been riddled with low wages and poor working conditions. Even today, much of the textile market is supplied by third-world countries where chemical exposure is common, working conditions are less than poor, and wages are no better. None of the major clothing companies have kept their hands clean when it comes to sweatshops. However, as the organic fiber market matures, producers are able to turn their attention to the manufacturing process, ensuring that workers have fair wages and healthy working conditions. Often, this comes through an affiliation with fair trade organizations.

Fair trade certification ensures that the clothing you buy supports workers, communities, and the environment through fair wages, equal employment, poverty reduction, sensitivity to native cultures, and sustainable production practices. Crafts and tropical foods such as coffee and chocolate currently dominate the available fair trade goods, but some clothing is also available, including shirts, T-shirts, scarves, and textiles. Fortunately, there are a number of small companies making pesticide-free, natural fiber, low-impact dyed, and sweatshop-free clothing. Because they are small, you may have to order online or through a catalog, but supporting fair trade ultimately supports us all. The Fair Trade Federation offers an online directory (www.fairtradefederation.com/mempro.html).

BEDDING AND DÉCOR

When you get comfortable at the end of the day and nestle underneath a comforter on the couch with a good book, the last thing you want to worry about is formaldehyde outgassing from the stain-resistant treatment on the couch or formaldehyde coming from fire retardants in the drapery. Neither do you want to worry that the polyester-filled comforter keeping you warm may be releasing phthlates that are being absorbed through your skin. Bedding and the textiles that make up the décor in your living environment can also be a source of toxins with the same chemicals found in clothing—often many times more concentrated.

Bedding

As a general rule, softer, breathable, natural fibers such as cotton and wool— even if they are not organically produced—are preferable to petrochemical fabrics like polyester. Polyester in sheets and blankets holds moisture next to your body all night, encouraging sweating and fungal problems. It's just like sleeping on plastic.

Also watch for fire retardants, mothproofing, and permanent-press treatments. When possible, choose bedding made of organic natural fibers. Although not always available in department stores, these items are available online. Read labels and ask manufacturers for details. As a precaution, wash all new bedding in hot water at least once (preferably twice) before use to reduce formaldehyde in fabric finishes. Although washing won't remove all chemicals, it can significantly reduce your exposure. A 1999 study found that a single washing of permanent-press fabrics reduced formaldehyde emissions by 60 percent.[234]

Drapes and upholstery

As with clothing and bedding, avoid drapery and upholstery textiles labeled permanent press, stain resistant, crease resistant, shrink-proof, stretch-proof, water repellent, and fire retardant. All will outgas formaldehyde.

Mattresses

Since 1973, the U.S. government has required that all mattresses and mattress pads meet requirements to reduce the risk of bed fires. To comply, mattresses and pads are treated with fire-retardant chemicals. The most widely used of these chemicals are the class known as polybrominated diphenyl ethers (PBDEs).

Today, the only way to purchase a cotton mattress without flame retardants is with a doctor's prescription verifying chemical sensitivities, or to purchase a mattress wrapped in a layer of wool (wool is naturally fire retardant).

Many mattress cores (the stuffing) contain polyurethane foam. These outgas volatile organic compounds (VOCs) associated with upper-respiratory problems and skin irritation. Natural latex mattress cores or cotton batting are preferred.

 (see Chapter 1: Volatile organic compounds)

The mattress foundation (the industry term for box springs) is either made of hardwood or less-expensive plywood or particleboard. Hardwood is preferred over plywood or particle board because those are treated with formaldehyde as a preservative.

 (see Chapter 10: Lumber)

The ideal mattress has a foundation made with natural, untreated, solid wood; a core of natural (not synthetic) latex or cotton batting; and it is topped with untreated, organic cotton and wool. Organic mattresses ensure against dioxins from the bleaching of both cotton and wool, and against dyes, color fixers (heavy metals such as chromium, copper, and zinc), and pesticides. There are many manufacturers that make high-quality organic mattresses (see sources).

SOURCES (in the order they appear in the chapter):

For a list of dozens of makers and retail outlets that sell organic, natural fiber clothing:
http://www.organicconsumers.org/btc/BuyingGuide.cfm

Soy clothing:
Of the Earth: http://www.vickerey.com/oftheearth
EnvironGentle: http://www.environgentle.com/

Colorgrown cotton:
FoxFiber™: http://www.vreseis.com/

Natural upholstery fabrics:
http://www.greensage.com/

Drapery fabrics:
White Lotus Home: www.whitelotus.net

Organic bedding:
Heart of Vermont: www.heartofvermont.com
Coyuchi: www.coyuchiorganic.com

Organic mattresses:
Naturepedic: http://www.naturepedic.com/
Nirvana Safe Haven: http://www.nontoxic.com/
Lifekind – www.organicmattresses.com

Chapter 10
HOME CONSTRUCTION AND REMODELING

✦

Lumber, insulation, floor coverings, paint/varnishes, lighting, and Feng Shui

The saying that epitomizes the green revolution is, *Think globally—act locally.* The construction industry is one area where implementing this philosophy can make a big difference for us all. Buildings have a profound effect on human health. Everything from the materials used in construction to the placement of walls, doorways, windows, and furniture can influence your health and the way you feel when you are inside. Buildings also have a substantial impact on the greater environment. For example, buildings use 40 percent of the total energy consumed on the planet every day, and construction waste constitutes 30 percent of our landfill space. The use of sustainable, nontoxic materials during construction can make a significant contribution to your health and to the health of the earth. Likewise, an understanding of energy flow can improve the energetic atmosphere of your home. This can further enhance your well-being.

Entire buildings have been condemned because of something called sick building syndrome, which is most often associated with newly constructed or remodeled buildings. This suggests that the chemicals used in construction products and furnishings are a major culprit. Construction materials are a major factor when it comes to indoor air quality. Lumber, vinyl, veneers, carpeting, adhesives, and sealants outgas volatile organic compounds (VOCs) for many months—often years. The VOCs in a new or remodeled home can be a tipping point for autism and multiple chemical sensitivity.

 (see Chapter 1: Sick building syndrome)

 (see Chapter 1: Volatile organic compounds)

Sustainable architecture or green home building refers to the design of buildings that enhance our living space without the use of toxic building materials. Sustainable architecture emphasizes the responsible use of resources, including land, energy, water, and materials. It focuses on nontoxic building supplies as well as those that do not pollute the environment, contribute to global warming, or deplete the earth's resources.

Sustainable building and remodeling can add a strong selling point for owners, designers, and contractors. It can often lower operating costs and reduce liability while contributing to the health, morale, and the productivity of occupants. Whether you are simply remodeling your kitchen or developing a commercial building, the use of nontoxic materials is a realistic option in today's world. In most cases, it is a matter of knowing there are choices.

A 2007 global survey estimated that the additional cost of building "green" was only 5 percent more than traditional building costs—with significant savings in energy efficiency that more than compensated for the additional up-front cost. As more people insist on sustainable materials, building codes will change, costs will go down, and the habitual use of toxic materials will eventually cease. Following the principles of *sustainable architecture* during construction, remodeling, or redecorating coupled with an understanding of energy movement can help you and your family enjoy a more natural living environment—one that is free of toxins as well as one that is energetically balanced.

LUMBER

The invention of pressed wood products was a boon to the construction industry and to the planet. It significantly reduced the amount of solid wood necessary for wood frame construction. Pressed-wood products offer many advantages. They can be made from almost any kind of wood and from all parts of the wood—there is little waste. Pressed-wood products— including plywood, oriented-strand board (OSB), laminated-strand lumber, particleboard, and medium-density fiberboard (MDF)—have the environmental advantage of being made from small-diameter, low-quality trees or waste from wood-processing operations, thus conserving higher-quality timber. MDF is actually made of sawdust. With these products, the wood is peeled into thin layers, chipped into small strands, or ground into wood flour. In each case, the pieces are then glued to produce a durable and stable lumber product.

But there is one significant drawback to pressed-wood products: they all require adhesives to bind the wood together—and the standard adhesives contain formaldehyde, a volatile compound that is classified as a known human carcinogen. Formaldehyde emissions can be recognized by the telltale sweet smell in most new kitchen and bath cabinets.

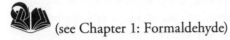 (see Chapter 1: Formaldehyde)

The adhesives in standard pressed-wood products contain either urea-formaldehyde (UF) resin or phenol-formaldehyde (PF) resin. PF resin is more chemically stable and water resistant than UF resin; it is used in pressed wood for outdoor use. UF resin is used in products for indoor use. Although UF binders are significantly less expensive than PF binders, they give off a lot more formaldehyde. For this reason, exterior grade plywood is sometimes more desirable for indoor applications. MDF—made from sawdust—contains a higher resin ratio than any other pressed-wood product. It is the highest formaldehyde-emitting wood product, resulting in long-term indoor formaldehyde emissions. Several particleboard products, including Roseburg, SkyBlend, and SierraPine Encore, use PF rather than UF binders in their pressed-wood production.

Because of concerns and in response to new California regulations that restrict formaldehyde emissions, the industry has begun to introduce other adhesive binders. Methyl diisocyanate (MDI) is a polyurethane binder that—once cured—is extremely stable with virtually no outgassing. However, it is extremely toxic during manufacture. Researchers at Oregon State University, inspired by the ability of mussels to form an extremely durable adhesion underwater, developed a formaldehyde-free, soy-based adhesive binder now used in Columbia Forest Products' PureBond hardwood plywood.

There are a number of alternatives to traditional plywood. One is to purchase pressed wood that is in conformance with American National Standards Institute (ANSI) criteria. These standards all specify lower formaldehyde emission levels. For particleboard flooring, look for ANSI grades PBU, D2, or D3 stamped on the panel. MDF should be in conformance with ANSI A208.2-1994. Hardwood plywood should be in conformance with ANSI/HPVA HP-1-1994.

There are also boards made from waste wheat or rice straw that are often stronger than MDF and just as workable. The pressure and heat during the process causes microscopic "hooks" on the straw to link together, reducing the need for adhesives. Particleboard made from straw uses MDI adhesives. Homasote, made of 100 percent recycled newspaper fiber, is another alternative that has actually been around longer than plywood. Its possible applications include structural roof decking, paintable interior panels, and concrete forms.

Wood is a renewable product and requires less energy than most materials to process into finished products. However, the logging, manufacture, transport, and disposal of wood products have substantial environmental impacts. Standard logging practices damage sensitive ecosystems, they reduce biodiversity, and they lead to soil erosion. The key to reducing these impacts is the minimization of wood use through material substitution, selection of wood from responsibly managed forests, and design and construction practices that control waste.

Forest Stewardship Council (FSC) certification is a widely recognized and respected standard for responsible forest management. FSC-labeled products are certified to be produced from responsibly managed forests. While not universally available, FSC certified wood is becoming easier to locate.

INSULATION

Like all glass products, fiberglass insulation is made primarily from silica. It is heated to high temperatures that require significant energy, and the process releases formaldehyde. Public health concerns from glass fibers are well documented, and short-term effects include irritation to eyes, nose, throat, lungs, and skin during installation or other contact. Longer-term effects are controversial, but fiberglass insulation is required to carry a cancer warning label. Binders in most fiberglass batts contain formaldehyde that is slowly emitted for months or years after installation, potentially contaminating indoor air.

There are *greener* options. Look for insulation that is free of formaldehyde, including the urea formaldehyde binders commonly used in fiberglass batts. Recycled cotton insulation insulates as well as fiberglass and offers superior noise reduction. Cotton insulation poses no lung cancer risk and is not irritating during installation. Cellulose (recycled newspaper) insulation also poses no risk of lung disease and offers superior insulation value (R-value). Both cotton and cellulose are treated with borate and make both materials more resistant to fire and insects than fiberglass.

If you use fiberglass, use recycled-content products, which save resources and landfill space. Recycled-content fiberglass insulation is becoming increasingly available (ask for minimum 25 percent postconsumer recycled content and minimum 50 percent total recycled content). Some products are designed with heavier glass fibers to reduce the fibers that can enter the lungs during installation.

FLOOR COVERINGS

The extraction, manufacture, and disposal of flooring material pollute air and water. Floor coverings (especially carpet, hardwood flooring, and vinyl) can also be major contributors to poor indoor air quality. This is due to the volatile organic compounds (VOCs) emitted from carpet backing, carpet padding, adhesives, and floor finishes. Since homes are now constructed more tightly in order to conserve energy, chemicals outgassing from flooring materials are more potent and harmful. Reducing the incidence of VOCs in the home can be achieved through alternative floor coverings.

The benefits of environmentally friendly flooring include reduced landfill waste, lower energy use, reduced impacts from harvest of materials (such as logging and the use of nonrenewable petroleum resources), reduced or eliminated outgassing, and easier cleaning. An excellent online resource for detailed information on many types of environmentally friendly flooring is http://www.greenfloors.com/.

Synthetic carpet

Carpet manufacture, use, and disposal have significant environmental and health concerns. Most carpet is synthetic—made of nonrenewable petroleum. Its manufacture requires substantial energy and water, and it creates harmful air contaminants during use. Synthetic carpet is not biodegradable. It is usually placed in a landfill at the end of its life. In 1999, roughly 2.4 million tons of carpet was discarded—enough to completely cover New York City.[235]

Synthetic carpet, backing, and adhesive typically outgas VOCs for many months. In addition to formaldehyde, carpet may contain numerous other chemicals, such as flame retardants, pesticides, toluene, benzene, styrene, and acetone. Besides the fact that carpet outgasses VOCs, babies and young children spend much of their time on the floor—later putting chemically contaminated hands into their mouths. Carpet backings of styrene butadiene rubber latex should be especially avoided.

If you must install synthetic carpeting, there are brands that are tested to emit fewer VOCs. Ask about the voluntary green label program for new carpet. The label tells consumers whether the carpet has been tested and passed green emissions criteria. There are also things you can do to limit your exposure during and after installation:

- Ask the retailer to unroll and air out the carpet in a well-ventilated area for at least a week before installation, or leave it in the sun a few days before you install it. If neither of these options is possible, consider turning up the heat as high as it will go for a week after installation. This will speed up the outgassing process. Leave the home during this period of time and air the house out before you return.

- Ask for low VOC-emitting adhesives if adhesives are necessary (see sources).
- During and after installation, ventilate the area with fresh outdoor air. Open all doors and windows.
- Use a carpet sealant called SafeChoice Carpet Seal made by AMF. It is designed to prevent the outgassing of harmful chemicals used in carpet backing (see sources).

Natural carpet fibers are an excellent alternative to synthetic carpet because they are renewable and biodegradeable. Options include jute, sisal, and coir floor coverings, as well as wool (see below).

Some carpet manufacturers have started recycling programs with their carpet products. At the end of the carpet's useful life, the manufacturer takes the product back and uses it to make new carpet. Synthetic carpets that are recycled can dramatically reduce the flow of carpet to the landfill.

Carpet tiles are another alternative to traditional wall-to-wall carpeting. They limit waste and are economically feasible because worn or stained tiles can be replaced without completely recarpeting the entire room. However, before you choose carpeting (natural or synthetic), consider the other options for flooring discussed in the remainder of this chapter.

Natural fiber carpet and rugs

There are many natural fibers now available for rugs and carpeting. They are rougher than synthetic fibers but have the advantage of being, renewable, biodegradable, and nontoxic.

Wool

Natural (organic) wool carpeting is extremely beautiful—especially when no dyes or unnatural elements are used during the manufacturing process. Wool is used extensively by those with chemical sensitivity. The primary backing is made of a combination of hemp (durable, strong, and mold and mildew resistant), and cotton. Organic wool yarns are locked into place with a natural latex adhesive derived from the rubber tree. This adhesive is completely biodegradable and nontoxic. Since wool is naturally flame resistant, no fire retardants are necessary. Both the carpet and the carpet pad are completely biodegradable. At the end of the life of the carpet, consumers are encouraged to use the carpet pad as a weed barrier or mulch in the garden during decomposition. Over a period of two to three seasons, the padding will completely disappear. A search for "organic wool carpeting" on the Internet will bring up numerous suppliers.

Other natural fibers

Sisal, seagrass, jute, and coir (coconut fiber) are all-natural plant fibers that can be used as wall-to-wall carpeting but are most often used as area rugs. They have a rougher texture than standard carpeting, but some of the weaves are amazingly beautiful and elegant. This Web site will get you started: http://www.fibreworks.com.

Hardwood floors

Hardwood floors are beautiful—and expensive. They also deplete a resource that is rapidly diminishing. Hardwood flooring can also be a major source of VOCs in the indoor environment—emitting high levels of formaldehyde. Not only is there formaldehyde in the wood itself, but standard hardwood finishes emit high levels of formaldehyde. In a study of the emissions of a wide variety of known indoor formaldehyde-emitting products, wood floor finishes were the highest.[236] If you have hardwood floors, choose a low VOC finish (see sources), and if you decide to use hardwood flooring in a remodeling or construction project, take into consideration the management practices of the source. Forest Stewardship Council (FSC) certification is a respected standard for responsible forest management. Columbia Forest Products recently released a line of formaldehyde-free, FSC-certified, engineered hardwood flooring to the commercial market (see sources).

There are also other *engineered* wood products on the market that utilize reclaimed wood. Flooring manufactured with salvaged wood is also an option to conserve resources; look for the SmartWood Rediscovered label. It may be necessary to plan ahead if large quantities are needed because availability can be an issue. Engineered wood rather than solid wood can also be used for flooring, especially if the product has a thick veneer (more than one-eighth inch thick) that allows for refinishing. Using shorter planks or parquet-style flooring makes use of leftover pieces.

Laminated wood flooring

Laminate wood flooring which mimics the appearance of a hardwood floor offers many possibilities for consumers looking for do-it-yourself flooring with the durability and look of hardwood. Many of the adhesives and coatings used in the manufacture of laminate flooring are water-based products, so laminate flooring comes free of solvents and wood preservatives. However, there are still some environmental concerns.

Look for products assembled with nonformaldehyde or non-urea-formaldehyde binders. Polyurethane binders such as MDI or PMDI are a better alternative. Also, look for low-VOC adhesives or choose floating options that snap together rather than use adhesives (see sources).

Vinyl flooring (polyvinyl chloride - PVC)

Vinyl (another name for PVC plastic) is common in flooring, siding, window frames, wall coverings, and roofing. It is pervasive because of its benefits: strength, durability, light weight, water resistance, and low cost. But the dramatic health and environmental liabilities of vinyl call for other options—especially in the indoor environment. Concerns with vinyl flooring include:

- Vinyl is derived from petroleum. Its manufacture is energy-intensive. It produces emissions of toxic air pollutants, and it generates hazardous wastes during disposal.
- Vinyl flooring tile and sheeting outgas VOCs.
- Plasticizers (such as phthalates) are required to make PVC flexible. Over time, phthalates can leach out or outgas, exposing building occupants to materials that have been linked with reproductive system damage and cancer.
- Chlorine is a key component of vinyl resin, accounting for more than half its weight. When PVC burns, its smoke contains dioxins—among the most toxic chemicals known to man.
- Lead, cadmium, and other heavy metals are also used in some PVC products. This can be a problem when vinyl floors are installed in homes with small children.

Vinyl poses so many problems during production, use, and disposal that many governments are banning its use.[237] Linoleum is a natural alternative to vinyl flooring that is nontoxic, biodegradable, and more durable.

ALTERNATIVES TO CARPET, VINYL, AND HARDWOOD FLOORING
Bamboo

Bamboo flooring is comparable to most hardwoods—in price, appearance, and durability. It also offers several advantages for conscientious, discriminating consumers. Bamboo flooring has been found to be harder than some oak and beachwood and more durable than most hardwoods. And unlike wood flooring, which can buckle or gap, bamboo is considered to have excellent stability; it can carry a warranty for up to twenty-five years.

Bamboo is a member of the grass family. It grows rapidly and matures in less than four years. Like grass, cutting bamboo does not kill the plant.

An extensive root system remains intact, allowing for rapid regeneration. This makes bamboo an ideal sustainable floor covering. Because bamboo floors can also be made with glues and finishes containing formaldehyde, look for bamboo flooring that is certified formaldehyde-free. Choosing a nonformaldehyde-based adhesive will also help to reduce the chances of outgassing (see sources).

Cork

Cork is another natural, sustainable choice. The renewable bark of the cork oak tree can be harvested every nine years without harm to the tree. Cork provides acoustical and thermal insulation, it is resistant to moisture damage and decay, and it is easy to clean. If you like walking barefoot in your home, you'll love natural cork flooring because cork feels warm and soft to the touch. Its quiet, clean surface is also extremely durable.

> **Properly cared for, a cork floor should last for decades, and prices are comparable to hardwood flooring.**

Natural cork flooring is different from the widely marketed cork-vinyl composite floor tile. Cork-vinyl products have a vinyl surface layer—little better than traditional vinyl flooring.

Linoleum

Linoleum, invented nearly 150 years ago, is resilient, natural flooring made of raw materials that are available in abundance: linseed oil (from flax), pine resin, wood flour, cork powder, limestone dust, natural pigments and jute. It is completely biodegradable, it is naturally antimicrobial, and it emits very low VOCs. Compared with vinyl flooring, linoleum is also more durable, lasting up to forty years.

Linoleum is inherently antistatic. It repels dust and dirt; occasional polishing is all that is necessary to maintain a glossy appearance. Waxes and chemical sealers are not usually necessary, but if you use a sealer, be sure to use a low VOC product (see sources).

CAUTION: Even though linoleum emits lower levels of VOCs than vinyl, the resins from linseed oil can cause difficulty for chemically sensitive individuals. Linoleum is also not recommended for large areas where children spend a great deal of time. Linoleum should not be placed in a basement. High moisture levels will seep up through the natural ingredients of the linoleum.

Tile

Tile continues to grow in popularity as an eco-friendly floor covering. It has a natural, handcrafted look that is durable and easy to care for. Design patterns are limitless when using all of the possible combinations of size, texture, and color. Recycled-content tile adds an additional advantage and makes use of otherwise wasted by-products utilizing glass, used tiles, granite dust, stone tailings, or unfired material from landfills. Manufacturers now offer more styles, sizes, and colors than ever before.

Many different kinds of tile are available including ceramic, porcelain, slate, stone, brick, saltillo, and terrazzo. All require sealants to protect them from moisture. When choosing a sealant, consider using only silicone sealants in interior areas. All other sealant types, especially the butyl sealants, emit VOCs and other toxic compounds. AMF makes a number of sealants for a variety of applications (see sources).

PAINT AND VARNISH

Paint, stain, and transparent finishes contain many toxins that release low-level toxic emissions into the air for years after application. In general, oil-based or alcohol-based paint contains higher levels of VOCs than latex or water-based paint. But even latex paint is highly toxic. It harms fish and wildlife; it contaminates the food chain, pollutes groundwater, and increases the cost of water treatment. Latex paint can also have an adverse effect on your health. If used in closed areas, its chemical components can irritate eyes, skin, and lungs and cause headaches and nausea. It can also contribute to respiratory problems, muscle weakness, and liver and kidney damage.

Until recently, VOCs were an inevitable consequence of the performance of paint. Today that does not have to be the case. Numerous nontoxic or low-VOC versions are available. Most paint manufacturers now produce one or more varieties of low-VOC paint. These new paints are durable, cost-effective, and less harmful to human and environmental health. There are three general categories of nontoxic (or low-toxic) paint: natural paint, zero VOC, and low VOC. Even zero-VOC formulations contain some small amounts of toxins.

Natural paint

Natural Paint is the safest for your health and for the environment. It is made from natural raw ingredients such as water, plant oils and resins, plant dyes, and essential oils; natural minerals such as clay, chalk, and talcum; milk casein, natural latex, bees' wax, earth, and mineral dyes. Water-based natural paint gives off almost no smell. Oil-based natural paint usually has a pleasant fragrance of citrus or essential oils. Allergies and sensitivities to natural paint are uncommon (see sources).

Zero-VOC paint

Any paint with VOCs in the range of five grams/liter or less can be called zero VOC according to the EPA. Some manufacturers may claim zero VOCs, but these paints may still use colorants, biocides, and fungicides with some VOCs. Adding a color tint usually brings the VOC level up to ten grams/liter, which is still quite low (see sources).

Low-VOC paint

Low-VOC paint, stain, and varnish use water instead of petroleum-based solvents. The level of harmful emissions is lower than solvent-based paint. These certified coatings also contain no or very low levels of heavy metals and formaldehyde. The amount of VOCs varies among different low-VOC products and is listed on the paint can. To meet the standard, these paints must not contain VOCs in excess of 200 grams per liter (g/L). Varnishes must not contain VOCs in excess of 300 g/L. As a general rule, low-VOC paint marketed by reputable paint manufacturers usually meets the 50 g/L VOC threshold. Paints with the Green Seal Standard (GS-11) are certified lower than 50 g/L. If you are particularly sensitive, make sure the paint you buy contains fewer than 25 g/L of VOCs. (see sources)

Although indoor paint is now virtually lead-free, older housing and furniture built before 1978 may still be coated with leaded paint. Often, lead paint is exposed during renovation projects. Under these circumstances, lead dust and fumes can permeate the air inhaled by both adults and children. Take precautions during renovation projects and call a professional if you suspect lead-based paint. Sealants are also available to seal older paint (see sources),

Remember to store paint away from the living area and to dispose of it properly. Contact your local environmental health, solid waste, or public works department to find out about household hazardous waste collection programs in your area. These programs have been set up to collect, reuse, and recycle leftover paint.

Painting tips

1. When selecting paint, look for:

- VOC content: Usually listed in grams per liter, this can range from 5 to 200.
- Solids content: Solids, or pigments, can range in concentration from 25 to 45 percent by volume. The higher the percent solids, the less VOCs in the paint.
- EPA, OSHA, DOT registrations: When a product has an EPA, OHSA, or DOT registration number, this means that it contains

toxic ingredients that must be monitored. One way to ensure that you are using a product that is safe, both for the environment and the applicator, is to seek out products that are not registered with these agencies.

2. Reuse turpentine and paint thinners. Allow used thinner or turpentine to stand in a closed, labeled container until paint or dirt particles settle to the bottom. Pour off the clear liquid and reuse.

3. Avoid cleaning brushes and rollers. Paint brushes and rollers used for an ongoing project can be saved overnight, or even up to a week, without cleaning at all. Simply wrap the brush or roller snugly in a plastic bag, squeeze out air pockets and store away from light. (This works for water and oil-based paints and stains. It does not work for varnishes or lacquers.)

4. Turpentine, made from the resin of coniferous trees, is an environmentally friendly solvent. It is excellent for cleaning brushes used with oil-based paints and for cleaning up small drips. Use a short, glass jar filled no higher than the bristles. Add a few drops of dishwashing liquid. After cleaning the brush, rinse with water.

5. You can reduce fresh paint odors by placing a small dish of white vinegar in the room.

6. Beware of old lead paint. Paint manufactured before the 1970s contains lead. If the paint is still in good shape, you can paint over it, or leave it—lead is only poisonous if ingested or inhaled. If paint must be removed in small areas, wet the surface and scrape carefully. Never sand dry lead paint. Clean up with trisodium phosphate. For large areas, call in a professional certified in lead abatement.

7. Leftover paint can be saved for months if stored properly. Make sure the lids are well sealed—then store the cans upside down. This prevents air from getting inside the can and causing the paint to thicken and dry.

8. Dispose of leftover paint responsibly. Contact your local waste management facility to find out what to do with leftover paint.

9. Consumers can help speed the development and lower the cost of nontoxic paints by choosing products that contain fewer hazardous ingredients. Choosing to use nontoxic, environmentally safe paints and stains can also greatly reduce the amount of toxins in the air, water, and soil.

WALL COVERINGS
Wallpaper

Conventional wallpaper outgasses VOCs and is often printed with toxic ink. It may contain vinyl (PVC), mold inhibitors, pesticides, and other chemicals. Wallpaper paste also contains harmful chemicals that may outgas for months. Combined, these can create toxic indoor air. Vinyl wallpaper is one of the worst.

Vinyl wallpaper

Because vinyl wall coverings form a moisture barrier, they encourage the growth of mold beneath the wallpaper. This is especially true where air conditioning or heating systems produce a significant temperature/humidity difference between the room and the air inside the wall. Some molds produce toxic substances that are suspected causes of respiratory and neurological problems. Vinyl has been cited as the interior building material most likely to facilitate the growth of these molds.[238] Numerous liability suits have been filed because of the growth of mold beneath vinyl wallpaper. There are numerous nontoxic wallpapers now being made—and a variety of choices in alternative wall coverings.

Nontoxic, sustainable wallpaper

Sustainable (Earth-friendly) wallpaper focuses on lower levels of energy use, waste reduction, recycling, eco-friendly packaging, and energy efficient distribution. Wood-based wallpaper can be sourced from sustainably managed forests. Many vinyl-free wallpaper choices are now available that will not outgas VOCs. Even silk-screened, cotton wallpaper made with water-based, nontoxic ink and water-based glaze is available (see silk-screened wallpaper in sources).

Wallpaper alternatives

In addition to the more traditional-looking wallpaper, many plant fibers are now used as wall coverings. Referred to as grasscloth, they can be made of a number of different grasses including arrowroot, bamboo, jute, seagrass, and sisal. This type of textured wallpaper is suitable for covering walls that have imperfections but not for areas with high levels of moisture. Natural grass wallpapers are sustainable and renewable resources that are harvested either biyearly or yearly and typically backed with recycled paper.

Wallpaper adhesive

Conventional wallpaper paste may contain polymers, mold inhibitors, pesticides, and other chemicals. Today, other options are available. Ask for a water-based, fungicide-free adhesive, or make your own following the recipe below:

Homemade Wallpaper Paste

1 cup flour (wheat, corn, or rice)
3 teaspoons alum
Water
10 drops oil of cloves (natural preservative)

Combine the flour and alum in a double boiler. (If you don't have a double boiler, set a smaller pan inside a bigger one that contains enough water that can be brought to a boil without overflowing). Add enough water to make a consistency of heavy cream; stir until blended. Heat, stirring constantly until the mixture has thickened to a gravy-like texture. Let cool. Stir in the clove oil. Pour into a glass jar with a screw top. Apply with a glue brush. Makes 1 cup. This recipe will keep in the refrigerator for 2 weeks.

LIGHTING

Light has been valued throughout history as a source of healing. Today, the therapeutic aspects of light are being reevaluated in major research centers around the world. At the same time, many people are concerned with the huge energy expenditure involved in lighting commercial buildings and homes. The use of fluorescent lighting to conserve energy and to reduce greenhouse gas emissions is being advocated by a growing number of people. There are many issues to consider when it comes to choosing lighting for your home or office.

Fluorescent lighting

Fluorescent lighting is about 65 percent more energy efficient than standard incandescent lighting. It can significantly reduce energy costs and reduce the emission of greenhouse gases. For these reasons, fluorescent lighting is becoming increasingly popular. The advent of compact fluorescent light (CFL) bulbs to replace incandescent lighting in homes has made the use of fluorescent lighting even more convenient. However, standard (cool-white) fluorescent light has been suspected for a long time of contributing to a wide variety of health problems—everything from eye strain to anxiety. In 1999, a team of scientists showed that fluorescent light caused free radical damage to the DNA of the eyes that could not be entirely repaired.[239] These scientists recommended limited exposure to fluorescent lighting.

Even before this research, it was widely known that the most harmful light for eyes is in the blue to violet range, with wavelengths from 430 to 440 nanometers (nm). Unfortunately, standard fluorescent lamps emit a large portion of their total energy in a narrow spike at 435.8 nm, precisely in the most eye-damaging region. Adult humans are somewhat protected from this damage because of yellowing of the retina with age, which filters out much of the blue and violet. However, these harmful wavelengths can freely penetrate into the more transparent eyes of children. They can cause an accelerated destruction of photoreceptors and a diminished ability to self-repair. This ultimately leads to the degeneration of the macula in later years.

The eye disease now known as age-related macular degeneration used to be called senile macular degeneration because people suffered from it only in their old age—typically in their eighties or nineties. Over the past two decades, this degeneration has begun to start earlier and earlier, to the point where millions of Americans now lose their central vision in their fifties and sixties. Age-related macular degeneration has become the most common cause of irreversible vision loss in the Western world. Many scientists believe this is due to indoor lighting—specifically the overabundant use of fluorescent lights. The issue has not been studied officially, so there is presently no proven link between the exposure to fluorescent light and the earlier appearance of macular degeneration. On the other hand, basic logic and prudence suggest the limitation of fluorescent lighting until its long-term safety can be established.

There is a movement to convert to the total use of fluorescent bulbs to save energy, but fluorescent light poses anther potential problem—mercury. Few people are aware of the small print on the inside of the package of fluorescent lighting, indicating that these bulbs/tubes contain mercury. According to California Assembly Bill 1109 (2007) Section (e):

> *Most fluorescent lighting products contain hazardous levels of mercury ... The hazardous materials in these products can be managed through recycling, but current recycling opportunities and levels are virtually nonexistent for most consumers.*

Fluorescent lighting products that deliver the same level of light and the same level of energy efficiency can have widely varying levels of mercury. Some fluorescent lamps have as little as 3.5 mg mercury, but some have as much as 40 mg. The average mercury content of a four-foot tube manufactured today is approximately 12 mg. Bulbs manufactured in the mid-1980s and earlier contained 40 mg. or more. Product labels are not required to designate the level of mercury so that consumers can pick the bulbs with the lowest level of mercury.

Low-mercury fluorescent lightbulbs/tubes contain less mercury than conventional fluorescent bulbs. They are labeled low mercury for identification by the consumer. Low-mercury fluorescent tubes are commonly called green-tips since they have green metallic ends to help distinguish them from conventional tubes. Even though these products contain less mercury than standard products, they are still considered hazardous waste and should be disposed of properly.

Consumers have not been educated as to the dangers of mercury, nor to procedures for clean up if they break. And perhaps more importantly, consumers are unaware of the danger to the environment. If the new energy-efficient CFLs replace incandescent bulbs and measures are not put into place for their proper disposal, they will contribute to the mercury already being placed in landfills.

According to a study released in 2003, between 17 and 40 percent of the mercury in broken low-mercury fluorescent bulbs is released to the air during a two-week period immediately following breakage, with higher temperatures contributing to higher release rates. One-third of the mercury release occurs during the first eight hours after breakage.[240] Every consumer using fluorescent lighting in their home should know what to do in case one of these lamps breaks:

Officially Recommended Handling of Broken Fluorescent Lamps[241]

> If a lamp breaks in your home, close off the room to other parts of the building. Open a window to disperse any vapor that may escape, and leave the room for at least 15 minutes. Carefully scoop up the fragments with a stiff paper (do not use your hands) and wipe the area with a disposable paper towel to remove all glass fragments. Do not use a vacuum as this disperses the mercury over a wider area. All fragments should be placed in a sealed plastic bag and properly disposed of.

Everyone, especially pets (who will pick up mercury and track it into other areas), should be removed from the area of the spill. The ventilation systems should be turned off from the area. Rubber gloves should be used to clean up the spill and shoes should be wiped off when clean-up is complete (and the paper towel placed with the debris for disposal). If a lamp is broken on carpet, contaminated items should be thrown away.

If you choose to use CFLs, make sure you and your family understand how to dispose of them properly. To find out if there are recycling options near you, call 1-800-CLEAN-UP for an automated hotline or visit www.earth911.org. (At the top of the earth911.org home page, enter your zip code and press "go." Click on the "Household Hazardous Waste" link, then the "fluorescent bulbs" link. This page will identify the nearest mercury recycling or disposal facility near you. If the page contains no specific information on CFLs, go back and click on the link for "Mercury Containing Items.")

A 2008 investigation conducted by the Environmental Working Group identified seven lines of CFL bulbs that were superior to the rest. These bulbs, listed in their Green Lighting Guide, which is available online, contain a fraction of the mercury allowed by Energy Star.[242] All the identified bulbs last longer than the Energy Star standard of six thousand hours, and all the recommended bulbs are energy efficient.

Full-spectrum lighting
Full-spectrum lighting can have therapeutic value on a variety of conditions, including depression, insomnia, fatigue, hyperactivity, osteoporosis, and metabolic imbalances. There is also growing evidence that light can impact circadian rhythms and that specific light wavelengths are necessary to promote optimal health.[243] However, most artificial lighting lacks the complete balanced spectrum of light naturally available from the sun. Among other things, this imbalance can interfere with the absorption of nutrients and can contribute to suppressed immune function and hyperactivity in children. During a study of first grade children, full spectrum lighting significantly reduced hyperactivity over the course of the semester. Children in classrooms with standard fluorescent lighting actually became more hyperactive as the semester progressed.[244]

 (see Chapter 17: Full-spectrum lighting)

Components of good full-spectrum light
In order to achieve natural balanced light, bulbs must emit a full spectrum of color. Additionally, true full-spectrum lighting should contain infrared and ultraviolet wavelengths. Although there are several incandescent bulbs marketed as full spectrum, the incandescent technology cannot produce a *true* full-spectrum emission. These bulbs are certainly a step in the right direction, and they may be a good choice for some applications (see sources). However, the new compact fluorescent bulbs are currently the best choice for full-spectrum light. This technology can come very close to true full-spectrum light. But just because a bulb says "full spectrum" doesn't mean that it is. Some brands are only marginally better than cool-white fluorescent bulbs.

The Correlated Color Temperature (CCT) rating is a general indication of the warmth of a bulb's light. Lamps with a lower color temperature (3500 Kelvin or less) have a warm or reddish-yellow appearance. Lamps with a midrange color temperature (3500K to 4100K) have a neutral or white appearance. Lamps with a higher color temperature (4100K or higher) have a cool or bluish-white appearance. Summer sunlight at noon on a clear day has a very cool appearance at about 5500K. Sunlight is saturated in green and blue wavelengths.

Another term to understand in evaluating the quality of full spectrum lighting is Color Rendering Index or CRI. This describes how a light source makes the color of an object appear to human eyes. CRI is expressed as a rating from 0 to 100—the higher the CRI rating, the better its color rendering ability. Standard cool-white fluorescent bulbs have a CCT rating of about 4200K and a CRI rating of about 62. Some fluorescent bulbs that are being marketed as full spectrum lights have CCT ratings between 3000–4100K, and CRI ratings between 80–85. While this is better than standard cool-white lighting, superior brands are available. Full Spectrum Solutions makes a line of fluorescent bulbs called BlueMax with CCT ratings between 5000–5900K and CRI ratings between 90–95 (depending o the type of bulb) (see sources). Balanced, full-spectrum lighting (the same wavelengths provided by the sun) can go a long way toward improving your indoor environment and supporting your health.

Light-emitting diode (LED) lighting

LED (light-emitting diode) lighting promises to solve both the energy and the pollution problems of traditional lighting. LED lighting is energy efficient; it burns with low CO_2 emissions; and it contains no mercury. These lightbulbs (originally only available for flashlights) are extremely bright and burn with little heat. A 10-watt bulb replaces a 100-watt incandescent bulb and will last up to fifty thousand hours.

Unlike fluorescent lights, which need time to warm up, LED lights turn on instantly when you flip the switch. They can also be turned on and off endlessly with no harm or degradation to the life of the bulb. One drawback to LED lights is that they are directional. They are not appropriate for use in lamps with lamp shades or other lighting applications where light needs to be emitted in all directions at once. However, the light pattern produced by LED lighting is remarkably smooth, with no shadows or hot spots. Even though LED lightbulbs are currently very expensive, in the long run they may still save money. The next several years will see these products come down in price. Watch for this technology to replace both incandescent and fluorescent lightbulbs (see sources).

FENG SHUI

Feng Shui is a Chinese term that means "the way of wind and water." It is part of an ancient Chinese philosophy concerned with understanding the relationship between nature, energy, and ourselves. Other cultures have different terms for similar concepts; Europeans use the term geomancy. Feng Shui has also been referred to as "the art of placement"—a tool for creating the energy in your environment to support balance and positive change.

According to Candace Czarry, author and professional in energy and environmental design, Feng Shui is a metaphor for conscious living. It is the art of choosing energy fields and vibrations to your benefit.[245] Feng Shui can be a very powerful tool. Architects have used the principles of Feng Shui for the layout and design of many powerful cities, including Washington DC. All the major buildings in Hong Kong are constructed using the principles of Feng Shui. Today, the same principles are used by large corporations in the design of buildings—to enhance sales and to improve productivity. Donald Trump and Merrill Lynch incorporate the principles in the design of their buildings.[246]

To the Western mind, Feng Shui can seem complex and almost superstitious. Many Westerners have shied away from the practice of Feng Shui simply because they have not understood the power of energy. However, those who have taken the time to apply the principles have generally been pleasantly rewarded. By recognizing the connection you have with your living environment and by making conscious alterations in that environment, you bring energy to your desires for such areas as greater harmony in relationships, career, and finances. A delightful and highly recommended way to learn Feng Shui while balancing the energy of your home is available online: http://www.artofplacement.com/FengShui/20MinuteFengShui.htm.

SOURCES (in the order they appear in the chapter):

Sustainable building material suppliers:
www.sustainableabc.com/

Environmentally preferable building materials:
http://www.oikos.com/

Carpet Sealant:
SafeChoice Carpet Seal made by AMF: http://www.afmsafecoat.com/index.php

Low VOC adhesives:
EnviroTech adhesive: www.environproducts.com
Titebond Solvent Free Construction Adhesive: www.environmentalhomecenter.com
Dri-Tac Flooring Adhesive for cork flooring: http://www.dritac.com/

Floor and lead paint sealants:
Safecoat Safe Seal (low-VOC sealer); MexeSeal, Paver Seal, and WaterShield (water- and stain-proofing): www.afmsafecoat.com
OS Hardwax Oil (finish): www.environmentalhomecenter.com

FSC-certified hardwood flooring:
Columbia forest Products: http://www.columbiaforestproducts.com/

Laminated wood flooring without adhesives:
Unilin Quick-Step: www.quick-step.com
Pergo Presto: www.pergo.com
KronoSwiss Crystal Clic also uses FSC-certified materials: www.kronoswiss.com

Bamboo flooring:
Plyboo: http://www.plyboo.com/

Natural Paint:
The Real Milk Paint Company: Nontoxic paint made with milk protein, lime, clay and earth pigments: www.realmilkpaint.com
Aglaia www.aglaiapaint.com
Livos: Organic paint with linseed oil and citrus oil, designed primarily for wood: www.livos.us
Auro: www.aurousa.com

BioShield (EcoDesign): www.bioshieldpaint.com

Weather-Bos: Natural oils and resins designed to adhere to wood: www.weatherbos.com

Silacote: For use on masonry, concrete, and wallboard; interior/exterior: www.silacote.com

Anna Sova: Natural paints from milk casein, titanium dioxide, and food-grade ingredients www.annasova.com

Green Planet Paints: Natural clay paints for interiors using Mayan clay pigments www.greenplanetpaints.com

Zero-VOC Paint

AFM Safecoat: Flat interior latex; semi-gloss interior enamel: www.afmsafecoat.com

Best Paint Company: Zero-VOC interior paints, primers, and specialty products www.bestpaintco.com

ICI Decra-Shield: Exterior zero-VOC paints

Devoe Wonder Pure: Odor-free interior acrylic latex paints: www.devoepaint.com

Ecoshield: Zero-VOC, low odor, ethylene glycol-free interior paints: www.dunnedwards.com

American Pride – Zero-VOC interior latex and acrylic enamel paints www.americanpridepaint.com

Sherwin Williams: Harmony line of zero-VOC, low-odor latex interior paints www.sherwin.com

Frazee Paint EnviroKote: Interior zero-VOC paints: semi-gloss, flat, and primer

Allied PhotoChemical: Zero-VOC, UV-curable paints, inks, and coatings to manufacturers. www.alliedphotochemical.com

Olympic Paint and Stain: Zero-VOC Olympic Premium interior line

Yolo Colorhouse: Zero-VOC, low-odor, premium interior paint: www.yolocolorhouse.com

Green Planet Paints: Zero-VOC, clay-based interior paints: www.greenplanetpaints.com

Benjamin Moore Pristine EcoSpec: Zero-VOC, semi-gloss finishes and a primer

Low-VOC paint:

Benjamin Moore Aura: Low-VOCs: www.myaurapaints.com

Benjamin Moore Saman: Water-based wood stains

Cloverdale Horizon: Flat, eggshell, semi-gloss interior enamels
Cloverdale EcoLogic: Low-VOCs flat, eggshell, semi-gloss interior
MAB Paints: Enviro-Pure interior latex zero-VOC line
Miller Paint: Acro solvent-free interior acrylic line
Vista Paint: Carefree Earth Coat line
PPG Architectural Finishes: Pittsburgh Paints Pure Performance line

Silk-screened wallpaper:
Mod Green Pod: http://www.modgreenpod.com/

Wallpaper remover:
Dif made by Zissner: http://www.zinsser.com/

Full-spectrum lighting:
BlueMax: www.fullspectrumsolutions.com
Incandescent full spectrum: http://bluesbuster.com/

LED lighting:
http://www.betterlifegoods.com/ProductDetails.
asp?ProductCode=LED%2DCAT21417

 Recommended Reading:
Optimum Environments for Optimum Health & Creativity: Designing and Building a Healthy Home or Office by Dr. William Rea, MD

Prescriptions for a Healthy House, by Paula Baker-Laporte, Erika Elliott, John Banta and Lisa Flynn

Chapter 11

HOW DOES YOUR GARDEN GROW?

The human race is undergoing a transition—especially when it comes to gardening. This transition reflects a partnership with nature rather than domination.

> We consider an environment to be "nature friendly" when ...
> humans understand that nature is a full partner in the design
> and operation of [the] environment.[247]
> —Perelandra Garden Workbook

A new consciousness has emerged among gardeners, both professional and amateur. Sensitivity to the earth is being cultivated on many fronts. Many people are returning to the natural, to the simple, and to the basic. Gardeners are recognizing that their participation with nature and their connection with the earth is as much a part of the process of gardening as the enjoyment of the vegetables and/or the flowers they grow. Today, more and more homeowners are collecting rainwater, composting their kitchen garbage, and learning to work with nature to produce a portion of their own food. Perhaps more importantly, they are stepping away from the toxic pesticides and inorganic fertilizers that poison the earth, upset the ecosystem, and destroy food value. Even the purchase of flowers now includes organic options.

This chapter discusses the difficulties with toxic pesticides and synthetic fertilizers and offers alternatives that will support the rebuilding of the soil and the balancing of the ecosystem.

PESTICIDES

Pesticides are poisons—intended to kill. They get into the human body and into the brain the same way they are designed to get into plants and insects. Because we are larger than insects, the effects appear to be harmless. But nothing could be further from the truth. The effects of pesticides are so insidious that they often go unnoticed until their effects creep up on the next generation.

Pesticides cause difficulties that were never considered possible. Only during the last decade have we begun to connect the dots and to discover the far-reaching consequences that pesticides are having on the human family. Pesticides are persistent. Like other synthetic chemicals, they do not break down easily. They quietly build up and slowly poison the environment and the human body.

Pesticides affect the growing fetus. Recent studies indicate that tiny amounts transferred from mother to unborn child cause birth defects—often the smaller the amount, the greater the effect. And worse, pesticides appear to affect children even before they are conceived—the result of genetic damage to the parents. In a study of over two hundred thousand live births in Minnesota between 1989 and 1992, pesticide applicators' children had a higher percentage of birth defects. The same was true of children born in the agricultural region of the state where pesticides were routinely used.[248]

Pesticides also affect childhood development. One of the most revealing studies was conducted in Sonora, Mexico, where preschool-aged children living in areas where agricultural pesticides were frequently applied were compared with children living in the foothills where pesticide use was avoided. Pesticide-exposed children demonstrated a decrease in stamina, eye-hand coordination, memory, and in the ability to draw. Children from the foothills drew figures with features—typical of normal four- and five-year-old children. The children exposed to pesticides lacked the ability to draw with any detail.[249]

A large proportion of all the pesticides used today are neurotoxic (toxic to the brain and nervous system). Recent experiments indicate that tiny doses of combinations of pesticides, equivalent to levels found in drinking water today, caused both aggression and learning problems in rats.[250] Could this be an explanation for the growing amount of violent behavior in our schools and on the road? Could it explain attention deficit? Some scientists think the answer to both of these questions is yes. Pesticides also affect the thyroid gland, which controls the brain, sexual development, numerous hormones, and immune function. The effects of pesticides are so broad that we may never know the full extent of the damage they have caused.

Unfortunately, it is hard to tell what dangers lurk in most of the pesticides available for homeowners. Not all the ingredients are listed. Pesticide labels typically list the active ingredients but not the inert ingredients. Research has found that the inert ingredients—the ingredients that often comprise the bulk of the product—can also be toxic. In fact, some ingredients listed as active ingredients in one product may be present (but unlisted) in others when they are not the main poison. There is little market testing of pesticide products before they are sold for home use and before they are widely applied on lawns and gardens.

It is impossible for anyone to keep up with the increasing number of new chemicals sold in so many formulations and combinations and under such a bewildering array of brand names. Many pesticides have been banned in recent years, but three of the most common pesticides still in use by homeowners are listed below:

> **Pests function in a similar way to some microorganisms— their job is to get rid of the dead and dying to make way for healthier populations. In this regard, pests are nature's way of maintaining balance. When we get rid of the pests, we get rid of one of nature's balancing mechanisms, and we may open the door to other potential problems.**

2,4-D

2,4-D is a weed killer found in most "Weed and Feed" products available in home and garden stores. It is commonly used for lawns and gardens but is also frequently applied on golf courses, playing fields, and parks. 2,4-D was the major ingredient in Agent Orange, the jungle defoliant used in the Vietnam War and later blamed for cancer and birth defects in Vietnamese people and in war veterans. Studies have linked 2,4-D to hormone disruption, breast and testicular cancers, learning disabilities, and birth defects. One study found that dogs whose owners regularly used 2,4-D on their lawns were twice as likely to get cancer.[251]

Malathion

Malathion is an organophosphate insecticide, a chemical family that functions by interfering with enzymes essential to nervous system function in insects and humans. Although it is one of the least poisonous of this family of pesticides, exposure to Malathion can cause respiratory distress, headache, dizziness, and nausea. It is used on all kinds of insects, from aphids to ants and mosquitoes. Malathion is also highly toxic to bees and other beneficial insects. This raises concerns about the long-term impact of its ubiquitous use. Malathion was used in Massachusetts and New York for aerial spraying of mosquitoes, after which hundreds of people reported nausea, headaches, and dizziness.

Pyrethrum/pyrethroids

Pyrethrum is one of the earliest insecticides—prepared from dried flowers of several species of chrysanthemum and sold under various trade names. Since it is naturally derived, it is often sold as a safe pesticide. Although it does break down more rapidly than other pesticides, it is still a poison. Pyrethrum causes a quick paralysis of insects. Resmethrin is a synthetic pyrethroid insecticide. It is the active ingredient in a product called Scourge, which is commonly sprayed from trucks to control mosquitoes. The following Web site contains detailed information on all pesticides, including some that have been banned: http://extoxnet.orst.edu/pips/ghindex.html

PESTICIDE ALTERNATIVES

Despite the fact that most people have pesticide residues in their bodies from the food they eat, families that use pesticides on lawns or in their gardens have even higher levels in their bodies. This applies not just to the pesticide applicator but to the whole family, because residues find their way indoors— on feet, pets, and on air currents. Studies with commonly used backyard pesticides demonstrate that indoor levels in house dust and air go up ten times after an outdoor application.[252] Needless to say, it is time to phase out the use of toxic pesticides—in any form.

Today, there are numerous methods of managing pests in the garden without having to resort to poisons. As with any of the subjects in this book, knowing that there are alternatives is the doorway to a new paradigm. When it comes to pest management, one of the best resources is the Web site http://www.stephentvedten.com/ with more than twenty-eight hundred safe and effective alternatives to pesticides. The wealth of information on this Web site, called Best Control II, may also be purchased on CD (see recommended reading). Two of the cornerstones of Best Control II are enzymes and food-grade diatomaceous earth—both are natural and nontoxic when used as suggested. Neither carries restrictions by the EPA.

Enzymes

Enzymes are catalysts that speed the breakdown of organic substances. They are "digestors" classified by the specific components they break down. For example: proteases, or proteolytic enzymes, break down proteins; carbohydrases break down carbohydrates; and lipases break down fats (lipids).

There are literally thousands of enzymes that function in biological systems. These same enzymes can be used to control pests in the garden.

Plants that digest their insect prey (e.g., Venus fly trap) do so with enzymes. Some spiders inject enzymes into their prey to predigest the contents of the insect's body. Insects even use enzymes to molt. In this case, enzymes create a chemical "zipper" so insects can crawl from their old skin. When you spray protein-digesting enzymes (proteases) on insects, they literally dissolve—no toxic poison and no devastating side effects.

Enzyme formulations have improved over the years. In 2004, a patent was approved for the use of enzymes to control pests.[253] Safe Solutions enzymes for gardens, lawns, orchards, and water (for algae) quickly and safely control virtually all insects, fungus, mildew, and mold (see sources).

CAUTION: Safe Solutions enzymes will kill all insects including beneficial insects, so use them with discretion!

Diatomaceous earth

Diatomaceous earth (DE) is another nontoxic pest control that works on insects of all species. DE physically controls insects through abrasive action, breaking down their outer skeleton (exoskeleton) so they die of dehydration. DE is composed of microscopic marine fossils called diatoms. Diatoms are tiny, single-celled plants that live in the sea by the billions, providing the foundation of the food chain for all marine life. As diatoms die, their exoskeletons drift to the bottom, building up large deposits of diatomaceous earth. Geologic changes have brought these ancient deposits to the surface, making them available for many purposes.

DE has long been used by farmers to protect their crops from insects. It is also commonly used as a food additive to eliminate intestinal parasites in livestock. Eating DE can have many health benefits for animals and humans alike, but it is important to consume food-grade DE—not all forms of diatomaceous earth are safe to use for organic gardening and agriculture. Some brands of DE advertised as insecticidal have pesticides such as pyrethrum. Safe Solutions offers a food-grade DE mined from uncontaminated fresh-water deposits (see soures).

> **The use of anything to eradicate insects is a form of pesticide— even though it may not be a toxic chemical. If it "kills," it is toxic to some life forms, and it is likely to upset nature's balance.**

CAUTION: Like enzymes, DE is a universal pest control method. It kills beneficial insects as well as those considered pests. When DE is used for organic gardening, care should be taken *not* to apply DE to the flowers of the plant, in order to protect the bees that will be needed for pollination. Eliminating just the pests (difficult to do) may cause an imbalance with broader consequences.

Perelandra gardening

The Perelandra method of gardening, developed by Machaelle Wright, takes into account the sacredness of all life and strives to maintain balance in the garden by respecting the elemental forces of nature. Where bugs are concerned, the Perelandra method advocates working with them directly— to have them find other areas to live. It may sound strange to the uninitiated, but the Perelandra gardening method has been proven over and over again to produce successful harvests. In fact, the Perelandra gardens in Virginia are some of the most productive in the world. Workbooks and many supporting materials are available at http://www.perelandra-ltd.com/.

Soil management

Growing healthy plants is much the same as maintaining a healthy body. If the terrain is healthy, disease cannot infiltrate. Insect infestations are most often a symptom of stress caused by poor soil that lacks the elements to grow healthy, vibrant plants. Pest management begins with healthy soil—soil that provides the terrain for a healthy plant. Healthy soil is a living community, full of microorganisms, enzymes, and minerals. It requires nurturing just as plants do. Soil-building practices, like composting, and remineralizing will improve the abundance (and flavor) of the harvest and will significantly reduce the need for harmful pesticides.

> **Insect infestations occur when plant populations are weak or stressed. Truly healthy plants rarely attract the kind of bugs that we consider to be "pests."**

Commercial agriculture has adopted the practice of *feeding the plant* rather than *feeding the soil*. Here again, it is similar to how the body works. Supplements are fine when real food is lacking, but the body responds best to whole-food nutrition because whole foods contain the full spectrum of vitamins and co-factors necessary for optimal health. Feeding the soil is the best way to feed plants. Primary foods for the soil are organic matter and minerals. The organic matter actually carries minerals into the plant. Together, organic matter and minerals provide whole-food nutrition for a healthy garden.

Compost versus fertilizer

Compost (mostly organic matter) is the ultimate garden elixir. It is the supreme soil conditioner that will improve air and water availability as well as provide the microorganisms and enzymes that make nutrients available to plants. The organic matter in compost not only conditions soil but acts as a slow-release plant fertilizer. This slow release of nutrients has many advantages over inorganic fertilizers.

Organic matter contains billions of microorganisms that "fix" nitrogen, making it available for plant uptake on an as-needed basis. Trace minerals that are held in organic matter are also available as necessary. On the other hand, when excessive amounts of nutrients are available to plants from highly soluble inorganic fertilizers, plants tend to take up more than they need. This creates lush, watery growth that is more susceptible to attack by pests and diseases. Aphids, for example, are attracted to plants with high levels of nitrogen in their leaves. Nitrogen is also the most expensive part of an inorganic fertilizer. It requires huge amounts of energy to produce—taking a toll on the environment even before it is used.

Inorganic fertilizers have a salt base which causes imbalances in the pH of most soils. Another disadvantage to highly soluble inorganic fertilizers is that they are easily washed away from the garden—threatening the health of nearby ground and surface water. Excessive nitrates are a hazard to human health and create a burden for water treatment facilities. Chemical fertilizers also destroy the beneficial microorganisms in soil.

The number one alternative to inorganic fertilizer has always been manure. Combining manure with other plant materials makes wonderful compost (food) for your soil. A diet of compost will replenish and increase the life in your soil and keep your plants in the best of health. The following Web site provides helpful information on a variety of gardening subjects including how to create a compost pile: www.theorganicreport.com

Soil remineralization

In addition to organic matter, soil must supply a well-balanced mix of micronutrients or trace minerals. Plants need only tiny amounts of micronutrients; too much of any of them can be harmful. On the other hand, when trace minerals are missing, the health of the plant can become compromised—the same is true of the human body. Organic matter, with the help of microorganisms, binds these minerals into chemical complexes that keep them from washing away; they are available as needed.

It is the minerals that have become depleted from our soils. Much of the organic matter we return to the soil is already depleted of minerals. Remineralizing the soil with rock dust containing a variety of trace minerals will help to condition the soil and improve the health of plants as well as their "healthfullness" when consumed as food.

Many forms of rock dust are helpful when incorporated into the soil. Azomite is a rock formation containing a particularly balanced variety of minerals and trace minerals. It is one of the best ways to remineralize soils—with amazing results (see sources).

Beneficial insects

Of the millions of insects in the world, less than 2 percent are considered pests. Beneficial insects such as bees, ladybugs, fireflies, green lacewings, praying mantis, spiders, and ground beetles keep harmful insects in check. They also pollinate plants and decompose organic matter. The indiscriminate use of pesticides kills beneficial insects too. Electric bug zappers destroy many more beneficial insects than harmful ones.

Depending on the nature of your "pest" problems, the use of beneficial insects and natural predators in the garden may help keep pests under control. Growing plants alongside or along with your garden can provide a safe haven for beneficial insects. The following plants attract beneficial, predatory insects to help control pests such as aphids, mealy bugs, mites:

- Alyssum
- Butterfly weed
- Caraway
- Clover
- Coriander
- Dill
- Fennel
- Marigolds
- Nasturtiums
- Wild carrot
- Yarrow

You can also purchase beneficial and predatory insects for your garden. This Web site contains an abundance of information to get you started: http://www.bugladyconsulting.com/

> **And don't forget the birds. Birds can also be very helpful for controlling insect pests in your garden. Trees, shrubs with berries, birdhouses, and water features all encourage birds to visit your yard. They may also eat your produce so pay attention and encourage those species that eat insects rather than those that will eat the fruits of your labors.**

LAWNS

Grass is a beautiful and enjoyable part of any garden but it is also the cause of environmental concerns. Watering lawns accounts for an incredible 40 to 60 percent of residential water consumption during the summer months, making lawn maintenance not only a chore but also a drain on finances and water supplies.

In the past, large lawns were the rule in many areas. Now, replacing part of the lawn with a low-maintenance ground cover may be desirable. Trees and shrubs grow better when the soil over their roots is covered with a mulch or ground cover rather than lawn—grass competes for nutrients and water. Ground covers are especially useful for filling in areas where maneuvering a mower is difficult or where grass doesn't thrive, such as under dense shade trees (see sources).

ONLINE GARDENING RESOURCES

The following online resources provide information that will help you to begin an organic garden or to make the transition away from the use of pesticides:

theorganicreport.com for organic garden suppliers
organicgardening.com for how-tos
gardensalive.com for organic fertilizers, soil-testing kits
planetnatural.com for rain barrels, biological pesticides thegreenguide.com/ doc.mhtml?i=95&s=seeds for sources of organic seeds

SOURCES (in the order they appear in the chapter):

Safe Solutions enzymes: http://www.safesolutionsinc.com/Enzyme_
Cleaner_Pest_Control.htm

Diatomaceous earth food grade:
http://www.safesolutionsinc.com/Diatomaceous_Earth.htm#de

Natural soil minerals:
Azomite: http://www.azomite.com/index.html

Ground covers:
http://www.ext.colostate.edu/pubs/garden/07230.html

Recommended Reading:

The Best Control II by Steven Tvedten. 2007. This is a huge resource that covers every aspect of safe pest control. It is updated regularly online: http://www.stephentvedten.com/

Peralandra Gardening Workbooks I and II, by Machaelle Wright. 1993.

Chapter 12

TOXINS IN YOUR TEETH

✦

Holistic dentistry

Dr. Benjamin Rush, George Washington's physician, was one of the first American doctors to recognize the connection between the teeth and the health of the rest of the body. He said, "I cannot help thinking that our success in the treatment of all chronic diseases would be very much promoted, by directing our inquiries into the state of the teeth in sick people."[254]

Based on Traditional Chinese Medicine, each tooth is correlated to an acupuncture meridian and to specific organs and tissues within the body. In essence, the health of the teeth can accurately pinpoint (and cause) problems in the rest of the body. This dental/body relationship has been acknowledged by holistic physicians for decades. It is referred to as the odontosomatic relationship.

Western medicine does not acknowledge the odontosomatic relationship. Hence, the clues present in the teeth go unnoticed by most doctors and dentists. Also unacknowledged is the fact that bacteria from points of seemingly benign dental infection can migrate to the heart, kidney, eyes, brain, arthritic joints, and countless other body tissues, causing serious secondary infections. Unfortunately, many dentists are in the dark when it comes to taking care of your teeth, and many of the processes employed in dentistry do more harm than good. Unknowingly, patients are exposed to numerous toxins and to a variety of toxic procedures in the dental chair; they can have an effect on much more than just your teeth.

Mercury Amalgam Fillings

Mercury is an acute neurotoxin (toxic to the brain). It is the most toxic nonradioactive element and the most volatile heavy metal. In recent years, it has been removed from all health care uses, with one exception—dental fillings. Despite the fact that the American Dental Association still endorses the use of mercury in dental fillings, more than 50 percent of dentists have chosen to eliminate its use.[255]

The term *amalgam* means mixture. Amalgam fillings contain between 49 and 54 percent mercury. They also contain silver, tin, copper, and zinc. Vast amounts of science have confirmed that these mercury-containing fillings release mercury far in excess of safe limits—and not just when the filing is first placed in the tooth. Mercury amalgam fillings release mercury vapors for the life of the filling, exposing the body to harmful amounts of mercury day after day. Children and pregnant women are especially at risk. In 1991, the World Health Organization acknowledged that the predominant source of human exposure to mercury was from dental fillings.[256]

A recent video presentation sponsored by the International Academy of Oral Medicine and Toxicology, available online at http://iaomt.org/, shows the amount of mercury that is visible against a phosphorescent background, vaporizing from a twenty-five-year-old filling. The amount released is more than a thousand times greater than the established safe limit for the air you breathe. When rubbed with a pencil eraser (simulating chewing or brushing), even more mercury vaporizes. Every time you eat or drink—especially hot or acidic foods—every time you brush your teeth or chew gum, if you have mercury amalgam fillings you breathe excessive mercury vapors for more than an hour.[257]

The history of the use of mercury fillings is a telling story. When mercury fillings were introduced in the United States by French entrepreneurs in 1833, reputable dentists considered the use of mercury in fillings to be the equivalent of malpractice. Any dentist who used the toxic mercury fillings was expelled from the American Society of Dental Surgeons. However, because these fillings were so inexpensive and so easy to use, dentists who were in favor of using the amalgam fillings left the society and formed the American Dental Association.[258] This same organization still maintains that mercury amalgam fillings are safe—despite overwhelming evidence to the contrary. The following points outline the evidence against mercury amalgam fillings:

- Every amalgam filling daily releases approximately ten micrograms of mercury into the body (i.e., 3,000,000,000,000,000 mercury atoms per day).[259]
- Mercury from fillings is distributed in all the organs and tissues, with heavy concentrations in the jaw, stomach, brain, kidneys, and liver.[260]

- More than two-thirds of the excretable mercury in humans is derived from amalgam fillings.[261]
- Mercury crosses the maternal placenta into the tissue of a developing fetus within two days. Fetal concentrations of mercury are higher than in the mothers.[262]
- Mercury is capable of inducing autoimmune diseases.[263]
- Mercury from fillings immediately and continually challenges the function of the kidneys.[264]
- Mercury promotes an increase in antibiotic resistant intestinal flora.[265]
- Sustained exposure to mercury from fillings increases the risk of lowered fertility.[266]
- Mercury causes neuronal degeneration in the brain and is now suspected of being one of the major causal factors in Alzheimer's disease.[267]

Besides the obvious dangers of placing mercury in your mouth, the placement of amalgam fillings is more destructive to the tooth. Large amounts of tooth must be removed (even for a tiny cavity) when amalgam fillings are put in place. This is necessary so that the filling will stay.

> **Mercury accumulates over time unless the body has extra antioxidants and natural substances to physically remove it.**
>
> (see Chapter 19: Mercury detoxification)

Methylated mercury

In the presence of bacteria (both the mouth and the intestinal tract are full of bacteria), mercury is methylated, which means that it is changed into a compound called methyl mercury. Methyl mercury is at least ten times more toxic than mercury—and much more difficult to remove from the body. Methyl mercury can rapidly destroy bone cells, invading weakened areas such as tooth abscesses and vulnerable parts of the jawbone. It accelerates the damage mercury causes and is a primary generator of dental infections.[268]

Dental galvanism

Galvanism is another known but ignored dental occurrence. Galvanism is defined as the phenomenon in which two or more different metals that have been used to restore or replace missing teeth produce the flow of an electric current in the mouth. Galvanism is dramatically increased when gold, nickel, aluminum, or other metal in fillings, inlays, crowns, bridges, or braces are placed near an amalgam filling. The electric current that is generated increases the release of mercury by ten to twenty times. Placing gold crowns next to amalgam fillings or on top of amalgam fillings can generate between a hundred and a thousand millivolts of electricity.[269] This causes anxiety, irritability, and other nervous disorders besides the increased release of mercury. Because amalgam fillings contain several metals, a certain amount of galvanism occurs with any amalgam filling and is amplified by the presence of other metals in the mouth.

Mercury and Alzheimer's disease

The effects of mercury are lethal to brain tissue. Scientists at the University of Calgary in Canada were able to show rapid degeneration of neurons in the presence of even small amounts of mercury. These damaged neurons form "neurofibrillary tangles" that are consistently found in the brains of Alzheimer's patients. This is illustrated in a video available on YouTube: http://www.youtube.com/watch?v=VImCpWzXJ_w. Further to this work, studies carried out at the University of Kentucky Center on Aging showed that tiny amounts of mercury block the synthesis of the major brain neural protein.[270] Most holistic dentists consider the connection between mercury amalgam fillings and Alzheimer's disease to be more than coincidence.

Mercury and the developing fetus

An unborn baby has no protection from mercury. Mercury is infinitely more toxic to the fetus and to a nursing baby than it is to an adult because there is no blood-brain barrier and there is no way for an unborn baby to eliminate mercury. In his book, *The Poison in Your Teeth,* Tom McGuire, DDS, explains that a child's first exposure to mercury from amalgam fillings occurs at the moment of conception and continues throughout the entire gestation period if the mother has amalgam fillings. If a mother with amalgam fillings is nursing, her baby will ingest mercury during the entire nursing period too. According to Tom McGuire, the most significant factor in autism and other developmental disorders is the mercury released from amalgam fillings in the mother.[271]

> **"The most potent combination of all is a child being exposed to large amounts of elemental mercury as a fetus and during nursing, and then to mercury from the full complement of vaccinations."**
>
> —Tom McGuire, DDS, The Poison in Your Teeth
>
> (see Chapter 13: Vaccines)

The mercury that is *stored* in a mother's body is tightly bound. It poses little problem for an unborn baby. But the mercury that a mother is exposed to while she is pregnant (like the mercury vapor continuously being released from fillings) is mobile in her body and is likely to become bound in the tissues of the developing baby. Women contemplating a family should consider the removal of amalgam fillings well before conception. Most mercury-safe dentists do not recommend the removal of amalgam fillings during pregnancy or nursing because of the amount of mercury that is released during removal.

Mercury and infertility

Mercury can also cause infertility. Most women with very high levels of mercury are infertile, yet following a mercury detoxification program they become fertile again.[272, 273] In men, mercury causes lower sperm counts, defective sperm cells, and lowered testosterone levels. In women, mercury causes menstrual disturbances, spontaneous abortion, miscarriage, and birth defects.

According to a 2001 report from the Centers for Disease Control, more than 10 percent of women of childbearing age had blood levels above the risk standard established by the World Health Organization. Those with levels above the risk standard were considered to be at significant risk of having children with developmental disabilities.[274] If you are unsuccessfully attempting to have children, have your mercury levels checked before you spend thousands of dollars on fertility programs.

Removing amalgam fillings

Those who are serious about removing toxins from their bodies should consider having all amalgam fillings removed and replaced with less-toxic materials. Only when this ongoing source of mercury is removed can the body fully sense and release its stores of mercury and other heavy metals. Unfortunately, the process of amalgam removal releases large amounts of mercury vapor and mercury particles; those who are already sick should be cautious. Especially if you are sick, work with a health professional who can help you prepare and follow up afterward. At a very minimum, do what you can to fortify your immune system before you begin to have amalgam fillings removed. Do one quadrant of your mouth at a time and wait at least two or three weeks in between appointments—longer if you experience difficulty after your first appointment. It is important to support the detoxification process for three to six months following the removal of amalgam fillings. Dr. McGuire's Web site is a good source of information: www.dentalwellness4u.com.

 (see Chapter 19: Mercury detoxification)

Select a holistic or biological dentist who will take the necessary precautions during amalgam removal, including the use of lots of water, chunking (the use of a special drill that allows large chunks to be removed rather than drilling the entire filling out), high-volume suction for the removal of vapor and filling material as quickly as possible, and an alternate source of breathable air during the procedure. Several online organizations have lists of holistic dentists from which you can choose (see sources).

If you cannot have your amalgam fillings removed right away, there are a number of things you can do to reduce the amount of mercury that is released.

- Don't chew gum—chewing stimulates mercury release for up to an hour.
- Don't drink hot liquids—warm temperatures increase the amount of mercury released.
- Reduce snacking between meals—any chewing stimulates mercury release.
- Reduce the number of abrasive foods you eat, like nuts and chips.
- Eliminate acidic foods, especially soft drinks.
- Change the way you brush your teeth to avoid the chewing surface; focus on the margins where fillings meet the tooth. Get a soft tooth brush.
- Rinse your mouth with cool water after eating and brushing: this reduces the temperature and slows the release of mercury.
- If you grind your teeth at night, have your dentist fit you with a teeth guard. This one thing can reduce mercury more than any of the above suggestions.
- Stop smoking.

OTHER DENTAL FILLING MATERIALS

Research and development during the last few years have produced dental materials that are not only more biologically compatible but that are stronger and can actually reinforce the tooth. There are now several hundred different polymers that are superior to amalgam materials. These include composite materials as well as ceramic and glass-ceramic materials that are superior in strength and function. In addition, small decayed areas can now be treated with pin-point lasers or air particle beams to reduce the damage to the tooth. Lasers allow the material to be fused to the tooth. These newer techniques preserve the integrity and the health of the tooth.

Composite fillings

Fortunately, today there are alternatives to mercury amalgam fillings. The placement of tooth-colored, composite fillings preserves much more of the integrity of the tooth. However, there is no perfect dental filling material. None can be considered completely nontoxic. Materials known as composites are the most inert to date.

There are a number of composite materials in use today. Manufacturers often change the names of compounds in dental materials, so discuss the most recent filling materials with a holistic dentist to determine the best option for your circumstances.

DENTAL OZONE

In 2003, a revolutionary new way of handling tooth decay became available in many parts of Europe. Researchers at the Queen's Dental Hospital and Belfast University, Ireland, pioneered a new technique that could virtually eliminate the need for dental drilling.[275, 276] Their research proved that ozone destroys bacteria in a decayed tooth. When caught early, no further treatment is necessary. Minerals from the patients own saliva are capable of remineralizing the treated, previously decayed area. Once hardened, the remineralized area is even more resistant to future decay.

Dental ozone is a completely new way of treating decay. The treatment is simple, inexpensive, and requires no drilling when decay is caught early. The correct operation of the technique meets all current health and safety regulations worldwide. Using modern dental diagnostic equipment available to most dentists, tooth decay can be caught at very early stages (before it is visibly seen). A simple sixty-second (average) burst of ozone, delivered to the isolated tooth, destroys all the bacteria that cause decay. Even if the area of decay is deeper, ozone can still play a role. Drilling may be necessary to remove the cover of enamel over the decay, but ozone can be used to sterilize the area without removing a large volume of tooth. When ozone is used to sterilize an area of decay, there is no sensitivity after the local anesthetic wears away. Ozone can even be used to eliminate sensitivity after new crowns or veneers are placed. Where the area at the neck of a tooth is sensitive, a simple forty-second application with ozone can often eliminate the sensitivity entirely. Ozone can also be used in the preparation of a root canal.

 (see Chapter 12: Root canals)

In the United States, Dr. Richard Hansen is using this new technique and has developed an educational training program for dentists. To find a dentist using this technique, visit www.functionaldentistry.org.

ANESTHETICS

There are many anesthetics used by dentists for numbing your mouth during dental work. Most are nerve toxins. The most common dental anesthetic used today is lidocaine.

In 1990, Dr. Alfred Nickel discovered that long-term numbness (paresthesis) experienced by some patients after dental procedures resulted from the breakdown of the local anesthetic into a known chemical poison—2,6 dimethylaniline. Lidocaine, as well as other dental anesthetics (including mepivacaine, bupivacaine, procaine), all break down in the body to compounds known as anilines.

Anilines belong to the chemical family of aromatic hydrocarbons. Other members of this family include the toxins benzene, phenol, hydroquinone, toluene, xylene, and napthalene. All of these are suspected carcinogens and have similar effects. Since the effect of anilines is cumulative, repetitive exposure can constitute a major, overlooked cause of cancer and other serious disorders. Dr. Nickel cites the following as support for this observation:

> *Our research team noted a curious and intriguing commonality among the thirty cancer patients evaluated at a recent meeting of the tumor board of one of the local hospitals. Each patient's dental history was visualized on the total body scans (crowns, fillings, etc. produce shadows on the film). The total body scans clearly demonstrated that each of the patients had undergone from twelve to twenty-eight crown and bridge dental procedures, necessitating extensive exposure to local anesthetics.*[277]

The amount of aniline resulting from routine clinical use of local anesthetics frequently exceeds the maximum daily occupational exposure (skin and lung exposure of 10 to 20 mg per cubic meter). A dentist may inject as much as 14 ml of lidocaine when doing a tooth extraction. This amounts to 140 mg of 2,6 dimethylaniline.

> **2,6 dimethylaniline is also one of the carcinogenic chemical components identified in tobacco.**
> **Injecting 1 cc of 2% lidocaine will result in the same aniline dose as smoking 94,000 unfiltered cigarettes!**

In view of the suppressed information that has now surfaced regarding aniline toxicity, the widespread use of aniline-based local anesthetics in medicine and dentistry should be seriously reevaluated. Today, there are safer alternatives to lidocaine.

Most dental anesthetic solutions also contain adrenaline (epinephrine), and preservatives (methylparaban and sodium metabisulfite). Both adrenaline and preservatives add to the body burden when undergoing dental procedures. Epinephrine is a vasoconstrictor used to prolong the action of the anesthetic. It increases heart rate and anxiety for many patients and can result in local tissue death. Sodium metabisulfite is a sulfite that may cause allergic reactions including anaphylactic symptoms for those allergic to sulfur. Methyl paraben is a common preservative in personal care products known to have estrogenic effects.

 (see Chapter 7: Paraben family)

Dr. Nickel developed an aniline-free dental anesthetic which was approved in 2000. It is known as articaine or septocaine. Unfortunately, it also contains epinephrine and sodium metabisulfite, but it is better for most people than lidocaine.

Another alternative is bupivacaine, which has been shown to have a lower aniline breakdown—by as much as 85 percent. Its effects last longer (your mouth may be numb for several hours longer than with traditional anesthetics), but it releases significantly less aniline. It is also available without preservatives or epinephrine and can be special ordered by dentists from Apothecure pharmacy (see sources).

ROOT CANALS

A root canal is the procedure where a hole is drilled and the pulp of the tooth is removed. The pulp is the tooth's connection with the life forces of the body. It contains nerves, blood vessels, and lymph vessels. Removing the pulp kills the tooth. The pulp chamber is then cleaned and filled with an inert material and sealed.

The problem with root canals is that it is virtually impossible to completely seal off and sterilize the inner chamber of the tooth, which has miles of tubules that fan out perpendicular to the pulp chamber. During the root canal procedure, bacteria that are normally found in the tooth are sealed inside. They multiply inside the tubules and release toxins from the tiny hole in the bottom of the root or from micropores in the tooth. This is why a good portion of root canals eventually fail, requiring further, more serious intervention.

Having a root canal is an open invitation for further problems. Even though you may never experience pain or an abscess, infection from a root canal can cause symptoms in other parts of your body. This was eloquently demonstrated by Dr. Weston A. Price, who is considered to be the father of holistic dentistry. A female patient of his with severe arthritis had a root canal that appeared perfectly normal and showed no infection on x-ray. Dr. Price suspected that her arthritis was caused by the tooth and received permission to pull it. After being confined to a wheelchair for six years with crippling arthritis, the woman was able to walk again and even to do fine needlework.[278]

More recently, Dr. George Meinig began his career as an endodontist (a dentist specializing in root canals). When he discovered Dr. Price's research on root canals and the efforts to dismiss his work, Dr. Meinig quit his profession and dedicated the rest of his life to exposing the root canal cover-up. His book *Root Canal Cover-Up* is a must-read if you are considering having a root canal.

Never consent to a root canal without consulting a holistic dentist. In many cases, a deep cavity can be sealed with an inlay, an onlay, or a crown. Sometimes a tooth is structurally injured by a poor bite and can be saved with an oral appliance. The recent availability of ozone for use in the preparation of the root canal may be a godsend. Ozone is the best way to sterilize the root canal before sealing the tooth. When a tooth is positively beyond repair, the decision for how to proceed can be difficult. There are several options.

1. **Traditional root canal**. In the traditional root canal procedure, a substance called gutta-percha is used to fill the root canal. This is a latex substance with zinc oxide, barium, and traces of heavy metals (lead and cadmium). One of the biggest difficulties with gutta-percha

is that it shrinks and allows bacteria to multiply and escape through the bottom of the tooth. Lead and cadmium may also escape.

2. **EndoCal10**. European dentists have been using a mineral compound to fill the root canal for more than thirty years. This compound is primarily composed of calcium oxide and zinc oxide and has the ability to expand into the dental tubules, sealing off these areas better than gutta-percha. This material, called EndoCal10, has also been shown to inhibit the growth of some anaerobic bacteria.[279] Because it expands, it must be applied extremely carefully so as not to fracture the root of the tooth.

3. **MTA**. Another more recent material called mineral trioxide aggregate (MTA) is medical grade, modified cement. It can be used to pack the terminal end of the root, providing a better seal, and then the rest of the root chamber is filled with Endocal10. This method shows the most promise, and bacterial growth is less likely.[280]

4. **Tooth extraction**. Although tooth extraction is not a comforting option, it is often the best option.

Dental Sealants

During the last fifteen to twenty years, a popular treatment for children's teeth has been the placement of sealants on the chewing surface. Sealants are intended to protect the tooth from decay by covering the tiny grooves and depressions where decay is most apt to begin. This procedure may initially prevent cavities. But there are things that parents are not told before they give consent to this procedure. Chances are your dentist may not even be aware of some of the risks.

Many dental sealants contain fluoride, which is released slowly in the mouth. Parents who have chosen <u>not</u> to have fluoride treatment for their children may end up getting it anyway, via the sealants. Some sealants are even intended to be recharged with fluoride. This is the case with the most popular sealant used today: UltraSeal XT plus.

Dental sealants also contain bisphenol A, known to have estrogenic effects. A study released in January 2000 reported that polymerization of sealants is not complete and that bisphenol A leaches into the mouth.[281] Even the tiny amounts that are released from these sealants are enough to cause biological effects in experimental models.[282]

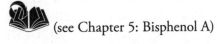 (see Chapter 5: Bisphenol A)

Sealants, and most composite filling materials, are made with dimethacrylate—known to cause contact dermatitis.[283] They are also suspected of neurological and respiratory damage. These sealants fall into the class of cyanoacrylate adhesives known as super glue. Their safety is being challenged when used in dental applications.[284] Little work has been done concerning the toxicity of dental sealants. Likewise, their metabolism is unknown.[285] Methacrylates have been shown to release toxic substances for at least two weeks.[286] Dentists are being warned about the occupational hazards of these substances. What about the children who walk home with these substances on their teeth?

Teeth are filled with a matrix of tiny micropores called dentin tubules. These microscopic channels reach to the surface of the tooth and allow circulation between blood vessels and lymphatic tissues—they carry nutrients and expel wastes in much the same way your skin does. Dental sealants literally seal off the natural ability of the tooth to breathe. Sealing off this capacity is similar to wrapping your body in plastic—then allowing toxins (fluoride, methacrylate, and bisphenol A) to leach from the plastic into your body with a reduced capacity to expel them.

But perhaps the biggest difficulty with dental sealants is that if they are not placed with great care, decay can grow *underneath* the sealant where it is invisible—even to x-ray. This is more common than most dentists are willing to admit. If the tooth is not completely dry when the sealant is placed or if the curing (hardening) process proceeds too rapidly, the sealant tends to pull away from the tooth—just enough to allow bacteria in. Bacteria then grow in a protected environment. Even x-rays do not detect the decay until it has progressed enough to be significant. It is also quite common for a dentist to place a sealant over a microscopic area of decay. Some dentists use lasers to detect decay that cannot be seen by the naked eye, but not all dentists have this capacity.

Far too many children's teeth have required root canals because the sealant gives a false sense of security. Progressive decay is not noticed until the damage is so severe that root canals are the only option. Be very careful if you decide to have your dentist apply sealants. In the long run, you may be better off teaching your children to stay away from sugar and to take personal responsibility for their health—especially their teeth.

TEETH WHITENERS

People are willing to go to great lengths for a white smile. Consequently, a vast array of pastes, gels, and strips are available to help you get the whitest teeth possible. Many of these products work at home; some are applied in the dentist's chair. Most use carbamide peroxide and other caustic substances that can cause sensitive teeth, irritated gums, and other problems.

Drinking red wine, coffee, and tea can discolor your teeth. Dark pigments in cigarettes, blueberries, and other foods can also discolor teeth. Much of this superficial staining can be taken care of by regular brushing. But over time, stains can penetrate into the enamel where they cannot be removed by brushing alone. The antibiotic known as tetracycline can also discolor children's teeth if taken during their early years when tooth enamel is still forming. Tetracycline is incorporated into the enamel and dentin of the tooth, leaving darker yellow and gray colors on the enamel. Many adults today have stained teeth as a result of antibiotics given when they were young.

To combat stains below the surface of the teeth, whitening gels containing hydrogen peroxide (H_2O_2) were introduced in 1989. Hydrogen peroxide can diffuse through tooth enamel and into the dentin in about fifteen minutes. A close inspection of the labels of many of the whitening products on the market shows that they contain carbamide peroxide—a 1/1 compound of urea and H_2O_2. The carbamide peroxide formulation allows products to have a longer shelf-life. It also provides a slower release of the H_2O_2.

The Material Safety Data Sheet (MSDS) on carbamide peroxide says it is very hazardous in case of skin contact (corrosive); that the amount of tissue damage depends on length of contact. As for data on carcinogenic effects, mutagenic effects, developmental effects, and developmental toxicity, no data are available—no one knows. Gels containing 10 or 20 percent carbamide peroxide are brushed directly onto teeth, or they may be delivered in a mouthguard-like tray, or embedded in an adhesive plastic strip that is stuck on the teeth. In professional procedures for teeth whitening, dentists use up to 35 percent H_2O_2. All of these procedures make some contact with the tissue of the gums.

Hydrogen peroxide itself is an oxidant; it releases free radicals as it decomposes. Free radicals can destroy healthy tissue. This is one reason why teeth whiteners cause gum irritation. It may also be the reason these whiteners cause tooth pain and tooth sensitivity. Several cases have been documented in which people have burned away excessive gum tissue by overusing tooth whitening products. Two clinical cases have been documented in dental literature where the use of an over-the-counter teeth whitener adversely affected the enamel of a person's teeth. These cases involved whiteners that had a high peroxide content, an acidic prerinse, or the whitener itself was acidic. The tooth damage caused by these whiteners was irreversible.[287]

The Cochrane Database of Systematic Reviews reviewed twenty-five scientific publications on the use of teeth whitening products. Their concluding comments indicated that side effects (gum irritation and painful or sensitive teeth) were correlated with the concentration of active ingredient in the product, and that there were no studies to evaluate the possibility of long-term harm.[288] Certainly this product, which is known to cause a high percentage of tooth pain, should be evaluated further before it is sold as safe and before it is made so widely available.

If you choose to use a tooth whitening product or to have your dentist apply one, choose one with the lowest concentration of H_2O_2. Stop immediately if you experience pain or sensitivity. Pain and sensitivity are signals from the body that something is wrong. They should not be ignored. Remember, the tooth is a living organ with a vital function beyond just chewing food.

Homemade Teeth Whitener

A much gentler homemade teeth whitener is made by diluting food grade hydrogen peroxide (see sources) with distilled water at a rate of 10 to 1. Mix the peroxide dilution with a mixture of 3 parts baking soda and 1 part sea salt to form a paste. Brush your teeth with this once a week. The whitening process will take longer, but it will not cause harm to your teeth, and it will help prevent decay.

GINGIVITIS AND PERIODONTAL DISEASE

Gingivitis is caused by bacteria and plaque that build up in the tissues surrounding and supporting your teeth. It can lead to bad breath, bleeding, and receding gums. Left unchecked, gingivitis can also lead to the more serious form of gum disease called periodontitis. This long-term infection can eventually cause deterioration of the bones in your jaw and eventual loss of teeth. Since gingivitis doesn't usually cause pain, it often goes unnoticed. Initial signs include:

- gums that bleed when you brush your teeth
- red, swollen or tender gums
- gums that have pulled away from the teeth
- chronic bad breath that doesn't go away
- loose teeth
- tooth aches
- a change in the way your teeth fit together when you bite

Gingivitis is often a sign of poor oral hygiene. It can clear up in less than a week when teeth are regularly brushed and flossed. Removing the sticky plaque that harbors bacteria is often all it takes to control bad breath, bleeding, and tender gums.

 (see Chapter 7: Mouthwash)

If gingivitis is not caught and taken care of early, bacteria may build up and cause the more serious periodontal disease, which can require dental intervention. Dentists may treat periodontitis by scaling and root planing (also called debridement) to clear away pockets of bacteria. When this is not successful, surgery is usually recommended. Surgery involves lifting back the gums, removing the hardened plaque buildup, and then stitching the gums back in place. There is a newer laser treatment called LANAP that is less painful and less intrusive.

Whole-food nutrition can play a huge role in dental health. Foods high in vitamin C, folic acid (most raw fruits and vegetables), and the supplement CoQ-10 all help clear up and prevent gingivitis.[289] Essential oils may also support the elimination of periodontal infection. A combination of peppermint oil and almond oil at the gum line may also help kill bacteria and restore healthy gums. You may want to consult a holistic dentist who can help you determine a specific program of dietary, lifestyle, and other therapies that may help with the deeper causes of dental problems.

Essential oils

Essential oils can be powerful tools for fighting infection—especially in the mouth where infections can weaken the immune system and can cause problems elsewhere in the body. Some dentists now use oregano, clove, thyme, and tea tree oils to kill infections rather than using antibiotics, depending on the severity of the infection. In fact, clove oil was used to sterilize surgical equipment over a hundred years ago.

CAUTION: Oregano and clove oil are quite strong, so be cautious if you choose to use these oils.

Oils for oral use include helichrysum, thyme, peppermint, eucalyptus, palmarosa, tea tree, and Niaouli. Bio Excel markets an essential oil blend called Dental Delight specifically for oral use (see sources). Essential oils can easily be added to a toothbrush, waterpick, dental floss, or mouth rinse. Using a cotton swab to dab essential oils on trouble spots can also be effective. Here are some suggestions:

- Dilute two to three drops of essential oils in a small cup of water. Dip your toothbrush during brushing.
- Add one to two drops of essential oil to the basin of your waterpick.
- Apply one drop of essential oil along the length of unwaxed dental floss.
- Add two drops of an essential oil or oil blend to each ounce of mouthwash or water.

- Dab undiluted oils on the infected area. Rinse about an hour later with helichrysum in water to heal and regenerate tissue.
- Following dental work, rinse your mouth with one drop of tea tree oil and one drop of helichrysum in a half-cup of warm water. This combination is anti-inflammatory and will promote new cell growth.

Sources (in the order they appear in the chapter):

Holistic dentists:
International Association of Mercury Free Dentists (IAMFD): www.dentalwellness4u.com
International Academy of Oral Medicine and Toxicology (IAOMT): http://iaomt.org/
Holistic Dental Association (HAD): http://www.holisticdental.org/
International Academy of Biological Dentistry and Medicine (IABDM): http://www.iabdm.org/

Apothecure Pharmacy: 1-800-969-6601

Essential oils:
Dental Delight and others: www.bioexcel.com

Food grade hydrogen peroxide:
Natural Health Supply: http://www.naturalhealthsupply.com/servlet/Detail?no=142

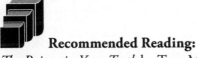 **Recommended Reading:**
The Poison in Your Teeth by Tom McGuire, DDS
Root Canal Cover-up by George Meinig, MD

Chapter 13

WHAT ABOUT VACCINES?

Mayer Eisenstein, MD, author of the book *Don't Vaccinate Before You Educate*, made this statement about childhood disease: "The greatest threat of childhood disease lies in the dangerous and ineffectual efforts made to prevent them through mass immunization."[290] His statement echoes the sentiment of a growing number of doctors and health professionals who have investigated the ills and the deceit behind the vaccination debacle.

A vaccine is defined as a preparation of weakened or killed bacteria or virus that is introduced into the body to prevent a disease by stimulating antibodies against it. Although the theory has merit, the truth is that a healthy body does not need immunization. Often, vaccines are more harmful than helpful. Vaccines, intended to "protect," end up taxing the immune system and the detoxification systems of the body to such an extent that they trigger allergies, learning disabilities, autism, and other chronic neuroimmune and neurodevelopmental illnesses. Children are at the greatest risk because their immune systems and their brains are still developing. Yet children are the ones who are targeted. They may receive dozens of vaccines during the first two years of their lives—often four and five at a time. Rather than attempting to create immunity, our efforts would be much better spent on building and fortifying the naturally protective functions of the immune system.

Vaccines carry an unpredictable risk of injury. By their very nature, they are an assault on the body. Every year, ten thousand to fourteen thousand reports of hospitalizations, injuries, and deaths following vaccinations are made to the federal Vaccine Adverse Event Reporting System. These numbers include one hundred to two hundred deaths and several times that number of permanent disabilities. Yet more than 90 percent of adverse reactions are never reported.[291] Since there is no requirement to report vaccine reactions, we have no idea of the degree to which vaccines are responsible for injury and death. Further, no long-term studies have ever been conducted to determine various degrees of health in vaccinated versus unvaccinated populations. The incidences of chronic, childhood, autoimmune diseases such as asthma, autism, and juvenile-onset diabetes continue to rise along with the quantity of vaccines our children receive.

There has been a moratorium on animal organ transplants in humans because of the concern for contracting latent animal viruses. Despite this fact, animal cells containing DNA and foreign proteins are still routinely injected via vaccines. After years of use, the polio vaccine was discovered to have one such virus because it had been cultured in monkey kidney tissue. This virus (SV-40) has since been determined to cause cancer and is carried into the genetic coding of future generations. Many of the children of those who were originally vaccinated have the virus, and it has been found in numerous tumors.

In 1986, Congress officially acknowledged the reality of vaccine-caused injuries and death by passing The National Childhood Vaccine Injury Act. In order to pay for injuries and deaths, a surtax was added to the price of vaccines. Now, when parents have their children vaccinated, a portion of the money they spend goes into a congressional fund to compensate families whose children are injured by vaccines. The act also narrowed the criteria for applying for compensation. Some symptoms have to occur within four hours in order to qualify for compensation. Others have to occur between five and fifteen days (not before five days and not after fifteen days). Even with this limited criteria, over $1.3 billion dollars had been paid out in compensation as of 2001. Thousands of cases are pending. According to the National Vaccine Injury Compensation Program, the state of Illinois alone had 216 claims during the period from 1990–1998. Forty-four of those were deaths. In addition, 2,173 cases were filed in Illinois for sudden infant death syndrome (SIDS).[292]

The truth is that vaccines have never been proven to be safe. The liability and the cost of compensation have increased so dramatically that a bit of language was carefully slipped into the recent Homeland Security bill. It granted immunity to a number of vaccine manufacturers. In other words, if vaccines caused harm, vaccine manufacturers would not be held liable. Fortunately, that portion of the bill was later rescinded.

Congressional hearings have raised eye-opening questions about safety standards, about conflicts of interest, and about huge gaps in scientific knowledge regarding how vaccines affect the body. Some children are at greater biological risk than others. Genetic factors play a big role. There are children who have genetically inherited weaknesses and who don't eliminate heavy metals or the other toxins from vaccines. The more toxins they are exposed to, the greater their risk. Given this emerging knowledge, the one-size-fits-all vaccination program makes little sense. It fails to acknowledge the risk of vaccine-induced injury for many children.

Every parent deserves to be given truthful, unbiased information about diseases and vaccines and to be allowed to make informed decisions. But unless parents have educated themselves, this is rarely the case. Unfortunately, the public is often misguided, with fear-based information about disease hazards without the balance of information on vaccine hazards. Even when parents know the risks, the decision is often not in their hands.

VACCINE INGREDIENTS

If the average American were aware of the common components of vaccines, they would think twice before consenting to them. Vaccines are made from the mucus of infected children (whooping cough), excrement from typhoid victims (typhoid), scabs and pus from calves (smallpox), and until recently, the diseased kidneys of monkeys (polio). They may also contain a variety of toxic preservatives, heavy metals, and other components:

Aluminum—As vaccine manufacturers have removed mercury from many vaccines, the level of aluminum has doubled. Five vaccines (hepatitis B, hepatitis A, pertussis, diphtheria, and tetanus) now contain more aluminum. Aluminum is used to amplify the effects of the active ingredients in vaccines. It accumulates in brain, muscle, and bone tissue and has been linked to cancerous tumors at the injection site.

Antibiotics—The antibiotics neomycin, streptomycin, and polymyxin are common components of vaccines.

Formaldehyde—Formaldehyde is a known carcinogen. There is no level that is considered safe, yet six vaccines (polio, hepatitis B, hepatitis A, pertussis, diphtheria, and tetanus) contain formaldehyde.

 (see Chapter 1: Formaldehyde)

 (also see Chapter 7: Formaldehyde)

Live Viruses—Some vaccines contain live virus. These vaccines include measles, mumps, rubella, polio, rotavirus, varicella (chicken pox), and the most recent vaccine, shingles. Live virus vaccines can sometimes cause the disease in the recipient and can even infect those in close contact with the recipient. This can put a pregnant mother or immunocompromised adult at risk by being around a recently vaccinated individual with a live virus vaccine.

More importantly, live viruses contain genetic material that can become incorporated into our genetic code in much the same way that genetic engineering transfers genes from one species to another. The resulting genetic imbalance may manifest as immunological impairment or brain damage.[293] It may take years before this is apparent, and it can be passed on to future generations.

Mercury—Mercury has been used in vaccines for many years as a preservative known as thimerosol. Only recently has it been removed from many vaccines. Before this, children who received a full schedule of vaccinations were injected with one hundred-seventy times the EPA safety limit of mercury. Mercury is a potent neurotoxin; it kills developing nerve cells. To see mercury-induced nerve damage, watch the online video:
http://www.youtube.com/watch?v=VImCpWzXJ_w

 (see Chapter 12: Mercury amalgam fillings)

The story of how thimerosol came to the attention of the public is an interesting one. In June 2000, a private conference was held at the Simpsonwood Retreat Center in Norcross, Georgia. The meeting included dozens of representatives from the FDA, Centers for Disease Control (CDC), and from the vaccine industry. The conference was held to discuss a disturbing study that raised alarming questions about the safety of thimerosol. According to the medical records of one hundred thousand children, thimerosol appeared to be responsible for a dramatic increase in speech delays, attention deficit disorder, hyperactivity, and autism. Some of the comments from the proceedings of that meeting are as follows:

- *There are just a host of neurodevelopmental data that would suggest we've got a serious problem.*
- *My gut feeling? It worries me. I don't want my grandson to get a thimerosol-containing vaccine until we know better what's going on.*
- *We are in a bad position from the standpoint of defending any lawsuits.*
- *We have asked you to keep this information confidential.*[294]

Following the Simpsonwood Conference, the CDC paid the Institute of Medicine to conduct a new study to whitewash the risks of thimerosol. And to thwart the Freedom of Information Act, the CDC handed its giant database of vaccine records over to a private company, declaring it off-limits to researchers and to other interested parties. In 2005, Robert F. Kennedy, Jr. published a lengthy examination of the suppressed data about the dangers of thimerosol. According to Kennedy:

> *The story of how government health agencies colluded with Big Pharma to hide the risks of thimerosol from the public is a chilling case study of institutional arrogance, power, and greed.*

In his paper, Kennedy stated that he became convinced about the reality of the thimerosol link to the rising epidemic of childhood neurological disorders after reading the Simpsonwood Conference transcripts, studying the leading scientific research, and speaking with many of the nation's authorities on mercury.

Autism and mercury poisoning have nearly identical symptoms. In 2005, pediatricians were diagnosing over 40,000 new cases of autism annually. Yet, until 1943, the disease was unknown. In 1943, autism was identified and diagnosed among eleven children born in the months after thimerosol was first added to baby vaccines.

Since 1991, when the CDC and the FDA recommended that three additional vaccines with thimerosol be given to infants, the estimated number of cases of autism increased from one in every 2,500 children to one in 166 children.

Prior to the removal of thimerosol from most childhood vaccines, a single day's vaccination regimen may have included forty-one times the level of mercury known to cause harm. Perhaps this is why the autism rate has mushroomed (nearly 8000 percent) over the past twenty years. Dramatic increases in autism followed the introduction of the MMR (measles, mumps, and rubella) vaccine in the early 1980s. England also had dramatic autism increases beginning in the 1990s, following the introduction of the MMR vaccine there.

Monosodium glutamate (MSG)—Monosodium glutamate, listed as *glutamate* on the ingredient list, is the notorious MSG used as a flavoring agent in foods. It is considered an excitotoxin, causing a number of allergic reactions as well as brain damage. R. Gordon Douglas, Jr., MD, president of the vaccine division of Merck (a pharmaceutical company responsible for making several vaccines), told the Illinois Vaccine Awareness Coalition that MSG was in all viral vaccines. When asked why it was only listed in the chickenpox vaccine, he said MSG didn't have to be listed in the ingredients.[295] MSG may be present in more vaccines than we realize.

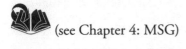 (see Chapter 4: MSG)

Phenol—The use of phenol (in 2-phenoxyethanol) in vaccine preparations introduces a poisonous and caustic substance into the body. Phenols in vaccines inhibit an appropriate immune response. Phenol is considered to be corrosive to the skin and is known to be a protoplasmic poison, toxic to all cells. Since it also inhibits phagocytic activity, it actually serves to hinder, rather than stimulate, the immune response. Phagocytes serve as the body's first line of defense against infection; they engulf and digest organisms and cause other elements of the immune system to become activated.

CHILDREN'S VACCINES

In 2008, children's vaccination schedules included thirty-one vaccinations before a child reaches eighteen months of age. This represents a huge onslaught of toxins for a developing immune system. Vaccine side effects range from infant high-pitched screaming, seizures, and severe joint pains to chronic fatigue, behavioral problems, and death. Side effects are most often labeled as coincidental. Furthermore, none of the eleven required childhood vaccines have been studied for the long-term or cumulative effects of combining vaccines together—a common practice, today.

> *A single vaccine given to a six-pound newborn is the equivalent of giving a 180-pound adult thirty vaccines on the same day.*
>
> —Dr. Boyd Haley, professor and chair, department of chemistry, University of Kentucky (2001)

Sudden Infant Death syndrome

Sudden infant death syndrome (SIDS) is, by definition, the sudden and unexpected death of an apparently healthy infant. It is also known as crib death or cot death. Many studies have shown vaccination to be a cause of SIDS. Peak incidence of SIDS occurs between the ages of two and four months in the United States—precisely when the first two immunizations are given. Studies show a clear pattern of correlation extending three weeks after immunization.[296] Of the 145 SIDS deaths in Los Angeles County between January 1979 and August 1980, 53 had received a DPT immunization within twenty-eight days of death. Six deaths occurred within twenty-four hours; 17 deaths occurred within one week of DPT immunization.[297]

Dr. William Torch, of the University of Nevada School of Medicine, found that two-thirds of 103 children who died of SIDS had been immunized with the DPT vaccine in the three weeks before their deaths, many dying within a day after getting the shot.[298]

Vaccinations place toxins in the body. They require additional nutrients (especially antioxidants) to neutralize the toxins. Studies in Australia have shown that vitamin C deficiency plays a big role in SIDS—that when children are given adequate amounts of vitamin C, the incidence of SIDS practically disappears.[299] If children must be vaccinated, make sure they are fortified with vitamin C and other antioxidants beforehand. This will give them a much better chance of dealing with the toxic overload.

Pediarix

Pediarix is the new five-in-one combination vaccine for diphtheria, tetanus, pertussis, hepatitis B, and polio. It was created in an effort to reduce the number of injections given to infants during the first several months of their lives. A review of the study that allowed this vaccine to be approved uncovers serious investigational flaws. Researchers concluded that "there were no vaccine-related serious adverse events in any group after any vaccine dose." But when the study was read carefully, evidence to the contrary was uncovered:

> *Two subjects withdrew from the study because of serious adverse events that were determined by the safety monitor to be unrelated to vaccination. One subject in Group A was diagnosed with a seizure disorder fourteen days after the first immunization. Another subject in Group B had a neuroblastoma detected six weeks after the first immunization. Six other reported serious adverse events involved hospitalizations for bronchiolitis/ pneumonia, meningitis and apnea and were also determined to be unrelated to vaccination.[300]*

According to a press release, the administration of Pediarix is associated with higher rates of fever relative to separately administered vaccines.[301] The list of inert ingredients in Pediarix includes, among others:

- Formaldehyde, a known carcinogen for which there is no safe level.
- Glutaraldehyde, a toxic chemical used for cold sterilization for which there is no permissible exposure limit.

- 2-Phenoxyethanol. The vaccine contains 2.5 mg of this phenol compound.
- Thimerosol, a mercury-containing compound used in the production of the hepatitis B fraction of the vaccine: up to 12.5ng (nanograms) remain in the final vaccine.
- Neomycin and Polymyxin B—antibiotics.
- Yeast protein.

Hepatitis B

The hepatitis B vaccine was the first recombinant DNA vaccine on the market in the United States. It does not contain live virus but it does contain genetically engineered proteins that have been known to trigger autoimmune reactions and neurological disorders including multiple sclerosis. Even though the hepatitis B vaccine is mandatory for newborns and is given at birth, infants have little chance of getting the disease. The virus is primarily transmitted among adults (sexually transmitted). There is also evidence that it can be passed through saliva and tears and from a mother to a child in the womb. Only a few cases of hepatitis B in children are reported each year.

> In 1998, following hundreds of reports of autoimmune and neurological disorders caused by the hepatitis B vaccine in France, a lawsuit was filed by 15,000 French citizens. The lawsuit accused the French government of overstating the benefits of the hepatitis B vaccine and understating the hazards. The French minister of health ended the mandatory hepatitis B vaccination program for all school children. Perhaps it is time to reevaluate its mandatory use in the United States.

Adverse reactions to the hepatitis B vaccine include arthritis, Bell's palsy, brain disease, diarrhea, drowsiness, ear ringing, edema, fainting, fatigue, fever, flu, Guillain-Barre syndrome, headache, irritability, hair loss, hives, liver enzymes elevation, lupus-like syndrome, multiple sclerosis, nausea, rash, sore throat, spinal cord inflammation, and upper respiratory infection. The hepatitis B vaccine contains hepatitis B colonies cloned into a genetically engineered strain of yeast. It is available with and without thimerosol. The vaccine also contains:

- aluminum
- formaldehyde
- soy peptone

Rotavirus

In February 2006, a new vaccine replaced the rotavirus vaccine called RotaShield, which was withdrawn from the market because it caused intussusception (intestinal twisting in which one segment of the intestine telescopes inwardly into another). The vaccine caused numerous hospitalizations, surgeries and several deaths. Only a year later, the new vaccine (RotaTeq) came under scrutiny for the same problem.[302] So far, there have only been warnings, but there is significant cause for concern—especially considering the history of the previous vaccine.

When RotaShield was pulled from the market, an investigation was instigated. The Association of American Physicians and Surgeons discovered that prelicensure trials of the vaccine had caused bowel intussusception at rates thirty times higher than normal. Why was it approved in the first place? The question has never been adequately answered. Is the current vaccine, which is administered to children at ages two, four, and six months of age, any safer?

RotaTeq is a liquid live virus vaccine that is given by mouth in three doses. Infants who received RotaTeq, when compared to infants who received a placebo during preapproval trials, were reported to experience diarrhea, vomiting, ear infections, runny nose, and coughing at slightly higher rates.[303]

Diptheria, tetanus, acellular pertussis (whooping cough) (DTaP)

Since the 1940s, the three vaccines (diptheria, tetanus, and pertussis [whooping cough]) have been administered together in the combined vaccine called DTP. The original pertussus vaccine (referred to as the "whole cell" vaccine) causes more noticeable side effects and is being replaced with the acellular pertussis vaccine (aP), although both are still in use.

Diptheria

The diphtheria vaccine is always given in combination with the tetanus vaccine. There are two forms: pediatric (D) and adult (d). The pediatric vaccine is called DT and the adult vaccine is referred to as dT. The distinction is made because the DT form contains eight times more diphtheria toxoid than the adult form. The pediatric vaccine is never given to adults or to children over the age of seven because of the increased likelihood of side effects. The reason the higher concentration is considered safe for smaller, younger children is unclear. Infants are given four doses of the DT form (as DTP or DTaP) during the first twelve months of life, resulting in thirty-two times the dose adults are given. The DT vaccine also contains:

- formaldehyde
- aluminum

Tetanus

Tetanus vaccines have not received the bad press as have many of the other vaccines. It is imagined that the risk of infection exceeds the potential risk of the vaccine. However, investigation by Dr. Sherri Tenpenny provoked the following commentary:

> *Discovering that most people recover from an acute bout of tetanus was unexpected, but it was disconcerting to find that many of the reported cases of tetanus were in "fully vaccinated" people ... In the Emergency Department, if the tetanus status of a patient is unknown, an additional shot is routinely given, because it is thought to be harmless. However, this is simply bad medicine. If the person doesn't need the tetanus booster, the vaccine can cause a severe allergic reaction referred to as an Arthus type, Type III hypersensitivity reaction. The reaction starts two to eight hours after a tetanus toxiod injection and occurs if the person has very high serum antitoxin antibodies due to overly frequent injections. Recommending "routine" tetanus boosters based on mathematical models of antibody degradation can result in severe complications and is risky business, indeed.*[304]

Tetanus differs from other childhood diseases because it is caused by a bacterium which cannot live and reproduce in the presence of oxygen and therefore is not contagious. In fact, the bacterium which releases the toxin that can cause tetanus can be found in our own bodies and yet not cause infection. Even if infection does develop, contrary to what you have likely been told, it usually doesn't end in death.

Prompt and adequate care of wounds is perhaps more important than vaccination in preventing tetanus disease. When a wound is allowed to bleed freely, oxygen is supplied at the site and the bacteria (unable to survive in oxygen) have less of a chance for survival. The application of hydrogen peroxide (3 percent drugstore dilution) is also very useful as it releases oxygen in high concentration. Other ingredients that are in the tetanus vaccine include:

- formaldehyde
- sodium phosphate dibasic, an eye and skin irritant
- aluminum
- thimerosol

Pertussis (whooping cough)

Before the pertussis vaccine, mothers who had had whooping cough as children were able to pass immunity on to their children before birth and via breast milk after birth. Antibodies supplied by the mother were capable of protecting children for the vulnerable first year of their lives, particularly if combined with breast feeding.[305] Most modern mothers have been vaccinated as children; they are not able to pass on the immune factors to their children. This is the biggest reason children are now vulnerable. As well, there are increasing numbers of teens and adults getting whooping cough, often in a mild form similar to a bad cold or flu. This is because immunity derived from the pertussis vaccine lasts only a few years. Adverse reactions to the pertussis vaccine include irritability; persistent, unusually high pitched crying; seizures; a shock-like hypotensive, hyporesponsive state; and encephalopathy.

Haemophilus influenzae type b (Hib)

When it was first discovered, Haemophilus influenzae type b (Hib) was thought to be the pathogen that caused influenza—hence its confusing name. Hib is actually a bacterium which can lead to bacterial meningitis. It is spread through coughing and sneezing and by direct or indirect contact. Despite the long list of illnesses possible from Hib, research has shown that it resides harmlessly in the noses, throats, and respiratory tracts of up to 90 percent of all healthy people. It is thought that most children have achieved immunity by the time they are five years old.[306]

The most common side effect of the Hib vaccine is meningitis—the primary disease it is supposed to protect against. Several studies have found that Hib-vaccinated children are six times more likely to contract Hib-meningitis during the first week after vaccination.[307]

Another side effect from the Hib vaccine that needs serious consideration is insulin dependent diabetes. In 2000, immunologist Bart Classen presented data that showed the Hib vaccine increased the risk of getting insulin dependent diabetes by 25 percent.[308]

Adverse reactions to the Hib vaccine include unusual, high-pitched or prolonged crying, diarrhea, drowsiness, ear pain, fever, fussiness, injection site abscess, seizures, upper-respiratory infection, and vomiting. The vaccine may contain:

- formaldehyde
- aluminum
- phenol
- soy
- yeast

Pneumococcal (PCV)

The streptococcal pneumonia vaccine (PCV) is one of the most recent vaccines. It was not routinely recommended until 2000. Streptococcal pneumonia can be caused by about ninety different strains of the bacteria; the pneumococcal vaccine contains only seven of these. In fact, as with the Hib bacteria, over half of the population harbors these bacteria their entire life with no problem. The most susceptible individuals are those with compromised immune systems; most healthy children are not at risk. Notwithstanding, four doses of the PCV vaccine are given; at age two, four, and six months and again at eighteen months. Side effects include wheezing, asthma, seizures, vomiting, diarrhea, decreased appetite, autoimmune disease, and SIDS.

Inactivated poliovirus (IPV)

Unknown to most people, the polio vaccine has been at the center of controversy since its initial use. Although it has been credited for virtually eliminating polio, polio had naturally declined in both England and the United States before mass inoculation began. After the vaccine was introduced, the number of reported cases nearly doubled.[309]

After years of use, it was discovered that a virus in the monkey tissue used to incubate the polio vaccine survived the formaldehyde in the vaccine and was given to between 30 and 100 million Americans. The virus (SV-40) can be passed from mother to child and has now been linked to cancer. In a study of fifty-nine thousand women, the children of mothers who received the initial vaccine had brain tumors at a rate thirteen times greater than children of mothers who had not received the polio vaccine. Even more incriminating is the fact that the monkeys used for this vaccine also harbored simian immunodeficiency virus (SIV), virtually indistinguishable from the human form of the disease (HIV). Several authorities believe that the SIV virus was capable of mutating into the HIV form through contaminated vaccines.[310]

More recently, the Centers for Disease Control admitted that *every* case of polio since 1979 has been caused by the oral vaccine. And from 1983 to 1991, not a single dose of polio vaccine met U.S. safety standards.[311] These statistics are incorrigible. Yet today, another "safer" polio vaccine is routinely given to children in a four-part series. Adverse reactions include anorexia, fever, pain, swelling, irritability, persistent crying, sleepiness, and vomiting. The vaccine contains:

- VERO monkey kidney cells
- newborn calf serum
- formaldehyde
- neomycin, polymyxin, streptomycin (antibiotics)
- 2-phenoxyethanol (phenol)

Influenza

In the United States, health authorities recommend that the influenza (flu) vaccine be given to children aged twenty-three months to six years old and also to anyone age fifty or older; to people with chronic health conditions; and to health care professionals. But the author of a 2006 review concluded that there is no good science to back the policies of influenza vaccination.[312] Dr. Tom Jefferson, coordinator of the Cochrane Vaccines Field in Rome, Italy, had this to say:

> *Influenza vaccines have little or no effect on many influenza campaign objectives, such as hospital stay, time off work, or death from influenza and its complications. We've got an exaggerated expectation of what vaccines can actually do. I'm hoping American and European taxpayers will be alerted and will start asking questions.* [313]

More recently, the American Thoracic Society's 105th International Conference, May 15-20, 2009, states: "The inactivated flu vaccine does not prevent influenza-related hospitalizations in children, especially the ones with asthma…In fact, children who get the flu vaccine are *three times more at risk for hospitalization* than children who do not get the vaccine."[314]

Influenza vaccines still contain thimerosol—the mercury-containing preservative.

Nutrition is the key when it comes to the flu. According to recent theory, the reason the flu is prevalent during winter months is because most people become vitamin D deficient during that time. Since the formation of vitamin D is dependant on ultraviolet rays from the sun, many people lack vitamin D in the winter. Supplementing with two thousand units of vitamin D_3 per day has effectively *nutritionally immunized* whole hospital wards from the flu.[315]

Measles, mumps, rubella (MMR)

In 1971, three vaccines (measles, mumps, and rubella) were combined. Now known as the MMR vaccine, it contains live viral colonies of each of the separate vaccines grown on chick embryos and human cells. Over the last few years, an enormous outcry has erupted over the safety of the MMR vaccine. Thousands of parents in Britain and the United States have reported autism-like disorders after the MMR vaccine. The development of autism and other conditions is closely linked to the time the vaccine is administered.

In 1998, the mothers of twelve autistic children with intestinal problems approached Dr. Andrew Wakefield, a gastroenterologist at the Royal Free Hospital in London. He determined that each of these children had what he called "leaky gut," where the intestinal wall becomes permeable. His study also found traces of the measles disease in the intestinal wall of these autistic children. Shortly after this study was published, Dr. Jeff Bradstreet conducted a study that found traces of the measles virus in the spinal fluid and the brains of almost two thousand autistic children who had received the MMR vaccine.

The Japanese health authorities withdrew the MMR vaccine in 1993 because of severe neurological problems and replaced it with separate vaccines. Since that time, there have been far fewer adverse reactions reported in Japan. Because the mumps vaccine may not be required in all states, these vaccines can still be given separately in the United States.

Adverse reactions to the MMR vaccine include arthritis, atypical measles, brain disease, convulsions, cough, diabetes, diarrhea, dizziness, ear infection and nerve deafness, edema, eye paralysis, fainting, fever, Guillain-Barre syndrome, headache, irritability, hives, meningitis (aseptic), sclerosis (brain), nausea, nerve inflammation, nose inflammation, pitting of abdomen and thigh, pneumonia, rash, seizures, sore throat, testes inflammation, upper-respiratory infection, visual disturbances, and vomiting. Components of the MMR vaccine include:

- live measles virus grown in chick embryo cell culture
- live mumps virus grown in chick embryo cell culture
- live weakened rubella virus grown in aborted human lung fibroblasts
- fetal bovine serum
- glutamate (MSG)
- human albumin
- neomycin (antibiotic)

Measles

Measles was officially declared eliminated in the United States in 2000. However, it remains a major illness in many other parts of the world. Measles is a highly contagious virus of the upper-respiratory tract that usually lasts ten to fourteen days. It causes a total-body skin rash and flulike symptoms, including a fever, cough, and runny nose. For healthy children, symptoms usually subside on their own without medical treatment. In parts of the world where nutrition is a problem, measles can be dangerous. According to

David Morley, who studied the connection between nutrition and disease, malnutrition is responsible for higher disease and complication rates:

> *Severity of measles is greatest in the developing countries where children have nutritional deficiencies … The child with severe measles and an immune system suppressed by malnutrition secretes the virus three times longer than does a child with normal nutrition.*[316]

Doctors and other health authorities often exaggerate the risks of measles. For example, vaccine pamphlets published by the Centers for Disease control claim that one out of every one thousand children who contract measles will get encephalitis, an infection of the brain. However, Dr. Robert Mendelsohn, renowned pediatrician and vaccine researcher, had this to say:

> *After decades of experience with measles, I question this statistic, and so do many other pediatricians. The incidence of 1/1,000 may be accurate for children who live in conditions of poverty and malnutrition, but in the middle- and upper-income brackets, if one excludes simple sleepiness from the measles itself, the incidence of true encephalitis is probably more like 1/10,000 or 1/100,000.*[317]

In 1990, the *New England Journal of Medicine* confirmed that vitamin A supplements significantly reduce measles complication and death rates.[318] In 1998, researchers in Japan determined that vitamin A supplementation shortened the duration of measles symptoms.[319] The biggest risk factor for measles is travel outside the United States. Undernourished young children and adults with compromised immune systems have a greater chance of complications.

> **The measles vaccine has a long history of causing serious adverse reactions. The pharmaceutical company responsible for producing the measles vaccine publishes an extensive list of ailments known to have occurred following the vaccination. These include: encephalitis, Guillain-Barre syndrome, convulsions, seizures, ataxia, ocular palsies, anaphylaxis, edema, bronchial spasms, atypical measles, thrombocytopenia, pneumonitis, deafness, otitis media, retinitis, optic neuritis, rash, fever, dizziness, headache, and death.**

Mumps

Mumps is a childhood disease that is rarely serious, and the need for medical intervention is also rare. The risks versus benefits are hard to justify when the vaccination may cause side effects that are more serious than the disease itself. This is one reason that the mumps vaccine is not required in many states. Adverse reactions to the vaccine include meningitis, encephalitis, diabetes, hearing loss, and anaphylaxis.

Rubella

For a number of reasons, the rubella vaccine has been seriously questioned. Rubella is a disease that is very mild, often showing limited or no symptoms in children. The only potential risk of rubella is when a woman contracts it during the early weeks of pregnancy. Unfortunately, that is precisely when the rubella vaccination (given at childhood) begins to wear off. Pregnant women cannot take the vaccine because the vaccine itself is capable of causing the disease, since it is a live vaccine. Rubella is of no risk to men. Essentially, we are vaccinating an entire population that is not at risk to provide limited protection for a tiny group.

Women are routinely tested for rubella immunity before marriage, and those susceptible are vaccinated if they are not pregnant. The Centers for Disease Control recommends that pregnant women found to lack rubella immunity be vaccinated during the postpartum period. This practice is also highly suspect. During one study, sixty rubella-susceptible mothers were revaccinated after they gave birth. Their children later received the MMR vaccine. Fifty-five of these women now have children diagnosed with either autistic-like symptoms, ADD/ADHD, or other developmental delays. Four women have children with other health problems, mostly immunologic.[320] These outcomes raise extremely serious concerns about the practice of postpartum vaccination and suggest that it may increase children's susceptibility.

Varicella (chicken pox)

Varicella (chicken pox) is considered by most experts to be a relatively harmless childhood disease. Serious problems in children are rare. In fact, before the chicken pox vaccine was introduced, doctors used to recommend exposing children to the virus while they were young because complication rates increase when the disease is contracted as an adult. One of the things the chicken pox vaccine does is put adults at greater risk because the vaccine may only last six to ten years. Since adults are rarely vaccinated, the vaccine only postpones vulnerability until adulthood, when complications are more severe. From the beginning, the FDA was aware that vaccinating children against chicken pox would also increase the risk of adult shingles, which is a reactivation of the chicken pox virus.

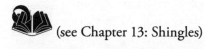 (see Chapter 13: Shingles)

The varicella vaccine is a live virus. Like many vaccines, it contains residual components of DNA and protein, which can cause serious side effects, including neurological disorders and immune system damage. There are many who wonder whether the vaccine is really effective. As recently as 2006, a community in Wisconsin experienced a 36 percent rate of chicken pox amongst vaccinated children.[321]

Hepatitis A

Hepatitis A is associated with poor hygiene and unsanitary conditions, usually transmitted through contaminated food and water in underdeveloped countries. Groups with the highest risk are those traveling to countries where sanitation is poor. Homosexual communities and intravenous drug users are also at risk. Children are not considered at risk—especially in the United States. Nevertheless, in order to reduce the overall incidence of the disease, children are vaccinated. Adverse reactions include encephalopathy, meningitis, and multiple sclerosis. The vaccine includes:

- bovine albumin
- formaldehyde
- aluminum
- phenol
- neomycin
- yeast protein

OTHER VACCINES

There were eleven vaccines on the recommended adult immunization schedule for 2008.[322] More than two hundred new vaccines, which are being developed for everything from cocaine addiction to sexually transmitted diseases, will be candidates for future mandates.

Anthrax

The anthrax vaccine is currently mandatory for some military personnel, although it has been highly contested. Canada relinquished the mandatory status for its military personnel. It has been estimated that 10–30 percent of all soldiers who have been vaccinated have developed some medical problem as a result of the vaccine. Many airmen have lost the ability to continue flying. Most soldiers who have been in the military for some time know of several people who became ill or disabled shortly after receiving anthrax inoculations. The most common side effects are new pains in muscles and joints, short-term memory loss, and periods of confusion. Fatigue and problems sleeping usually accompany these symptoms. Some people develop inflammatory bowel disease. Some develop autoimmune disorders like lupus, multiple sclerosis, and reactive arthritis. Rashes and thyroid disorders are also common. Even though you may be in the military, no one has the right to immunize you against your will. You do not give up your constitutional rights when you join the armed forces.

Human papillomavirus (HPV)

In July 2006, the FDA approved Gardasil as a vaccine for women ages nine to twenty-six to protect against cervical cancer caused by infection with human papillomavirus (HPV). Makers of the vaccine spent $250,000 for a legislative push to make the vaccine mandatory for school-aged girls in Texas. The cost of the vaccine? The series of three shots costs an average of $360, making Gardasil the most expensive vaccine on the market.

HPV (human papillomavirus) is a common virus that is spread through sexual contact. There are more than one hundred twenty strains of HPV—most do not cause problems. However, certain strains of HPV can lead to cervical cancer. Other strains may cause genital warts. According to the Centers for Disease Control and Prevention: In 90 percent of cases, your body's immune system clears the HPV infection naturally within two years. This is true whether the infection is the type that can cause warts or cancer.

The HPV vaccine contains only four strains of HPV. The vaccine literature says that it does not protect women against some nonvaccine HPV types. This is by no means protection against cervical cancer from HPV. As with other vaccines, it comes with numerous side effects and no long-term studies to guarantee its safety.

As of October 2007, 3,779 adverse reactions and eleven deaths had been filed with the FDA's Vaccine Adverse Event Report System (only about 10 percent of adverse reactions are ever reported). According to the National Vaccine Information Center's Health Policy Analyst, Vicky Debold, RN, PhD:

> *The most frequent serious health events after Gardasil shots are neurological symptoms. These young girls are experiencing severe headaches, dizziness, temporary loss of vision, slurred speech, fainting, involuntary contraction of limbs (seizures),*

*muscle weakness, tingling and numbness in the hands and feet
and joint pain. Some of the girls have lost consciousness during
what appears to be seizures.*[323]

The best way to reduce your risk of getting HPV is to follow safe-sex practices and to keep your immune system in top shape.

Shingles

Shingles occurs when the latent chicken pox virus becomes reactivated. It is generally a disease of the elderly that is triggered by stress (emotional, physical, or chemical). A 2002 letter to the editor of the *Journal of the American Medical Association* pointed out that the FDA was aware that vaccinating children against chicken pox would increase the risk of adult shingles.[324] Now a vaccine is recommended for adult shingles.

The shingles vaccine (Zostavax) contains live chicken pox virus. Prior to its acceptance in 2006, the vaccine was only tested on caucasians over the age of sixty; it worked just 50 percent of the time. According to FDA drug reviewer Dr. David Markovitz, researchers still don't know how it may affect other races, and they still don't know how long immunity may last after vaccination.[325]

Yellow Fever

Several vaccines are considered voluntary when traveling overseas. The only vaccine that is not voluntary is the yellow fever vaccine, which is mandatory when traveling to countries that are known to have the disease (some South American countries and some African countries).

Yellow fever is a viral disease that is transmitted to humans through the bite of infected mosquitoes. Illness ranges in severity from an influenza-like syndrome to severe hepatitis and hemorrhagic fever. Because of recent reports of deaths due to yellow fever among unvaccinated travelers to yellow fever-endemic areas, yellow fever vaccination of travelers to high-risk areas has been encouraged as a preventive. However, severe adverse events can follow yellow fever vaccination. Some physicians have been advised to administer the vaccine only to people who are truly at risk.

A serious adverse reaction syndrome has been described within the last ten years among recipients of the yellow fever vaccine. Since 1996, twelve cases of YEL-AVD, a disease that is clinically and pathologically similar to naturally acquired yellow fever, have been reported in the United States. An additional twenty-four suspected cases have been identified worldwide as of August 2006. All U.S. cases required intensive care. Seven were fatal. Even though this vaccine may be mandatory in several countries during some months of the year, waivers can be obtained.

 (see Chapter 18: Vaccinations—travel)

 (see Chapter 7: Insect repellants)

H1N1 (Swine flu)

The H1N1 vaccine is the largest and fastest vaccination program in world history. The fact that the vaccine took less than a year to develop, test, and mass produce, raises some serious questions about its safety. The vaccine was only tested on a small scale and for an extremely short period of time. (The product insert for the H1N1 vaccine states that safety was evaluated in 31 children ages 6-26 months of age.)[326] Safety information for the vaccine uses the data from another vaccine made using the same process—not the H1N1 vaccine. Long-term effects (as with all influenza vaccines) are unknown and no data exist for pregnant women or for developing fetuses. At the publication of this book, large numbers of adverse reactions are being reported on a regular basis.

The National Vaccine Information Center has a wealth of information on the swine flu vaccine and other vaccines. Visit: http://www.nvic.org/vaccines-and-diseases/h1n1-swine-flu.aspx. Also read the Vaccine Action Letter Web site: www.vaccineactionletter.blogspot.com. According to the Vaccine Action Letter Web site:

> *The best way to be protected from any flu including the H1N1 live virus swine flu is to have a healthy immune system by living a natural, earth-connected way of being, which includes: organic, plant-source-only foods, supplements including nano-silver, vitamin C, A, and D, medicinal immune-building mushrooms and herbs, and specific aromatherapy oils...These healthy approaches have been historically proven to be far more safe and effective than generated vaccines, which have truly never been scientifically proven to be either safe or effective except for building the economic pockets of the vaccine companies.*[327]

EXEMPTIONS

Most states currently allow for medical and religious exemptions. Unfortunately, you may not be told this when you go to a pediatrician. You may simply be told that you have to vaccinate. But that is not true. It is important for you to know the legal requirements of the vaccination laws in your state and to understand the difference between a legal requirement and a recommendation. Vaccine policymakers recommend certain vaccines, but they may not always be legally required. There are many exemptions unknown to most parents. Exemptions may be philosophical, conscientiously held beliefs (religious), and medical. You may call or write your state representative and ask for a copy of the immunization laws in your state. Making this available is part of his/her job, and it will be sent promptly.

Philosophical exemption

Currently, eighteen states allow exemption to vaccination based on philosophical, personal, or conscientiously held beliefs:

- Arizona
- Arkansas
- California
- Colorado
- Idaho
- Louisiana
- Maine
- Michigan
- Minnesota
- New Mexico
- North Dakota
- Ohio
- Oklahoma
- Texas
- Utah
- Vermont
- Washington
- Wisconsin

In some of these states, individuals must object to all vaccines in order to use the philosophical or personal belief exemption. Many state legislators are being urged by federal health officials and medical organizations to revoke this exemption to vaccination. If you object to vaccination based on philosophical or personal conviction, be aware that public health officials are seeking to change state laws to eliminate this exemption. (See sources for individual state Web sites where forms and instructions can be found.)

Religious exemption

The religious exemption is intended for people who hold a sincere religious belief opposing vaccination to the extent that if the state forced vaccination, it would be an infringement on their right to exercise their religious beliefs. Some state laws define religious exemptions broadly. Other states require an individual who claims a religious exemption to be a member of The First Church of Christ, Scientist (Christian Science), or another religion whose written tenets include prohibition of invasive medical procedures such as vaccination. The religious exemption is granted based on the First Amendment of the Constitution, which is the right to freely exercise your religion. All states except Mississippi and West Virginia allow a religious exemption to vaccination.

Medical exemptions

All fifty states allow medical exemption to vaccination. Proof of medical exemption must take the form of a signed statement by a medical doctor (MD) or doctor of osteopathy (DO) that the administering of one or more vaccines would be detrimental to the health of an individual. Most states do not allow doctors of chiropractic (DC) to write medical exemptions to vaccination. Some states will accept a private physician's written exemption without question. Other states allow the state health department to review the doctor's exemption and revoke it if health department officials don't think the exemption is justified.

Proof of immunity

You also have the option in most states to be exempted from vaccination or re-vaccination if you can show proof of existing immunity. Immunity can be proven if you or your child have had the natural disease or have been previously vaccinated. Private medical laboratories will take blood and analyze it to measure the level of antibodies. If the antibody level is high enough, you may be able to use this for an exemption to vaccination. Check your state laws to determine which vaccines can be exempted if proof of immunity is demonstrated. A blood test that measures antibody levels will cost $60 or more, depending on the disease.

ADVICE FOR PARENTS

The decision to vaccinate—or not—is an extremely important one. Parents may want to read the books in the recommended reading section at the end of this chapter. Parents may also want to confer with a holistic doctor besides their pediatrician, and to visit several Web sites for further information. The Web site www.thinktwice.com is an excellent resource.

In most instances it is better to have single vaccinations rather than combination doses of vaccines. It is also better to wait as long as possible in between vaccinations. When making an informed vaccination decision, consider whether one or more of the following factors will affect the safety and effectiveness of a particular vaccine or combination of vaccines your child may receive:

- child's age
- state of health at the time of vaccination
- number and types of vaccines to be given simultaneously
- past history of acute vaccine reactions or serious health problems following vaccination
- family history of vaccine reactions, severe allergies, or autoimmune or neurological disorders

In many cases, parents may find themselves in a position to accept vaccination for either themselves or their children. In such cases, there are things that can be done to mitigate some of the symptoms of vaccination.

Nutritional support

Too much can never be said for a good diet—especially before and following vaccination. It is well known that vaccinating a malnourished child encourages far more complications than vaccinating a well-nourished child. A good whole-food supplement is essential in today's world. Focusing on supporting the immune system provides much better long-term protection than vaccines have ever been proven to produce. Especially during the vaccination time frame (first two years of your child's life), stay away from pasteurized milk products, cheese, and refined gluten-containing grains (wheat, oats, barley, and rye). For more information on a variety of nutrient-dense whole foods visit www.wyntersway.com.

> **If mothers breastfeed their babies, the risk of death from childhood disease is dramatically reduced. If children (and adults) eat a proper diet, the risk of disease is significantly reduced.**

Regardless of the vaccine, the elimination of their toxins can be supported by algae and seaweed. Chlorella, spirulina, and other forms of algae given after vaccination can be of tremendous help. These foods are known to bind to heavy metals and to other toxins, eliminating them from the body.

Alginate Plus by Rx Vitamins is an excellent liquid algae formulation (see sources). Take these supplements for at least several weeks after vaccination. To download a free book on these superfoods, visit: http://www.chlorellafactor.com/

Cod liver oil with vitamins A and D has also been shown to improve learning disabilities, attention deficit, hyperactivity, and autism following vaccination.[328] Children with these problems should consider a regular program of supplementation that includes cod liver oil or other naturally high sources of vitamins A and D.

Magnesium and Vitamin B-6 have also been shown to support those with vaccine-induced autism and developmental disabilities. Dr. Bernard Rimlaud, director of the Autism Research Institute, has said that vitamin B-6 and magnesium beat any drug available for autism.[329] Magnesium supports the nerves and muscles often affected by vaccinations. Supplementing with magnesium before and after vaccination can tone down the neuromuscular degeneration sometimes experienced with vaccination. Whole-food sources of magnesium include most fresh fruits, vegetables, and raw chocolate (not to be confused with most chocolate confections available today.

Vitamin B-6 is involved in more bodily functions than almost any other single nutrient. It is required by the nervous system for brain function and for making RNA and DNA, which contain the genetic instructions for normal cellular growth. Whole-food sources of vitamin B-6 include carrots, eggs, meat, nuts, whole grains, and leafy vegetables.

Vitamin C and other antioxidants also help to neutralize the toxins in vaccines. Early medical literature identified vitamin C as the treatment of choice in all toxin-mediated diseases.

Proteolytic enzymes

Because most vaccines contain foreign proteins from cows, chickens, monkeys, guinea pigs, and from aborted fetuses, protein digesting (proteolytic) enzymes can be beneficial. These enzymes work to remove foreign proteins from the body—the quicker, the better, before allergic reactions have time to become too severe. These are available in most health food stores.

Homeopathy

Tautopathy is the term for a homeopathic remedy made from a medicine, to counteract the adverse effects of that medicine. Tautopathic remedies are available for each vaccine in many health food stores in the 30C potency. For example, if parents choose to vaccinate for Hib, then by giving the Hib Vaccine 30C tautopathic remedy, some common side effects may be overcome. A homeopathic physician can also determine what is known as a constitutional remedy. This may also have ameliorating effects following vaccination.[330]

Sources (in the order they appear in the chapter):

Algae:
Alginate Plus (Rx Vitamins): www.rxvitamins.com

Exemption information by state:
http://www.vaccinerights.com/stateexemptionlaws.html

 Recommended Reading:

Don't Vaccinate Before You Educate by Mayer Eisenstein, MD

Vaccine Safety manual by Neil Z. Miller

Vaccine Guide: Risks and Benefits for Children and Adults by Randall Neustaedter

Chapter 14
AUTOMOTIVE POLLUTANTS

Albert Einstein said, "One cannot solve a problem with the same kind of thinking that created it." That statement describes the current world situation as it relates to the petrochemical industry. We cannot solve the fuel crisis or global warming by refusing to look for alternatives.

Automobiles are the single greatest source of pollution on the planet. Emissions from over a billion vehicles combine to create huge pockets of toxic fumes in every major city. Exhaust from the unrestrained use of combustion engines produces adverse effects on the health of every living creature. Even if you roll up the windows, the synthetic materials used in the manufacture of automobiles will outgas volatile organic chemicals from a new car for many months, collecting on the inside of windows and on the inside of your lungs. Automobiles also leave behind oil, antifreeze, chemical coolants, tires, and a variety of petrochemical products that endanger animal, plant, and aquatic life. As long as we remain dependant on oil and the petrochemical status quo we will continue to pollute the planet and our own bodies.

Global gasoline use is expected to increase exponentially in the next decade, driven by increased use in developing countries like India and China. Shortages are inevitable in the very near future. Many countries have aggressive plans in place to reduce the need for oil and to move to more efficient fuel options. China's 2009 fuel efficiency policy is way ahead of our own.

The Energy Independence and Security Act of 2007 requires the Corporate Average Fuel Economy (CAFE) standard to reach thirty-five miles per gallon by the year 2020.[331] We have proven in the past that we can do much better than that. During the energy crises of the 1970s and 1980s, fuel economy made much greater jumps. Using *current* technology, the United States could dramatically reduce its oil consumption by 3.4 million barrels a day just by improving fuel efficiency and achieving a minimum of forty miles per gallon (mpg) in cars and light trucks.[332] In their book *Freedom from Mid-East Oil,* authors Brown, Brutoco, and Cusumano suggest tax credits and other simple incentives for manufacturers who provide energy efficient vehicles and credits for citizens who use more efficient fuels and more efficient vehicles.[333]

Now is the time for global citizens to demand and support renewable energy resources. In the U.S., it will be the consumer who will ultimately dictate better fuel economy by demanding it in the marketplace. Supporting companies who develop alternate sources of fuel and those who create energy-efficient cars will send a needed message to the marketplace. Limiting your personal use of an automobile will also contribute to your health and to a safer outdoor breathing environment.

Toxins "Inside" Your Car

Most people think about cars causing outdoor air pollution. However, breathing the air and dust *inside* your car may be even more dangerous—especially if your car is new. New cars outgas so many vapors that in some models warning labels have actually been displayed on the inside of the windshield. Keeping the windows rolled up in the hot sun leaves a visible residue on the inside of the windows. From the formaldehyde-laden new carpet and foam seat cushions, to the new vinyl or leather-treated interior, the fumes in new automobiles pose serious problems for the chemically sensitive. They are equally damaging to those who do not exhibit sensitivities—including children who begin to build up these toxins in their bodies. One analysis of the air in a new 1995 Lincoln Continental revealed the presence of more than fifty volatile organic chemicals (VOCs).

Volatile organic compounds

The term "volatile" means that a compound will vaporize, or become a gas at room temperature. At higher temperatures or in humid environments, these compounds vaporize more rapidly. VOCs in new cars are emitted from carpeting, vinyl, adhesives, fabric treatments, foam cushions, and solvents. Because cars are often exposed to extremely warm temperatures, they outgas more than do normal interior environments. Breathing VOCs at levels emitted from new cars has been associated with sensory irritation and impairment of performance and memory in controlled exposure studies—all are important car safety issues as well as occupant health and comfort issues.[334]

An Australian study of the VOCs in three new car interiors determined that VOC levels decrease approximately 20 percent each week after manufacture. Their data indicate that it takes about six months before indoor air quality standards are met.[335] Since adequate ventilation is the easiest and most effective way to maintain air quality when VOCs are present, leaving the windows open for the first six months after purchasing a new car is advisable whenever possible. Purchasing a used car may be an even better option.

 (see Chapter 1: Volatile organic compounds)

> **If you have left the windows rolled up in a new vehicle, be sure to air out the car before you get in. Make sure your air-conditioning system is set to bring in fresh air from outside— rather than recirculating the air in the car as you drive.**

Plastic

Most cars are about 9 percent plastic—everything from the dashboard to armrests, trim, and steering column. One of the components of that "new car smell" comes from phthalates in the plastic. Phthalates are plasticizers used to give flexibility to plastics. They leach continually from the plastic with age—especially in warm temperatures. Most of the plastic in car interiors is vinyl (PVC), a normally rigid plastic. PVC requires considerable phthalates in order to become flexible. Several studies have found dangerously high phthalate levels inside new cars.

 (see Chapter 5: Phthalates)

> **One of the reasons the dashboard becomes more brittle as a car ages is because phthalates are slowly migrating into the car's interior. As they sweat out from the plastic, residue enters the air, or it can be directly absorbed through the skin.**

PBDEs

Polybrominated diphenylethers (PBDEs) are fire retardants used on many textiles, including those on the interior of automobiles. These chemicals (now banned in Europe and parts of Asia) are persistent in the environment and bioaccumulative—they build up in your body over a lifetime and may cause liver toxicity, thyroid toxicity, and neurodevelopmental toxicity.[336] PBDEs impair attention, learning, and memory in laboratory animals at surprisingly low levels.[337]

 (see Chapter 9: Fire retardants)

A recent study conducted by the Ecology Center in Detroit found that solar exposure in cars can be five times higher than in homes or offices. Ultraviolet exposure from parking in the sun creates a favorable environment for chemical breakdown, causing PBDEs to become even more dangerous.[338] Some manufacturers are reducing the PBDEs in car interiors. The 2006 study by the Ecology Center showed which car models are the best. The Swedish manufacturer Volvo had the lowest level of PBDEs and phthalates together. Volvo has been working for years on creating a clean car interior.[339]

Gasoline Pollutants

Air pollution produced by combustion engines consists of tiny solid and liquid particles that can be inhaled deep into your lungs. Most particles are microscopic, but you can see the smog that forms when millions of these particles create a haze that blocks sunlight in many cities. These pollutants cause inflammation in your lungs and brain. They trigger reactions that can also affect heart function. Statistics show that as levels of fine particulates in the environment rise, so does the death rate from lung cancer and cardiopulmonary disease. The combustion of gasoline produces hydrocarbons, nitrogen oxides, carbon dioxide, carbon monoxide, and water. The only by-product of gasoline combustion that does not have serious consequences for the earth or its inhabitants is the water.

Hydrocarbons—Hydrocarbon emissions are fragments of fuel molecules that are only partially burned. Hydrocarbons react in the presence of nitrogen oxides and sunlight to form ground-level ozone, a major component of smog. Hydrocarbons in smog irritate the eyes, damage the lungs, and aggravate respiratory problems. A number of exhaust hydrocarbons are toxic and have the potential to cause cancer.

Benzene is a hydrocarbon found in gasoline and in exhaust fumes. The U.S. Department of Health and Human Services has determined that benzene is carcinogenic. Long-term exposure may affect normal blood production, possibly resulting in severe anemia and internal bleeding. In addition, human and animal studies indicate that benzene is harmful to the immune system, increasing the chance for infections and lowering the body's defense systems.

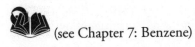 (see Chapter 7: Benzene)

Nitrogen oxides—Under the high pressure and temperature conditions in an engine, nitrogen and oxygen atoms react to form nitrogen oxides. Nitrogen oxides, like hydrocarbons, are precursors to the formation of ozone and they contribute to acid rain. Nitrogen oxides make up about 7.2 percent of the gases cited in global warming. Vehicles with catalytic converters produce nearly half of that nitrogen oxide.

Carbon monoxide—Carbon monoxide (CO) is a by-product of incomplete combustion. CO binds to hemoglobin in red blood cells two hundred times more strongly than oxygen. Thus, CO poisoning is a form of suffocation. CO can also exacerbate cardiovascular disease. In urban areas, the passenger vehicle contribution to CO pollution can exceed 90 percent. In major cities, we are literally suffocating ourselves.

Carbon dioxide (CO_2)—Carbon dioxide is a greenhouse gas that traps the earth's heat and contributes to global warming. The EPA originally viewed carbon dioxide (CO_2) as a product of "perfect" combustion. Now the EPA views CO_2 as a pollution concern. There is a fine balance between oxygen (released by vegetation and used by higher organisms) and CO_2 (released by higher organisms and used by plants). That balance has tipped so far in the direction of CO_2 that oxygen depletion has become a serious concern on the planet.

Diesel fumes—Diesel fumes represent an even greater threat to our health than normal automobile exhaust because diesel engines generate ten to one hundred times more particles than normal combustion engines. Diesel emissions also contain larger particles of soot. Those who work around diesel exhaust not only have a higher risk of respiratory problems, they also come home with a layer of soot on their skin and clothes. What happens on the inside of their lungs is similar to what happens for smokers.

Inhaled diesel exhaust triggers a stress response in the brain that may interfere with normal brain function and information processing. During a study released in 2008, volunteers were placed in a room filled with diesel exhaust. After thirty minutes, brain wave patterns displayed a stress response, and inflammation developed due to oxidative (free radical) damage.[340] Free radical damage is implicated in the development of neurodegenerative diseases such as Parkinson's and Alzheimer's disease. This kind of stress is the cause of headaches, "burnout," and traumatic brain injury. During this same study, researchers found that beta brain waves were adversely affected in the presence of diesel fumes. Beta waves are generated when your brain is actively engaged in mental activities, indicating that diesel exhaust may impair mental functions.

In another study, inhalation of diesel exhaust caused a three-fold increase in the stress of the heart during exercise. The body's ability to release a "guardian" protein known to prevent blood clots was also reduced during diesel exposure.[341] These studies help explain the growing incidence of heart disease. They may also explain the increasing incidence of malaise following the morning and afternoon drive to and from work in major cities.

Tips at the Fuel Pump

Besides limiting the amount of fuel you use, there are a few things you should know about gasoline that will help you get the most from the fuel you buy:

1. In the petroleum business, the specific gravity and the temperature of the gasoline, diesel, ethanol, or other fuel plays an important role. The specific gravity increases when the temperature is lower. This means that cool temperatures increase the density of the liquid and the amount of gasoline you get in a gallon. In the petroleum industry, gas is sold according to temperature, but service station pumps do not have temperature compensation. If you fill up your vehicle in the early morning when the ground temperature (gasoline is stored underground) is still cold, you will get more gasoline. The colder the ground is, the greater the amount of gasoline you get per gallon; buying in the afternoon or in the evening means that your gallon is not really a full gallon.
2. Keep your tank over half full. The reason for this is that the more gas you have in your tank, the less air you have occupying empty space. Gasoline evaporates faster than you can imagine. In the petroleum industry, gasoline storage tanks have an internal floating roof to minimize evaporation; your car does not have this feature.
3. When you fill up at the service station, use the slower trigger speed. In slow mode you minimize the vapors that are created while you are pumping. All hoses at the pump have a vapor return. If you are pumping in fast mode, more vapor goes back into the storage tank and you get less gasoline.

BIOFUELS

Biofuels have a proven track record of success. They are widely used and have completely eliminated the dependence on foreign oil in Brazil.[342] Biofuels can be classified into three major categories: biologically produced alcohols, biologically produced gasses, and biologically produced oil. The dominant biofuels are ethanol and biodiesel—both already in use to a great degree in many countries.

Ethanol

E85 is the term for a fuel blend of 85 percent ethanol alcohol and 15 percent gasoline. Ethanol burns cleaner than gasoline; it is completely renewable, and it can be made from corn or sugar cane. E85 vehicles reduce harmful hydrocarbon and benzene emissions when compared to vehicles running on gasoline alone. Ethanol also degrades quickly in water and therefore poses much less risk to the environment than oil or gasoline.

Ethanol can be burned in most combustion engines with little modification. In fact, most car manufacturers already have flexible-fuel vehicles on the market, and more than fifteen hundred filling stations of the one hundred seventy-six thousand in the country already provide E85. Flexible-fuel vehicles have the capacity to use either gasoline or ethanol mixtures. Many questions about ethanol are answered on the National Ethanol Vehicle Coalition's Web site: http://www.e85fuel.com/e85101/questions.php

Biodiesel

Biodiesel is another alternate fuel that is already available. It can be used with no major modifications and can be used alone or as a blend with regular diesel fuel. Biodiesel is made from a variety of plant and vegetable oils, including recycled restaurant oils. It is the only alternative fuel to have fully completed the health effects testing requirements of the Clean Air Act. The use of biodiesel results in a substantial reduction of unburned hydrocarbons. Exhaust emissions are nearly 50 percent less than for diesel fuel. Europe has already established a robust market for biodiesel. Even American sales of biodiesel boomed in 2006.

Make Your Own Biodiesel

Biodiesel is easy to make if you use recycled restaurant oil. Backyard production facilities are popping up everywhere. Several Web sites outline the process.

A professor of chemistry at Polytechnic University is taking the process one step further by turning plant oils into "bioplastic." When the plastic has fulfilled its purpose, rather than throwing it away, a naturally occurring enzyme is used to break down the plastic into biodiesel fuel. The Pentagon recently committed over 2 million dollars for further research.[343] Innovations like these have the potential to release us from our dependence on oil.

High-Tech Cars

Advancing technology is ushering in a new era in passenger vehicles. These technologies have the potential to make combustion engines obsolete. Electric cars, hybrids, plug-in hybrids, lightweight cars, and hydrogen-powered fuel cell vehicles are already on the freeway. Before you buy another car, consider the options.

Flexible-fuel vehicles

Flexible-fuel vehicles are already here. They are not really high-tech but they represent a big step in the right direction, and they can easily reduce the U.S. consumption of gasoline while we prepare for the switch to even more efficient fuel options. Flexible-fuel vehicles are designed to run on alcohol fuels or gasoline or a mixture of both. The fuel mixture is detected by sensors in the system that signal the engine control unit to adjust the fuel injection rate and spark timing for optimal performance, fuel economy, and emissions. In 2008, more than six million flexible-fuel vehicles were already on the road.

Hybrid electric vehicles

Hybrid electric vehicles have already gained widespread acceptance. Sales continue to increase as gasoline prices rise. According to the 2005 rankings by the EPA and the Department of Energy, the three top-rated vehicles for fuel economy are hybrid electric cars. They all get between fifty-five and sixty-five mpg.

Hybrid vehicles combine combustion engines with electric motors that run on an electric charge drawn from the engine or from the braking system—or both. The latest innovations replace bulky battery packs with capacitors that charge and discharge more rapidly than batteries, providing quicker response and quicker acceleration.

Plug-in electric vehicles

Like standard hybrid vehicles, plug-in hybrid electric vehicles are powered by both gasoline and electricity. Plug-ins offer the additional advantage of being chargeable directly from an electrical outlet. Since the average trip length for American households is less than ten miles, the plug-in hybrid (with a twenty-mile-range battery) could satisfy some households with a much reduced need for gasoline. With flexible fuel options (biofuels), the need could be even further reduced.

Fuel cell vehicles

Hydrogen fuel cells represent one of the most promising and innovative technologies to meet our future energy needs. Switching from a hydrocarbon economy to a hydrogen economy is the ultimate goal—and a very real possibility for the not-to-distant future. It will revolutionize the world economy, and it will go a long way toward the elimination of greenhouse gas emissions from out-dated, oil-based technology. Most people's concern is that hydrogen is flammable, but the truth is that it is far safer than gasoline. It is much less explosive, it burns at a lower temperature, and it generates lower amounts of radiant heat than gasoline.

Hydrogen is by far the most abundant molecule in the universe. It can be thought of as a gaseous form of electricity. It is clean, sustainable, and does not contribute to global warming. While it is still expensive, hydrogen generates twice as much energy as oil. Analysts have declared that with the price of oil skyrocketing, hydrogen is highly competitive in cost.[344] As an inexhaustible source of clean, safe energy, hydrogen will enhance human health, protect the environment, and provide an advanced source of power—not just for the automotive industry but for all energy needs.

In 2005, General Motors made headlines with the release of a prototype hydrogen vehicle that traveled three hundred miles on a single tank of hydrogen. BMW, Ford, and Mazda are all developing a variety of hydrogen-powered vehicles. Honda is now powering vehicles with hydrogen made from tap water in small, stationary units that drivers can keep in their garage. In 2007 Honda reported:

> *Honda's FCX was certified by the U.S. Environmental Protection Agency and the California Air Resources Board (CARB), making it the first and only fuel-cell car in history to be approved for commercial use. CARB and the EPA have also certified the FCX as a Zero-Emission.*[345]

Advanced materials vehicles

Super lightweight, super efficient vehicles made with advanced composite materials are being referred to as advanced materials vehicles (AMV). These vehicles could, in theory, raise fuel efficiency to more than ninety mpg. Hypercar, Inc. was founded in 1994 to research and capture the synergies of ultralight construction, low-drag design, and hybrid-electric drive. AMV cars will eventually be powered by fuel cells running on hydrogen.

Compressed-air vehicles

India's largest automaker is already producing an air-powered vehicle. The Air Car uses compressed air to fuel zero-emissions cars that were made available in India in 2008. One of the models, the CityCAT, has a range of 125 miles and can be refueled at any gas station equipped with compressed air. And what if you run out of air? You can plug into an electrical outlet, and the car's built-in compressor will refuel in four hours.[346] The manufacturer has signed agreements to bring the design to twelve more countries, including Germany, Israel, and South Africa—but not the United States.

CAR CARE AND MAINTENANCE

Since automobiles are an indispensable part of our lives, using the most environmentally friendly car maintenance products or at least recycling the petroleum-based products we use can play an important role in maintaining a clean and healthy environment for ourselves and for future generations.

Motor oil

About 2 billion gallons of motor oil are used every year in the United States simply to keep our car engines lubricated. This translates into an equivalent amount of used oil that is discarded in landfills, re-refined, or lost in accidental oil spills. Conventional petroleum-based motor oil is an indisputable environmental hazard.

Most of us are familiar with the recycling of newspapers, aluminum cans, glass, and plastic bottles, but you may not be aware of the significance of recycling used motor oil. Motor oil can be reprocessed and used in power plants to generate electricity. It can also be re-refined into base oils for automotive use. If you take your car to an automotive service outlet, you can be fairly certain that they recycle the oil. If you change your own oil, be sure to take it to a collection center for recycling. If you recycle just two gallons of used oil, it can generate enough electricity to run the average household for almost twenty-four hours. Better yet, there are emerging oils made from plants and animal fats that are completely biodegradable and renewable.

Green motor oil

Green Earth Technologies announced a completely biodegradable motor oil in 2007 called G-Oil, which is the first bio-based, high-endurance motor oil to provide superior performance. The oil comes from the tallow in cows—a waste product from the beef industry. Not only is the process highly efficient (one barrel of animal fat can yield one barrel of G-Oil), it is completely biodegradable. When mixed with an enzyme formulation, the used G-Oil can be converted into soil.

G-Oil exceeds API requirements for gasoline and diesel engine standards. The smokeless G-Oil is nontoxic; it reduces hydrocarbons by 32 percent; it cuts the emissions of carbon monoxide by 48 percent; and it cuts nitrogen oxide by 80 percent, according to Green Earth Technologies.[347] *PopularMechanics* magazine recently chose this motor oil for the Editors Choice Award[348] (see sources).

Synthetic oil

Synthetic oils aren't really synthetic. They are still made of petroleum. So-called synthetic lubricants are synthesized, hydrocarbon chains with molecular uniformity not found in traditional motor oils. They are significantly more expensive, but they represent a reduction in the wear and tear on your car and may need to be changed less often. Both can have a positive impact on the environment.

Vegetable-based lubricants

Vegetable oil–based lubricants are emerging as another high-performance, environmentally preferable alternative to petroleum products that can perform as well as or better than petroleum oils. They are biodegradable, much less toxic, and they offer numerous safety advantages (see sources).

Engine coolants

Most modern automobiles use a mixture of antifreeze and water as a coolant. Ninety-five percent of these are made of ethylene glycol—a nonrenewable resource produced from natural gas. Although ethylene glycol is technically biodegradable, it is poisonous to animals and small children. Waste antifreeze may also contain heavy metals such as lead, cadmium, and chromium in high enough levels to make it a regulated hazardous waste.

Propylene glycol can also be used as a coolant. It is biodegradable and requires no special disposal costs or procedures in most areas. Above all, its lower toxicity limits the threat to children, pets, or wildlife. Amsoil makes a coolant using propylene glycol rather than ethylene glycol. It can be used for seven years or 250,000 miles in passenger cars, light-duty trucks, vans, and recreational vehicles (see sources). Engine Ice is another alternative to ethylene glycol. It is a high-performance coolant that is also biodegradable and nontoxic.

SOURCES (in the order they appear in the chapter):

Web sites for how to make biodiesel:
http://journeytoforever.org/biodiesel_make.html
http://make-biodiesel.org/

Vegetable-based lubricants:
Renewable Lubricants: http://www.renewablelube.com/
G-Oil: Green Earth Technologies: http://www.getg.com/products/products.
php?CategoryID=1&ProductID=1
Eco-Oil: http://www.treehugger.com/files/2006/04/vegetable_motor.php

Engine coolants:
Amsoil antifreeze with propylene glycol: http://www.amsoil.com/storefront/
ant.aspx
Engine Ice: http://www.engineice.com/

 Recommended Reading:

Freedom from Mid-East Oil by Jerry B. Brown, Rinaldo S. Brutoco, and James A. Cusumano

Chapter 15

TOXINS AND MAN'S BEST FRIENDS

It has been said that the purity of a person's heart can be measured by how they treat animals. That statement ought to be required daily reading for everyone involved in the pet industry. Sadly, it is not reflected in the products that are commercially available. Just as with products designed for humans, the products created for pets can pose health hazards—and not just for pets. The adults and children who play with them and care for them may often be at risk as well.

PET FOOD

If you are in the habit of checking the ingredients on grocery store foods, you probably know that the list of ingredients doesn't always tell the whole truth about what's in the package. The same goes for pet food. Behind innocent-sounding words like meat by-products and meat meal are manufacturing practices that most people would rather not know about. "Most commercial pet foods are garbage," says Ann Martin, author of *Foods Your Pets Die For.*

Ninety percent of pet health problems are the result of poor nutrition at some point in an animal's lifetime. Considering the increasing number of pet health problems, the nutritional value of commercial pet food must be seriously questioned. Not only do pet foods contain slaughterhouse wastes, including up to 25 percent fecal matter, they also contain road kill, euthanized pets, 4-D (dead, diseased, disabled, dying) livestock, and preservatives not legal in human food. They may also contain artificial coloring agents and appetite stimulants (salt, sugar, propylene glycol, and phosphoric acid).

Protein

The major protein source in most commercial brands of pet food is meat by-products or meat meal. Both refer to the leftover parts of animals (head, feet, entrails, brain, bones, and blood) after meat has been stripped away. Rendering plants that produce meat meal receive shipments that must be denatured before they arrive. Carcasses are denatured using toxic chemicals such as carbolic acid (phenol) or creosote. According to federal meat inspection regulations, fuel oil, kerosene, crude carbolic acid, and citronella are the approved denaturing materials. In the case of a whole animal, the denaturing product is injected into the entire carcass before it is shipped to a rendering plant.

Phenol is derived from the distillation of coal tar. Creosote is derived from the distillation of wood. Both substances are very toxic. Creosote was used for many years as a preservative for wood power poles. Its effect on the environment proved to be so detrimental that it is no longer used for that purpose—yet it is still used to denature pet food.

 (see Chapter 7: Common Toxic Chemicals in Personal Care Products: Phenol)

Rendering facilities are not government controlled. Any animal can end up at a rendering plant. If an animal is diseased and declared unfit for human consumption, the carcass is still acceptable for pet food. Euthanized cats and dogs often end up in rendering vats along with other questionable material to make meat meal. This can be problematic because sodium pentobarbital (the drug used for euthanization) can withstand the heat from rendering. It is not broken down and remains in the end product. In other words, the poisons designed to kill pets are the same ones being fed to them. It is also common for collars, I.D. tags, and plastic bags to become part of the material called meat meal.[349]

At the rendering plant, animal parts are ground, cooked, then centrifuged (spun at a high speed), and the grease rises to the top. The grease becomes the source of animal fat in most pet foods. The heavier protein material is dried and pulverized into a brown powder—about a quarter of which consists of fecal material.[350] The powder is used as an additive to almost all pet food as well as to livestock feed. In the livestock industry it is called "protein concentrate."

> **A lot of pet food manufacturers say that their meat is inspected by the USDA.** *All* meat is *inspected*—but whether or nor it is *approved* is another matter. The claim that it is inspected is meaningless.

Grains

Cheap grain fillers and cellulose are used by most pet food manufacturers as bulk. In fact, most pet foods are primarily processed grain (particularly rice), which contributes to animal diabetes. Dry pet foods are entirely upside down when it comes to amounts of protein, fat, and carbohydrate. A cat's or dog's natural diet is high in animal protein (between 45 to 70 percent), moderate in fat (about 15 to 40 percent), and very low in carbohydrates (0 to 5 percent). Contrast this with the breakdown of most dry pet foods: 10 to 30 percent protein, 10 to 25 percent fat, and very high carbohydrate from processed cereals (35 to 50 percent). If your cat or dog is overweight, consider that this is the most logical reason.

> **Dogs and cats were never meant to eat carbohydrates. Cats in particular do not have the enzymes to digest carbohydrates. Hundreds of thousands of cats needlessly have diabetes because of the carbohydrates in dry pet food.**

Preservatives

Most pet food contains much higher levels of fat than human food. Fat spoilage (rancidity due to oxidation) decreases the nutritional quality of the food, makes it less palatable, and can even make it unsafe to eat. Canned pet food is protected from rancidity, but dry food must have preservatives. The most common preservatives used by the pet food industry are artificial: ethoxyquin, butylated hydroxytoluene (BHT), and butylated hydroxyanisole (BHA).

Animal tests have shown adverse kidney, liver, reproductive, brain, behavioral, and allergic reactions to BHA and BHT. These chemicals used to be on the GRAS (Generally Recognized as Safe) list because there were no known negative effects. However, in 1991 they were removed from the GRAS list. Some European countries now ban the use of these preservatives for human use.

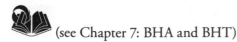 (see Chapter 7: BHA and BHT)

Ethoxyquin is perhaps the worst pet food preservative. It is a lethal herbicide. Although ethoxyquin has been used in animal feed for more than thirty years, it has been linked to immune deficiency syndrome; spleen, stomach, and liver cancers; and allergies.[351] The FDA currently allows only a trace amount of ethoxyquin residue (.5 to 5 ppm) in human-consumed foods, yet it allows high amounts (150 ppm) to be used in pet food and livestock feeds. In 1997, the FDA made a request to the pet food industry to voluntarily lower ethoxyquin levels in pet foods to 75 ppm. To date, there is still no mandatory requirement to meet this voluntary request. Rather than listing it as an ingredient on the packaging, some pet food manufacturers simply print "E" to represent ethoxyquin. And when it is added at the rendering plant and not by the manufacturer, ethoxyquin is not required to be listed on the pet food label.

Propylene glycol (first cousin to antifreeze, ethylene glycol) is used mostly in canned pet foods. It inhibits bacterial growth—but it also inhibits the growth of friendly flora in the digestive tract. Propylene glycol contributes to hard, dry stools by pulling moisture from the digestive tract.

Natural antioxidant preservatives used in pet food are vitamins C and E. Neither is as effective as the artificial preservatives. Therefore, when these natural alternatives are incorporated, food will not keep as long. Vitamin C is not naturally found in a carnivore's diet. Its addition to pet food can sometimes cause allergic skin reactions.

Appetite stimulants

Salt, sugar, and phosphoric acid are often heavily used in pet food as appetite stimulants to overcome the poor quality of the food itself. None of these are a part of an animal's normal diet and can cause kidney, liver, and colon stress.

Mad cow disease

Mad cow disease has been found in cows, deer, sheep, goats, mink, elk, cats, and humans on an increasing basis. The production of rendered feed for cattle is considered the reason for the spread of mad cow disease. Because 4-D meat (dead, diseased, dying, and disabled) can legally be rendered and used in pet food, the chances that pet food contains mad cow disease are quite large. The U.S. government believes it is safe to render diseased cattle for use in pet foods because this practice does not affect humans. But that is the same faulty logic that has been responsible for other disastrous consequences. Rendering diseased cattle and road kill for pet food perpetuates a growing problem and endangers our animal companions. This is already happening in Europe.[352]

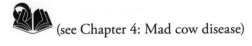 (see Chapter 4: Mad cow disease)

Food allergies

Allergies in pets are becoming more common. According to York Test Veterinary Services in England, most allergies in pets are caused by pet food because animals are eating ingredients nature never intended them to eat. The signs of an allergy can vary from one animal to another, including skin problems such as scratching and hair loss, or digestive problems which include vomiting. Just as with some children, allergies can manifest as behavioral problems. The veterinary approach to allergies is to treat the symptoms. A vet may prescribe steroids, antibiotics, tranquilizers, and antihistamines, when the real problem is most likely diet.

Real pet food—how to know

Pets today are not starving for food—they have plenty of that. But they are literally starving for nutrition because commercial pet food is rarely wholesome. Even many so-called natural or premium pet food products are made with ingredients of questionable quality. The nonprofit Consumer Wellness Center has posted a detailed nutritional review of more than five hundred pet food ingredients, available at: http://www.naturalnews.com/Report_pet_food_ingredients_1.html. When choosing a pet food, consider the following:

- The first five ingredients listed on any pet food product make up the bulk of the product.
- Don't be fooled by the words natural or wholesome on pet food product packaging. There is virtually no regulation of pet food health claims.
- Watch for artificial coloring and chemical additives—especially in pet treats.
- Never buy pet food in a big-box store, grocery store, or convenience store. These retail outlets usually offer the worst pet food products. Only health food stores, natural stores, and online retailers offer healthy pet food. Even pet specialty stores sell junk pet food.
- Avoid feeding your pet refined grains or sugars.
- Augment packaged pet food with real food that you make in your kitchen. Even the best pet food in the world is not a substitute for home-prepared meals for your pets.

Several recommended pet food brands are: California Natural, Timber Wolf, Innova, Wellness, Canidae, Pinnacle, Merrick, Solid Gold, Nature's Variety, and Avoderm. Not only do these contain high-quality protein sources, most also contain beneficial flora for healthy digestion.

Raw food diet

Pet food companies give huge funding to veterinary schools and even allow pet food companies to teach nutrition to veterinary students. This is why they graduate not knowing that dogs and cats have lived on raw food for most of their evolutionary lives. Some veterinarians tell clients that it is dangerous to feed raw food to pets, even though raw food is the most appropriate food for cats and dogs.

The best and most wholesome diet for animals is the one that most closely imitates their natural diet. If you are serious about having your pet eat the best food possible, stick with raw food. The ten-year study done by Dr. Francis Pottenger with more than nine hundred cats clearly illustrated this fact. Dr. Pottenger found that feeding cats cooked meat caused numerous problems, while feeding raw meat kept the cats healthy.[353]

A carnivore's intestines are nowhere near as long as a human's. Carnivores produce digestive enzymes in their stomachs which, with the high acidic level, give them the ability to digest raw meat and even bones. Raw meat helps to stimulate the highly acidic digestive system of a cat or dog. Raw meat is also an excellent source of B vitamins—cooking destroys many vitamins.

Cats and dogs do need vegetables, but how they get them in nature is to eat the contents of the stomach and intestines of the animals they kill. If you've ever watched a nature movie, you'll recall that's the first thing a carnivore will eat. These vegetables are partially digested and therefore able to be assimilated by a carnivore's digestive system.

Pet food—making your own

Homemade pet food does not need to take a lot of time. Meats should be raw; vegetables should be finely chopped or grated. A carnivore's digestive system is designed to eat one animal protein at a time. One type of meat should not be combined with another type of meat. Animals, because they are color blind, choose their foods by smell. Most dogs like gamey flavors best: liver, fat, garlic, horsemeat, lamb, beef, and fish. Cats enjoy chicken, liver, fish, turkey, lamb, and prefer fresh to aged flavors.

> **Carnivores drink very little water in the wild—that's because they get their water from their food. Homemade food should be the consistency of gravy to simulate their natural diet.**

Supplements are also necessary for your pets for the same reason they are needed in the human diet—because our soils have become depleted and many minerals are missing from foods. Calcium is the single most important supplement you can provide your pet. Carnivores need lots of calcium. In nature, a carnivore gets the majority of its calcium from blood. This can be hard to provide. The best source of calcium for your pets is ground-up egg shells. They supply a better ratio of calcium to phosphorous than bone meal.[354] Pets can also benefit from trace minerals, enzymes, and green food supplements. An excellent source of information about making homemade pet food is included in a free e-book available online. Every pet owner should read this simple 130 page book: http://www.pet-grub.com/. Another excellent source of information specifically for cats is *The Complete Guide to Holistic Cat Care* (see recommended reading.).

FLEAS AND TICKS

More than a billion dollars every year is spent on flea and tick products. Many Americans believe that the commercially available pesticides found in pet products are tightly regulated. They are not. In fact, only recently (1996) has the EPA begun to examine the risks from pesticides in pet products.

Probably thousands of pets have been injured or killed through exposure to pet products containing insecticides. The EPA allows the manufacture and sale of pet products containing hazardous insecticides with little or no demonstration that a pet's exposure to these ingredients would be safe. The other thing to consider is child safety. What child does not handle or hug his/her pet? The EPA calculates that a child's exposure to individual organophosphates in pet products on the day of treatment alone can exceed safe levels by up to five hundred times.[355] According to the Natural Resources Defense Council Report:

> *The EPA has never received adequate toxicity tests for these pesticide products. Of the seven chemicals that are the focus of this report, only one—chlorpyrifos—has been fully tested for its impact on a child's brain and nervous system. And, when the nervous-system testing for chlorpyrifos was recently completed, the results were so disturbing that the manufacturer itself took virtually all indoor uses of the chemical off the market.[356]*

Flea collars

A pesticide flea collar is a poison necklace around your pet's head. It emits a continuous toxic cloud that your pet inhales. You and your children are also exposed every time you hug your pet. Cats are particularly vulnerable, since they lack enzymes for metabolizing or detoxifying pesticides and because they are constantly grooming themselves.

The EPA's preliminary estimate concluded that toddlers exposed to pets wearing flea collars containing the pesticide dichlorvos would be exposed to twenty-one times the safe level just from inhalation. Flea collars containing the pesticide called Naled would expose toddlers to ten times more than the EPA's safe level. A toddler exposed to a dog wearing a collar containing chlorpyrifos could get more than seven times the level the EPA considers to be safe merely from hugging or petting a dog. Other pesticides contained in pet collars are tetrachlorvinphos and diazinon—they are no safer that those specifically tested.

As an alternative to the poison necklace, herb-based flea collars with natural flea repellants include combinations of eucalyptus, lavender, cedar, citrus, and sesame oils. The herbs don't actually kill fleas, but they can repel them. Another flea repellant for dogs (cats don't like the smell of lemons) is lemon oil, which can be made from lemons at home.

Homemade Lemon Flea Repellant for Dogs

Gently simmer 2–3 cut lemons in a quart of water. Strain and cool the liquid and apply liberally to the coat of your pet while brushing. You can also use this as a spritz to renew the scent regularly. Spritz bedding as well.

Flea and tick dips, sprays, powders, foggers, and bombs

Foggers and bombs poison the atmosphere so pervasively that they should be completely avoided. Cats that were regularly treated with flea powders and sprays have been found more likely to have hyperthyroidism. A statistically significant association between exposure to topical flea and tick dips and the occurrence of bladder cancer in dogs has also been found. One flea-and-tick repellent caused twenty-six known pet deaths in 1987 and at least two hundred dog and cat poisonings. The EPA forced the manufacturer to list warnings about tremors and vomiting on the label, but this has not kept consumers from using these volatile pesticides on their pets.[357]

Inert ingredients in pesticides can be almost as toxic as the pesticides themselves. What doesn't appear on labels, due to "trade-secret" laws, are solvents and petrochemicals that can make up to 90 percent of a pesticide's bulk. These toxic substances include xylene, methyl bromide, benzene, DDT (a by-product of the manufacture of certain pesticides), and toluene. Never use a dip, powder, spray, or fog directly on an animal.

Shampoo

What about insecticidal flea and tick shampoos? Labels warn you not to get them on your skin, to use rubber gloves, and to wash your hands. Yet the instructions also tell you to work them into your animal's coat, where they absorb into your pet's skin and are licked! Signs of pesticide overdose in your pet can include vomiting, diarrhea, trembling, seizures, and respiratory problems.

Pesticide shampoos are overkill since simple soap and water will kill fleas if the soap is left on for about ten minutes. Combing and other methods will remove ticks. Bathe pets with gentle herbal shampoos. Stay away from the same chemicals in personal care products that are harmful to humans. Fleas detest the scent of lavender, mint, citrus, and rosemary. Buying shampoos with these essential oils or adding them yourself will go a long way to controlling fleas. Safe Solutions has an enzymatic shampoo called Pet Wash that kills fleas and ticks by breaking down their outer exoskeleton. It is an excellent alternative to insecticidal shampoos (see sources).

 (see Chapter 7: Shampoo)

Alternatives for flea and tick protection

Adding garlic (not onions—never feed onions to cats) to homemade food is an excellent way to repel fleas and ticks. The garlic gets into the dog's system and creates an odor that fleas and ticks avoid. And don't worry, your dog won't smell like garlic. Humans usually don't detect the garlic odor. You can use real garlic or garlic juice sprayed on your pet's food.

Diatomaceous earth (DE) kills fleas by drying them out. DE is composed of microscopic marine fossils called diatoms. It is not recommended to be put directly on your pet as it can be a lung irritant. Safe Solutions offers a food-grade DE mined from uncontaminated fresh water deposits (see sources).

A flea comb is a good method of removing fleas and flea eggs. It works by catching the fleas in the narrow gaps between the teeth or by forcing them to jump off. After each run of the comb, dunk the comb in soapy water and remove hair and flea eggs. Flea traps provide another way to reduce the number of fleas in a home. They work with a small, incandescent lightbulb that attracts fleas to sticky paper. They may be effective at attracting between 10 to 50 percent of a flea population (see sources).

WORMS AND OTHER PARASITES

Several different kinds of worms can infect cats and dogs. Some are more serious than others and can cause harm to humans. Although this is an important concern (both to pets and for human caregivers), so are the deworming agents used to get rid of the worms. All deworming medications are dangerous and potentially toxic. Many pet owners have either caused serious illnesses or killed their pets by indiscriminately or incorrectly using these drugs. It is best to work with a vet and to determine from stool samples whether or not your pet really needs a deworming treatment. If natural treatments (garlic and DE) are used on a regular basis, deworming may not be necessary.

> **Most vets agree: Pets that are in good health generally are not threatened by worm infestations. If they are, they show fewer symptoms. This is more evidence for good nutrition.**

Panacur (Fenbendazole)

There are numerous deworming treatments for pets. Panacur (fenbendazole) is one of most widely used. It is recommended for the treatment of many parasites including roundworms, hookworms, whipworms, and tapeworms. It is also used in the treatment of flukes and giardia. It is considered to be safe, yet a look at the Material Data Safety Sheet (MSDS) says that information on carcinogenicity and developmental toxicity is not available. This means that tests have not been conducted to determine the possible cancer-causing effects or developmental effects. The MSDS also indicates that fenbendazole causes mutations in somatic cells.[358] A 2006 study of the effects of fenbendazole on marine bacteria was not entirely positive either. The compound was toxic to several marine life forms.[359]

Garlic

Besides helping to keep insects from your pets, garlic will help to keep them free of worms. Garlic juice is easily sprayed on their food, and most dogs and cats love it. Garlic juice keeps dogs from having worms and gets rid of worms that already exist. It also keeps fleas and ticks at bay while it supports good heart function. Besides a good diet, the use of garlic may be one of the most important things you can do for your pet (see sources). Recommended daily dosages are as follows:

5–20 lb. dogs—four sprays or one-quarter ounce in food daily
21–50 lb. dogs—six sprays daily
51 lbs. and over—eight sprays daily

Diatomaceous earth

Diatomaceous earth (DE) is another natural way to control worms and other intestinal parasites. It has been used for many years for that purpose. Add a spoonful of DE to your pet's food on a regular basis to eliminate and control worms. Be careful not to breathe any floating particles (see sources).

 (see Chapter 11: Diatomaceous earth)

PETS AND GARDEN PESTICIDES

Pet owners who use lawn and garden pesticides not only endanger their pets, but they also endanger themselves and their children. Pets spend much of their time outdoors. They cannot "take off their shoes" before entering the house, and they cannot bathe on a daily basis. Furthermore, cats do not have efficient ways of metabolizing and removing complex, synthetic chemicals from their bodies. They endlessly groom themselves, and any chemical which contacts their fur or their feet is carefully removed and swallowed.

Animals, like children, are more sensitive and are more easily poisoned by conditions which seem safe to adults. Numerous pesticides cause harm (cancer, reproductive problems, birth defects, central nervous system disorders, liver, kidney, and thyroid damage) to pets on a regular basis. Dog owners who use 2,4-D four or more times during the season double their dog's chances of suffering lymphoma.[360]

 (see Chapter 11: Pesticides)

VACCINES

A discussion of animal vaccines follows similar logic to the discussion of human vaccines. Especially for dogs and cats, too frequent vaccination may actually cause more harm than good. Most animals need only what are known as core vaccines: those that protect against the most common and most serious diseases. In dogs, the core vaccines are distemper, parvovirus, hepatitis, and rabies. In cats, they are panleukopenia, calicivirus, rhinotracheitis (herpesvirus), and rabies—as required by law.

Veterinarians have suspected for years that annual re-vaccinations for cats and dogs weren't always necessary. In fact, the most accepted veterinary text states that the practice lacks scientific validity. Initial vaccination produces an immunologic memory that often remains for years. Re-vaccination with most viral vaccines actually interferes with existing antibodies.[361] However, because vaccine manufacturers (interested in sales) arbitrarily recommend annual vaccinations, most veterinarians continue to concur.

According to the most recent research, even a rabies vaccine can last up to seven years. Annual re-vaccination for rabies is overkill.[362] Pet owners might want to ask their veterinarians to perform vaccine antibody titer tests which test antibody levels to determine whether re-vaccination is really necessary.

SOURCES (in the order they appear in the chapter):

Pet Wash :
Enzymatic shampoo (Safe Solutions): http://www.safesolutionsinc.com/

Flea traps:
Springstar: www.springstar.net
Woodstream: www.victorpest.com

Garlic Juice:
http://www.garlicvalleyfarms.com/

Diatomaceous earth, food grade:
Safe Solutions: http://www.safesolutionsinc.com/

 Recommended Reading:

The Complete Guide to Holistic Cat Care by Celeste Yarnall, PhD, and Jean Hofve, DMV

Pets Need Wholesome Foods Also by Jesse. Available online, free: http://www. pet-grub.com/

Food Pets Die For by Ann N. Martin

Chapter 16
TOXIC THOUGHTS AND EMOTIONS

Spiritual leader Marriane Williamson said, "Our past is a story existing only in our minds." She also said, "The only thing you need to recover from is a fractured self." "Fracturing" occurs early in life. Such moments set the stage for limiting beliefs—the foundation of toxic thoughts and emotions.

No matter how devoted you are to a proper diet and to a nontoxic lifestyle, there are other toxins in the form of toxic beliefs, thoughts, and emotions that may sabotage your progress toward a healthy, vibrant life. Your habitual thoughts and perceptions may ultimately be more important than any nutritional program, any detoxification protocol, or any attempt to shield yourself from harmful energy. Doing everything you can to eliminate the negative belief patterns that give rise to toxic thoughts and emotions will augment the other recommendations in this book and will go a long way to clearing the pathway for health and vitality.

The most powerful force in the universe is the power of your own thoughts. They send out magnetic vibrations that attract similar vibrations back into your life. You are like a broadcasting device that sends and receives messages all day long. Positive, empowering, outgoing messages attract positive, empowering, incoming life experiences. On the other hand, negative, self-defeating thoughts are toxic. They can only attract the same kind of vibrational circumstances back into your life.

It is quite well known that when groups of people pray or meditate for a specific purpose, measurable changes take place. But it is not as easy to accept the fact that we participate in shaping our own reality and that our own life experiences are the result of our underlying beliefs, thoughts, and emotions.

In his groundbreaking book *The Biology of Belief*, Dr. Bruce Lipton provides the science showing how, on a cellular level, our thoughts are the signals that control the expression of our DNA—not the other way around.

His work provides a whole new perspective for understanding that our bodies can be changed as we retrain our thinking.[363] As it turns out, science is proving that positive thoughts and empowering beliefs are a requirement for a happy, healthy life. This chapter discusses numerous methods for correcting your limiting beliefs.

BELIEFS

Beliefs are neither good nor bad. They just are. They can either support you or they can limit you. As the saying goes: *If you believe you can, you can. And if you believe you can't, you can't.*

Most beliefs—usually subconscious—are the result of experiences and programming from our early lives. The part of the brain that is responsible for logic and reason (the prefrontal lobe) does not become functional until the age of six or seven. Before this time children can't logically evaluate the experiences they have. They tend to feel responsible for everything that goes on around them. If something bad happens, they assume it was their fault. Usually, the beliefs we carry into adulthood are developed before the age of six—before we are capable of evaluating circumstances in a logical manner. That's why so many beliefs make no logical sense.

Common Beliefs

- I don't deserve to be happy.
- If I'm happy now, I won't be motivated to change.
- You have to do some things you don't want to do in this life.
- People who are optimistic aren't realistic.
- I can't change—it's just the way I am.
- I have to have [love, sex, or money] in order to be happy.
- Life is hard.
- You can't have your cake and eat it too.

When parents quarrel; when children make mistakes; when adults lose their temper; and especially during traumatic events, it is easy for children to accept beliefs like "I don't deserve to have the things I want," "I'm not good enough," "I'm unlovable," or "The world is not a safe place to live." These decisions, made during emotionally charged events, become the beliefs that eventually govern how we live our lives. Sometimes they are so illogical that they become buried beneath mounds of compensating behaviors. As an adult, we may not even know they exist. But as long as they remain the undercurrent beneath our thoughts and actions, we will continue to experience disappointment, ill health, or lack of zest for life.

Sometimes, we adopt beliefs directly from our parents. If our parents believed in working hard to attain the things they wanted, chances are we will also believe that we have to work hard to accomplish our desires. Yet that's only really true if you believe it. There are many people who effortlessly create wealth and joy in their lives. Their beliefs are usually based on ease and abundance.

Our beliefs form our attitudes and perceptions of the world. They are the foundation for our thoughts and emotions affecting every area of our lives. They affect where we live and work; they affect our relationships; they affect our health; and they effect our financial circumstances. Many times, even though we think we are clear about what we want, we don't always get the outcome we desire. This is because our subconscious beliefs do not support our conscious intentions. A person may say they want to lose weight, yet within the subconscious realms of their mind are fears about smallness, sexual advances, or being accepted for who they are. Sometimes people hold beliefs to prove something to their parents or to some other significant person in their lives.

Unfortunately, many of us aren't aware of the beliefs we acquired as children. We can live our whole lives unaware of how our beliefs are affecting our feelings, thoughts, and actions. But just imagine what you could create in your life if you updated your beliefs and if you were able to eliminate the toxic thoughts and emotions that keep you from your highest intentions.

In a recent television interview, Joe Vitale, participant in the widely acclaimed movie *The Secret*, identified five steps to realizing your financial goals. These steps apply to everything you want to accomplish, whether it is losing weight, regaining your health, or making money. The third step, and possibly the most important, is to clear your limiting beliefs.

Joe Vitale's Five Steps to Financial Freedom
(from an interview on the television show, *The Big Idea*)

1. Know what you don't want—this provides a springboard to step #2.
2. Check your intention—this realigns your body and mind for what you *do* want.
3. Get clear—clean up your beliefs.
4. Feel what it would be like to already have your desire.
5. "Let go" while taking inspired action.

Talk therapies that were popular in the past rely almost exclusively on motivation and will power—they seldom create real and lasting change. Positive affirmations have similar limitations. The most effective methods for change have been developed recently in response to the frustration with typical counseling and self-help techniques. These methods rely on accessing the subconscious mind—where beliefs are held—and on reprogramming the mind. There are numerous ways to go about it. The methods suggested below represent a few of the newer, more widely used techniques. They represent ways to accomplish step three in Joe Vitale's five-step program: Get clear—clean up your beliefs.

Emotional Freedom Technique (EFT)

Emotional Freedom Technique (EFT) is an emotional version of acupuncture. It is based on tapping specific acupuncture points while thinking about a problem or symptom and while repeating this phrase:

> *Even though I* (state the negative emotion or belief), *I deeply love, accept, and forgive myself.*

Tapping releases energetic blockages surrounding negative emotions, traumas, and beliefs that were instilled during childhood. The critical element in EFT is to be emotionally "tuned in" to the problem; in other words, to be really feeling it during the process. This is the access to the subconscious mind. Often the issues that need to be healed the most are the ones that are the most deeply hidden. Trained practitioners can help you to uncover these hidden traumas and beliefs; they can often see things that are not obvious from your perspective. However, with basic knowledge, many people can work on themselves.

Questions That Might Help to Uncover Hidden Issues in Your Life

- If you could live life over again, what person or event would you prefer to skip?
- When was the last time you cried and why?
- Who/what makes you angry and why?
- What is your biggest sadness or regret?
- What is missing to make your life perfect?
- Name three fears you would rather not have.
- What do you wish you had never done?

EFT is simple to learn. The basic EFT manual is available as a free download from the Internet, and there are many helps and resources on the EFT Web site to get you started: http://www.emofree.com/.

Psych-K

Psych-K is another powerful way to change outdated subconscious perceptions and beliefs that may be sabotaging your goals in life. It is a simple process that helps you communicate with your subconscious mind. Psych-K has been described as a user-friendly way to rewrite the software of your mind in order to change the printout of your life.

Psych-K creates a receptive state of mind that dramatically reduces resistance to change at the subconscious level. When right and left hemispheres of the brain are in simultaneous communication, the qualities and characteristics of both hemispheres are available to maximize the full potential in your life. This state is also ideal for changing beliefs at the subconscious level. Psych-K is designed to engage and activate the inner resources of the subconscious. The approach also honors the power and responsibility of the individual in making changes.

Psych-K uses muscle testing to help zero in on specific beliefs that are in need of updating. It is easy to learn and to apply in your daily life. Seminars are taught in many locations (see sources). You may also find skilled practitioners in connection with the Web site: http://psych-k.com/home.php

ZPoint

The ZPoint process was developed by a Canadian hynotherapist, Grant Connolly. It was designed to break the connection between the emotion and a belief or thought. Since the emotion is the power source, when it is disconnected, the thought or belief transforms and drops away. The first step is to choose a simple cue word—something unique and memorable.

The next step is to set up a healing program for the subconscious mind. This only has to be done once—by reading the following script:

> *I hereby set a powerful intention within you, my subconscious mind, to effect the best of all possible outcomes by this clearing, and that each time I notice a pattern or patterns I wish to eliminate, as I say or think my cue word, you will eliminate all such patterns and components of patterns completely and safely. Each time I repeat my cue word in sequence, you will access deeper and deeper layers and all parts and all aspects of my being.*

After setting the healing intent, every time you identify an emotion or belief that is disempowering, say the following statements in your mind:

1. I clear all the ways that I feel (angry, sad, resentful, lonely, etc.). Repeat the cue word several times.

2. I clear all the patterns connected to those ways. (CUE)
3. I clear all the emotions connected with those patterns. (CUE)
4. I clear all the ways I feel (_____) whenever ... (leave the sentence open ended so your subconscious mind fills in all that is appropriate. (CUE)
5. I clear all the ways I feel (_____) because ... (let your subconscious fill in). (CUE)
6. I clear all the ways I feel (_____) if ... (let your subconscious fill in). (CUE)
7. I clear all the ways hidden and other parts of me don't want to release this. (CUE)
8. I clear all the ways hidden and other parts of me don't want to let this (_____) go. (CUE)
9. I clear all the ways these parts don't want to let this (_____) go because ... (CUE)
10. I clear all the ways these parts get a benefit from holding onto this (_____). (CUE)
11. I clear all the ways these parts wouldn't feel safe if I let this (_____) go right now. (CUE)

Much more detailed information, including several videos, is available on the Internet at the ZPoint Web site: http://www.zpointprocess.com/. This is a process you can easily learn and do yourself. Using it regularly can produce tremendous benefits.

Hypnotherapy

Hypnosis also works at the level of the subconscious mind. It is recognized as a powerful tool for accessing and changing disempowering beliefs. The major difference between hypnotherapy and the other methods suggested above is that during hypnosis the conscious mind is out of the way.

Neuro-linguistic programming (NLP)

Neuro-linguistic programming refers to the use of the language of the subconscious mind to alter beliefs and patterns in your life. NLP has been shown to benefit a variety of health and emotional conditions. There is a very powerful NLP technique for correcting beliefs which is outlined on the following Web page: http://www.nlpu.com/Patterns/pattern3.htm. Some knowledge of NLP may be required to optimally complete the process. You may also be better served by an NLP practitioner (see sources).

Neuro-emotional technique (NET)

Neuro-emotional technique (NET) was developed by a chiropractor who wanted to understand why some patients held their adjustments better than others. He discovered that hidden emotional issues were often responsible. Other factors—toxins, nutritional needs, and structural misalignments—can also be addressed. Using muscle testing, a trained practitioner can help identify the specific emotion as well as the time it first occurred. While the client mentally holds the emotional memory (which allows the body's physiology to replicate the pattern formed in the subconscious mind by the original event), a gentle physical correction in made. Annoying behavioral and emotional patterns are often immediately resolved (see sources).

Eye movement desensitization and reprocessing (EMDR)

Eye movement desensitization and reprocessing (EMDR), as well as the related therapy known simply as rapid eye therapy, can help to reprocess how traumatic events are perceived. During EMDR, a person focuses on the memories and sensations associated with the trauma for brief periods of time while simultaneously focusing on an external stimulus. Therapist-directed eye movements are the most commonly used external stimulus, but a variety of other stimuli including hand-tapping and audio stimulation are often used. EMDR helps access the traumatic memory network so that new associations can be made between the traumatic memory and cognitive insights. This enables a person to reprocess how they perceive and respond to what happened in the past and to replace limiting thoughts and emotions with more positive, congruent alternatives. EMDR has been very helpful for people with posttraumatic stress disorder and has been shown to achieve resolution of deep-seated emotional issues related to trauma.[364] (see sources).

EMOTIONS

Most of us intuitively know that if we are carrying around anger, resentment, guilt, shame, and other negative emotions it will have physical consequences. If someone is angry, their stomach is tight, their blood pressure rises, and adrenaline is released, affecting many physical functions.

In an experiment conducted by the Institute of HeartMath, twenty-eight vials of DNA were given (one each) to twenty-eight trained researchers. Each researcher was instructed to generate and feel feelings and strong emotions. Changes in the DNA were monitored during the experiment. The outcome? The DNA changed its shape according to the feelings of the researchers. When the researchers felt emotions like gratitude, love, and appreciation, the DNA responded by relaxing, and the DNA strand actually unwound and became longer. When the researchers generated feelings of anger, fear, frustration, or stress, the DNA responded by tightening—and some DNA functions were shut down.[365]

This experiment illustrates how the tension we feel also exists at the molecular level and how it affects all the functions in our bodies. Hanging onto resentments, guilt, anger, grief, and other negative emotions can cause stress to be present all the time. After a while, many people are so used to the stress that they become unaware that these emotions are being held. This is the case with the traumatic events in our lives—especially traumatic events from our early childhood that have been long forgotten.

When emotions get "stuck" and are unable to be released, whole areas of your body can be walled off as though they were frozen in time. These areas do not receive the same amount of nourishing energy and are prime areas where disease develops. Learning to release anger, resentment, guilt, and other negative emotions in appropriate ways is critical for a healthy, emotional life. Discovering and releasing the long-held emotions from our early life is also important for real balance in everyday living.

Candace Pert, former chief of the section on brain biochemistry at the National Institute of Mental Health, and author of *Molecules of Emotion*, was one of the first to provide research showing that emotions are linked to specific chemical processes taking place throughout the body. These chemicals, called peptides, were eventually found to affect the functioning of all the systems of the body—particularly the immune system. In essence, our emotional state affects whether or not we get sick.[366] Unreleased and long-held emotions can literally make us sick.

Part of healing requires the recognition and release of negative emotions. The same techniques for discovering and correcting negative beliefs can help to identify and release hidden emotions. You may be attracted to one of the methods outlined above—or you may find another that is better suited to your circumstances. Finding someone you trust to help you identify and release beliefs and emotional traumas is important: It is the authors' opinion that as soon as you take action to find help, the right technique or facilitator will manifest.

THOUGHTS

Rev. Michael Beckwith, who contributed in the movie *The Secret,* said, "Every time an individual has a thought or a prolonged chronic way of thinking, they're in the creation process. Something is going to manifest out of those thoughts." We all think thousands of thoughts every day, and every thought is linked with an emotion. If the thought is empowering, then the emotion will also be empowering and the actions that result will lead in the direction of your desires. But if the thought is negative or restricting, then it is linked with a negative emotion, and it results in actions that are disempowering.

As Candace Pert documented in the book *Molecules of Emotion,* emotions are linked with specific processes that affect numerous functions in your body. Regular negative thinking and the corresponding negative emotions are just as toxic as any other environmental toxin—perhaps even more so—because they come from within and because they affect every cell.

One of the laws of the universe is that you attract what you focus on. If you focus on fear, you send a strong message to the universe to send you what you fear. But if you shift your focus to feelings of joy, love, appreciation, and gratitude, you will bring that into your life—you will manifest a different outcome from the ones that already exist in time and space. What that means in terms of health is that you can prevent sickness by staying in a positive emotional state.

Thinking is a habit—a learned response. Even if we are in the process of regularly updating negative beliefs and releasing hidden emotional traumas, we still need to break the habit of negative thinking. Like any habit or behavior, thinking patterns can be unlearned or changed. Making a conscious decision to catch yourself in negative thinking will have a direct impact on your life experiences. Find something to be happy about every day, even if only for a few minutes. This is the easiest and best protection against illness you have. If you find yourself dwelling on negative thoughts, consider one of the following ways to practice "thought stopping":

- Create a bank of positive thoughts and images to replace negative or self-defeating thoughts. When you become aware of an uncomfortable feeling or thought, intercept and replace it from one of the thoughts and images in your positive thought bank.
- Eliminate "I can't" thinking. When you find yourself thinking something is too difficult, take a moment to stop and see (and feel) yourself doing what you choose to do.
- Take a couple of moments a few times every day to repeat an empowering affirmation or to review a loving image. This is a boost to your immune system and a spiritual reconnection.
- Take responsibility for your reactions to events and stop blaming others. This approach will awaken you to your ability to create your life's circumstances rather than feeling helpless or victimized.

- Your body lives everything you think. Focus on all of the healthy, supporting systems of your body. If you are healthy, then express gratitude to your body on a regular basis.
- Take time to de-stress daily. Even a couple of ten-minute breaks during the day can have enormous benefits for your mind, body, and spirit. Deep breathing, short meditations, or regular stretching will relax your nervous system, calm your mind, and put you back in touch with your body.

Know (and feel) what you want

To the subconscious mind, focusing your thoughts on your destination rather than on the things you are unhappy about makes all the difference in the world. It is like getting into a taxi cab and telling the cab driver you *don't* want to go to the park. The park is the only option because you have not told the driver where you *do* want to go. To tell your subconscious mind that you don't want to be depressed, anxious, uncertain, or sick isn't the same as telling it what you *do* want—that you are happy, calm, confident, and healthy. Think about everything in terms of what you want in your life rather than what you don't want. For example: "I am well-off" as opposed to, "I don't want to be poor."

When you catch yourself thinking in negative terms, take a moment to "feel" what it would "feel like" to experience what it is you do want. Feeling the feeling of having your desires creates a vibration that literally attracts what you want. Feeling the feeling of longing for it is quite another thing and sets up the vibration of longing, rather than the vibration of having. They are quite different. The first will keep you in longing; the other is positive and will attract your desires.

Gratitude

Developing a spirit of gratitude is one of the most important aspects to finding success in your physical, financial, emotional, and spiritual life. Being grateful and expressing gratitude in all areas of your life literally sends molecules of gratitude throughout your body in the form of peptides that support health and happiness.

> **Begin each morning, and take time during the day to express gratitude for something. This sets the stage for everything in your mind and body to be receptive to more of the same.**

Find ways to be grateful for everything around you. No matter how bad things have been in the past, you can be grateful to be alive today and for the potential of a more fulfilling and happy future that exists for everyone who will seek it.

DEPRESSION

Beliefs, thoughts, and emotions affect brain chemistry (neurotransmitters). If a person experiences stresses or traumas early in life (or inherits negative beliefs), brain chemistry is affected and can cause depression, anxiety, or panic disorders. But when people are able to correct their beliefs, their thoughts, and their emotions, depression sometimes resolves naturally.

The medical answer for depression and anxiety is antidepressant drugs. But antidepressants often cause the problems they are intended to cure. Until recently, these side-effects have been whitewashed and withheld from public knowledge. In 2005, the FDA finally required new language to accompany antidepressant medications. The following black box must now appear on these drugs:

> **"Patients, their families, and their caregivers should be encouraged to be alert to the emergence of anxiety, panic attacks, insomnia, irritability, hostility, aggressiveness, impulsivity, akathisia (psychomotor restlessness), hypomania, mania, other unusual behavior, worsening of depression, and suicidal ideation, especially early during antidepressant treatment and when the dose is adjusted up or down."**

Exercise is recognized as a factor in resolving depression. Some evidence suggests that exercise raises the levels of certain mood-enhancing neurotransmitters in the brain. Exercise may also boost feel-good endorphins, release muscle tension, and help you sleep better, and it may reduce levels of the stress hormone cortisol. All of these mind and body changes can improve sadness, anxiety, irritability, stress, fatigue, anger, and hopelessness. It may take at least thirty minutes of exercise a day, three to five days a week, to significantly improve the symptoms of depression, but smaller amounts of activity—as little as ten to fifteen minutes at a time—can improve mood in the short term.

Another big factor in overcoming depression is nutrition. Supplying the body with the amino acids and minerals it lacks can cause brain chemistry to shift enough for depression to lift. Many have made near miraculous turnaround with nutritional support.

Environmental toxins play another important role. When the body is burdened with toxins, maintaining balanced brain chemistry is much more difficult. Detoxification (especially heavy metals) may help the body to find chemical and emotional balance.

 (see Chapter 19: Detoxification)

In the DVD *Curing Depression, Anxiety and Panic Disorder*, Burton Goldberg brings a variety of experts together to discuss alternatives to antidepressant drugs—everything from amino acid therapy to the role of hormones, toxins, and biofeedback. To help you or someone you love walk away from depression visit www.burtongoldberg.com.

HEALING THOUGHTS

In a recent program entitled Healing Hearts/Healing Nations: The Science of Peace and the Power of Prayer, Gregg Braden discussed the results of numerous experiments that defy conventional laws of time and space. He explained that time is not just linear (past, present, and future) but that it also has depth. The depth of time consists of all the possible outcomes that could ever exist. Essentially, all our hopes and dreams already exist, and all our prayers have already been answered. We activate the circumstances we are living through our thoughts and emotions. This is how we create our reality—by choosing it with our thoughts and feelings.

According to Braden, when thoughts and emotions are in complete harmony, we have direct access to creative healing forces. In his workshops Braden discusses the true mode of prayer which he describes as focused thoughts and feelings—as though the outcome already exists. This mode of prayer is more like a celebration. He uses a video from a hospital in Beijing, China, where this kind of prayer heals a cancerous tumor inside a woman's body. The video displays a real-time ultrasound image of the cancerous tumor dissolving in less than three minutes while the woman is fully awake and conscious. Some would describe this as a miraculous healing. Braden says that focused thought allowed a new outcome to be chosen.

Ho'oponopono

In his book *Zero Limits*, Joe Vitale tells about meeting a Hawaiian shaman who was able to cure criminally insane patients without ever seeing them. The shaman, Dr. Ihaleakala Hew Len, was also a psychologist. He used a Hawaiian healing process called, ho'oponopono. He would study each inmate's chart and then look within himself to see how he had created that person's illness. As he improved himself, the patient also improved. He simply repeated the following: *I love you. I'm sorry. Please forgive me. Thank You.* This same phrase can be used to overcome your own negative thinking. When you encounter negative circumstances or thoughts, repeat the phrase.

Loving yourself is possibly the best way to attract your dreams. It also has a tremendous effect on the rest of the world—the perfect illustration that we are all part of the same whole. Whenever you want to improve anything in your life, the place to start is within—with your own beliefs, thoughts, and emotions. And when you look, remember to look with love.

ENERGETIC SUPPORT

Mother Nature has provided a plethora of energetic tools that will help bring awareness and the release of toxic thoughts and emotions. These tools utilize the subtle energy of plants and minerals abundant on the earth. Many people find that flower essences, essential oils, and the earth's minerals are enough to help break through stubborn patterns and emotional issues. Others use these energetic tools in conjunction with the emotional release techniques outlined earlier. When used together, emotional healing often blossoms into spiritual awakening. Nature's energies are wonderful for children and for older people who may have a difficult time connecting with emotional issues. They are also wonderful for depression, PMS, and menopause. All are safe, nontoxic, and nonaddictive.

Flower essences

Flower essences, called "remedies," are made from the vital energy of flowers. Each flower addresses a particular emotional/psychological condition. Because they work on the vibrational level, flower essences bypass the conscious mind and "speak" to the energy that causes emotional blockages, transcending disharmony. When a person takes the appropriate flower remedy, negative thought patterns and behaviors tend to drop away as the individual becomes aware of new ways of being and new ways of accomplishing an outcome. Flower essences are widely available at most health food stores.

Essential oils

Essential oils, also widely available, are another gift from Mother Nature's plant kingdom. They are the distilled essences of plants that can directly impact emotional states through the sense of smell. According to Carolyn Mein, DC, compounds found in high levels in essential oils increase the oxygen in the brain which unlocks the DNA and allows emotional baggage to be released from cellular memory.[367] Aromas are sensed and analyzed in the reticular system of the brain stem where emotions and memories are accessed. Essential oils can be very therapeutic for a wide variety of conditions.

Crystals and gemstones

The earth's mineral kingdom is also full of vital, supportive energy. Every ancient civilization has used the properties of crystals and other stones to promote and support healing. In our modern day, whole books have been written on the healing and awakening properties of stones.[368],[369] Wearing jewelry with specific combinations of crystals and other stones can be very powerful as a person seeks to resolve and release the toxic thoughts and emotions they have accumulated throughout a lifetime. Crystals and other stones are subtle, but they can open the doorway to awareness and to new ways of being. Most people can benefit from the gentle energy supplied by crystals and other stones as they work through emotional issues. Energy Muse has created a wide variety of exquisite jewelry designed to support emotional well-being and conscious evolution (see sources).

SOURCES (in the order they appear in the chapter):

Emotional Freedom Technique:
http://www.emofree.com/

Psych-K:
http://psych-k.com/home.php

Z-Point Process:
http://www.zpointprocess.com/

Human Software Engineering:
http://www.GlobalPlayersInc.com/ and
http://www.greatlifetechnologies.com/

Hypnotherapy:
The American Society of Clinical Hypnosis: www.asch.net
American Association of Professional Hypnotherapists: www.aaph.org
The National Guild of Hypnotists: www.ngh.net

Neuro-Linguistic Programming (NLP):
www.nlpco.com

Neuro-Emotional Technique (NET):
www.netmindbody.com

Eye Movement Desensitization and Reprocessing (EMDR):
EMDR Institute www.emdr.com

Energy Muse jewelry:
www.wyntersway.com

 Recommended Reading/viewing:

The Biology of Belief by Bruce Lipton

Zero Limits by Joe Vitale

Secrets of the Lost Mode of Prayer by Gregg Braden

Molecules of Emotion: The Science Behind Mind-body Medicine by Candace Pert, PhD

Curing Depression, Anxiety and Panic Disorder by Burton Goldberg. Available at www.burtongoldberg.com

Chapter 17

WHAT ABOUT SCHOOLS?

The English poet Joseph Addison said, "What sculpture is to a block of marble, education is to the soul." Given this soul-shaping task, every parent, every teacher, and every school administrator needs to understand the impact that environmental toxins have on the learning and cognitive ability of our children. At a time when we are committed to raising academic performance and to honoring each child's potential, we have an obligation to reduce their health risks at school. This includes adopting healthy school facility design standards. It also includes stringent standards for indoor air quality, the use of safer cleaning and maintenance products, the use of nontoxic pesticides, incorporation of quality lighting, wholesome food, and safe outdoor spaces. Convincing research indicates that improving these factors in schools will improve attendance and academic performance. What will it do for the soul? It's time we found out.

Health standards for children's exposure—especially in schools—do not exist. According to a statement made to the U.S. Senate Environment and Public Works Committee Hearing in May 2007, an estimated 32 million children are at elevated risk of health and learning impairments and secondary disabilities due solely to the conditions of their schools.[370]

Children are uniquely vulnerable to environmental contaminants. They eat, drink, and breathe more per pound of body weight than adults. This exposes them to more toxins. Children also metabolize and assimilate materials faster than adults. Their organs and brain are still developing, and their immune systems are less capable of fending off toxins. Children's behavior also exposes them to more environmental risks, and they are often too young to be able to identify toxins or to protect themselves. Until stronger federal protections are passed, the biggest share of the burden to safeguard children from environmental hazards in schools will continue to fall on local shoulders. Parents can take an active role in supporting their school district's efforts—especially if they know what to look for. This chapter will help you understand how you can make a difference.

When to Suspect an Environmental Problem in the School

1. Your child starts most days healthy but develops headaches or other symptoms during the day.
2. Your child regularly comes home sick, tired, itchy, or angry.
3. Your child shows new or worsening health or learning problems as the school heating season starts.
4. Your child uses more asthma medication on school days.
5. Your child comes home with odd odors clinging to his or her clothes.
6. The building is new or newly renovated and still smells like paint, varnish, or glue.
7. The building smells damp or musty.

BUILDING DESIGN

The Collaborative for High Performance Schools (CHPS) is a *green* school building program that combines project management, building criteria, and third-party assessment to ensure that a school project is designed and built to the highest performance standards. The CHPS program was originally developed for California, but schools across the nation have adapted the building criteria for their own circumstances. The CHPS guide is available online and outlines design and construction requirements (see sources).

Across the country, many communities are building to the CHPS standards. Both California and New Jersey now have requirements for schools to be built *green*. CHPS manages a member directory of green school building services and products and a directory of certified low-emitting materials for school construction. CHPS also offers online trainings and detailed information. Design strategies include daylighting, energy efficiency, indoor air quality, acoustics, sustainable materials, waste reduction, preventive maintenance, site protection, and water conservation. If your community is considering a new school building or renovation, make sure the school board is aware of the CHPS program.

AIR QUALITY

The EPA has estimated that up to half of all schools have problems with indoor air quality. Both children and teachers are affected by poor ventilation, the use of inappropriate cleaning chemicals, pesticides, mold, and so on. School indoor air is a contributing factor to asthma, which is the leading cause of school absenteeism. Asthma is also the leading occupational disease of teachers. Other effects of poor indoor school air quality include poor concentration, rashes, headaches, and nervous disorders. Almost any child can be affected by aerosols, contaminated dust, and chemicals.

Clean air in our nation's schools begins with the use of nontoxic building materials that do not outgas volatile organic compounds. Clean air is also influenced by ventilation equipment, which ensures adequate air movement and controls humidity levels to keep mold problems from developing. Easy-to-clean floors are a must. Indoor air quality can also be supported by using safe cleaning and maintenance products and by implementing safety standards in art and science classes as well as in vocational training programs. CHPS maintains an up-to-date list of materials specifically for schools.

Art and craft supplies

Generally speaking, art supplies are not treated with the level of caution that their ingredients deserve. Until the 1970s, the toxicity of art materials was virtually unregulated. Some of the worst products have been removed from the market, but there are still toxic chemicals in many art supplies. A federal law passed in 1990 requires art materials to contain labels that list toxic ingredients and to provide warnings whenever needed. The AP symbol on art supplies means that it is an approved product and will cause no harm, even to a small child. The CL designation means that an art material is certified as properly labeled. It does not mean that it is safe. The following areas of concern should be a consideration in any school art program:

Paints—Oil-based paints still contain many volatile solvents and should be avoided in the classroom. Powdered paints should not be mixed in the classroom; airborne particles can be inhaled. Spray paint should also be avoided. Use only water-based paints—especially for younger children.

 (see Chapter 1: Paint for artists)

Glues—Children should only use water-based glues like library paste or glue sticks. Any glue that is solvent-based, like rubber cement, should be avoided. These contain volatile compounds including xylene and heptane.

Markers and crayons—Many markers are solvent-based. They emit volatile compounds that can cause respiratory and neurological damage—especially for young children. Use only water-based markers. Most crayons today are nontoxic and therefore not a problem.

Adhesives and fixatives—Adhesives and fixatives are used for matting framed pictures or for coating a piece of artwork to make it smudge-proof. These are aerosols which leave tiny particles in the air, and they contain solvents. They should only be used outdoors or in a well-ventilated area, not the classroom.

Pottery and ceramic glazes—Working with clay leaves a dust residue even after cleaning efforts. Direct damage to the lungs may result from silica or asbestos present in dry earth clays. Small children should not work with ceramic clay. Many ceramic glazes contain lead and should be avoided in the school environment. Kilns can also release volatile airborne contaminants and are best operated after school hours and only in a well-ventilated area.

Printing, lithography, and silk screening—The ink and pigments used in printing and silk screening contain solvents and can release lead, cadmium, and chromium. Children should not be directly involved with these processes. Use only water-based inks in well-ventilated areas.

Papier-mâché—Instant papier-mâché may contain asbestos, lead, or other metals from pigments in colored printing inks. Any papier-mâché used in the school environment should be made from black-and-white newspaper and library or white paste (or flour and water paste).

Vocational education

High schools with vocational training programs need to be concerned with the hazards inherent in each program. These classes provide an excellent opportunity to teach about the environmentally friendly options becoming available today:

- **Engine repair**—Automotive repair requires lubricants, oils, and fuels, all of which are currently toxic. This setting provides an excellent opportunity to introduce safer options.

 (see Chapter 14: Automotive pollutants)

- **Woodworking**—Dusts created by sawing and sanding can be very irritating to respiratory tissues. Common dust masks are not very effective. Wood finishes contain VOCs and should be used only in well-ventilated areas. Even water-based wood coatings contain some VOCs. AMF makes low-VOC wood finishes (see sources).

- **Auto body**—The paints and epoxy used in auto body work also contain VOCs. Good ventilation is a must.
- **Photography**—Film developing chemicals need to be handled in well-ventilated areas. Some chemicals are corrosive; proper protective equipment should always be provided.
- **Science labs**—Many dangerous chemicals, including benzene, mercury, formaldehyde, and hydrochloric acid can be found in chemistry and biology labs. These areas of the school should contain exhaust hoods to vent toxins out through the roof. Proper safety equipment should be provided in these classes, including safety goggles and gloves. Science classes provide a good platform for the discussion of how chemicals affect various body functions. When proper cautions are taken, children (and adults) learn to respect the harmful nature of chemicals.

ELECTROMAGNETIC INTERFERENCE

Children are often especially sensitive to electromagnetic (EM) fields. These foreign energy fields radiate from electrical equipment, from older fluorescent light ballasts, from Wi-Fi networks, cell phones, and even from the electrical wiring behind walls. Just being in close proximity to these objects induces current onto the body, which can have serious effects on the delicate electromagnetic frequencies that govern many bodily functions.

 (see Chapter 3: Electromagnetic pollution)

EM fields affect the electrical systems of the body. They can cause misfiring of nerve cells, which are associated with diabetes, multiple sclerosis, asthma, and many brain functions. This is especially significant in the school environment where children spend the majority of their day.

> **Wi-Fi networks are installed in most schools. These networks literally bring antennas into the school; each computer becomes a receiver and the frequencies are distributed throughout the entire school on the "network."**

Stetzer filters are a combination of capacitors and resistors that short-out high frequencies on incoming electrical wiring. They have effectively been used in many schools and have eliminated symptoms of asthma, fibromyalgia, and multiple sclerosis for both students and teachers[371] (see sources). Other devices can offer protection from the frequencies radiated with Wi-Fi connections as well as other abnormal frequencies found in the home and school environment. Many of these are intended to protect large areas and can be used effectively in schools (see sources). These protective devices can make a huge difference, especially if your child is having trouble concentrating or dealing with stress.

If your child's school does not use any of these devices, consider having your child wear a personal protection device to school (see sources). If your child carries a cell phone, make sure the phone has a protective device (see sources).

CUSTODIAL CLEANING SUPPLIES

Schools are several times more densely occupied than commercial office spaces. Because they are so densely occupied and because children are not known for cleanliness, schools need to be cleaned more often than most buildings. But the cleaning agents themselves should not contribute to the problem.

The cleaning agents used in schools can be a big factor, contributing to asthma, allergies, headaches, rashes, nosebleeds, nasal congestion, and a whole host of other symptoms. The Responsible Purchasing Network maintains a current list of safe industrial and commercial cleaning products available for use in schools (see sources). Make sure your child's school knows about this resource.

PESTICIDES

Children are among the least protected population group when it comes to pesticide exposure, according to the National Academy of Sciences report. Most parents would be appalled to discover the number of pesticides that are applied in classrooms and on playgrounds and playing fields. Communities across the country are acting in increasing numbers to protect children from pesticides used at their schools, yet there are no national standards set for children. Surveys indicate that a majority of schools in most states still use pesticides that are known to cause cancer or to adversely affect the nervous, hormone, and reproductive systems.

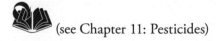 (see Chapter 11: Pesticides)

Federal legislation entitled School Environment Protection Act (SEPA) was first introduced in 1999 but was never passed. The act called for basic levels of protection for children and school staff from the use of pesticides in public school buildings and on school grounds. This important piece of legislation would have required schools to implement safer approaches to pest management that rely on a range of nonchemical and chemical alternatives and would have required notice be provided to parents and school staff when pesticides were used. SEPA was reintroduced in 2001—then again in 2003 and again in 2005. At this time it has still not passed. For a summary of the bill and for sample letters to write to your representatives to encourage their support of the act, visit http://www.beyondpesticides.org/schools/sepa/SEPA_summary.htm

Integrated pest management

Most integrated pest management (IPM) programs being introduced to schools have one thing in common—they continue to use some registered pesticide poisons. As with the home and garden environment, the tools to control school pests without using toxic chemicals are available nationwide and have proven to be effective and economical. Get Set, Inc. has developed a program that has been successfully implemented in over 350 schools—without *any* toxic chemicals. They call the program "Intelligent Pest Management." Much of the program is available online at http://www.getipm.com/

LIGHTING

The best lighting for schools (and elsewhere) is natural sunlight. That's why the CHPS guidelines recommend daylighting in schools wherever possible. Since, for the most part, schools only operate during daylight hours, daylighting is both an energy-saving and a health-promoting proposition. In many classrooms, students spend their day beneath cool-white fluorescent lights. These ordinary fluorescent lights cause bodily stress, anxiety, hyperactivity, attention problems, depression, and eyestrain. They lead to poor learning and poor performance.

 (see Chapter 10: Lighting)

Full-spectrum lighting

Significant research has revealed that full-spectrum fluorescent lighting in the school environment creates less stress and anxiety; it improves behavior and attitudes; it improves health and attendance; and it increases performance and academic achievement. In 1973, John Ott studied four classrooms in Florida. Two classrooms had full-spectrum, radiation-shielded fluorescent light fixtures. The other two classrooms remained with the traditional cool-white fluorescent bulbs. Children in classrooms with cool-white fluorescent lighting demonstrated hyperactivity, fatigue, irritability, and attention deficit. In the classrooms with full-spectrum lighting, behavior and classroom performance, as well as overall academic achievement, improved markedly within one month. Several learning-disabled children with extreme hyperactivity calmed down and seemed to overcome some of their learning and reading problems while they were in the classrooms with full-spectrum lighting.[372]

In an extensive 1995 study, Canadian psychologist Warren Hathaway demonstrated that full-spectrum lighting produced other benefits for school children. Students under full-spectrum lighting with ultraviolet supplements benefited the most, with higher rates of achievement and greater physical development. These students also had better attendance.[373]

In 1999, as an elementary school principal, William Titoff conducted research for his PhD dissertation and discovered that the level of depression in fourth grade students was reduced with full-spectrum lighting. When the project was completed, Titoff reported, "The teachers with the full-spectrum lighting refused to let me take it out and put back the old-style fluorescent bulbs."

In order to achieve natural balanced light, bulbs must emit a full spectrum of color. Additionally, true full-spectrum lighting should contain infrared and ultraviolet wavelengths. Full Spectrum Solutions makes a line of fluorescent bulbs/tubes called BlueMax that are energy efficient, full spectrum, and low-hazard risk for the school environment. The other advantage of the BlueMax line of fluorescent bulbs is that the mercury in them is a mixture of mercury and other metals. This reduces the vaporization of mercury if lamps are broken and greatly reduces their risk (see sources).

> **The new compact fluorescent lights are currently the best choice for full spectrum lights in the school environment. This technology can come very close to true full-spectrum light.**
>
> **(see Chapter 10 Fluorescent lighting)**

Disposal of fluorescent light tubes

Although fluorescent lighting technology has improved greatly during the past decade, these bulbs and light tubes contain mercury. They represent a contamination problem if they are broken. If they break at home or in the school environment, they release mercury vapor into the air. Anyone in the near vicinity should be evacuated and the ventilation system should be shut down so that vapor does not permeate the whole building.

 (see Chapter 1: Mercury Clean-up)

Taking care of these lamps at a landfill poses similar problems. Even if they *arrive* intact, (highly improbable), they release mercury into the soil, water, and air when they are broken. All fluorescent lamps should be recycled. Special facilities can remove the mercury for reuse, but only if they are taken to a proper facility. Especially in schools and commercial buildings, recycling programs should be in place. Schools should purchase only from vendors that offer collection and recycling programs (many do).

SCHOOL LUNCHES

Good nutrition contributes to better education. Children who get good nutrition have improved learning ability, better attention and memory, superior brain development, enhanced cognitive function, an improved sense of well-being, and they score better on standardized tests. These improvements ought to be enough to convince legislators and school administrators to take a closer look at the National School Lunch Program. Unfortunately, school lunch programs are a target for profit-driven corporations, just like our grocery stores—but children can't read the labels or choose what they get.

The National School Lunch Program is a federally assisted meal program that began in 1946 and is now operating in more than 99,800 out of 120,000 elementary and secondary schools in the country. In many areas, the school lunch program is little more than a fast food restaurant, with French fries, burgers, corn dogs, pizza, and fish sticks being standard fair. Read, or re-read the chapter on food to understand the myriad of problems with the typical American diet.

If you want your child to eat healthy, most school lunch programs are not in a position to help. Most school lunches contain the same preservatives, food colorings, additives, and genetically modified, irradiated, and bar code foods that are found in the grocery store.

 (see Chapter 4: Food preservatives)

 (see Chapter 4: Food colorings)

 (see Chapter 4: Food additives)

(see Chapter 4: Genetic modification)

 (see Chapter 4: Food irradiation)

 (see Chapter 4: Barcode foods)

Unless you work with your local school district and lobby for changes, you are probably better off providing a home lunch for your children. For ideas on creating healthy home lunches visit http://greenlivingideas.com/ kids/tips-for-packing-a-nutritious-waste-free-lunch.html.

Irradiated meat

On May 29, 2003, despite thousands of comments from parents, teachers, students, and concerned citizens, the USDA chose to include irradiated ground beef for federal nutrition programs. These programs include the National School Lunch Program. Food service directors and school officials in each district can now choose whether or not to purchase irradiated ground beef for their schools, without notifying parents.

Irradiation kills pathogens by splitting chemical bonds in food. When food is irradiated, ionizing radiation reacts with water in the food, causing the release of electrons and the formation of highly reactive free radicals. The free radicals interact with vitamins in ways that can alter and degrade their structure and activity.[374] Irradiation also produces elevated levels of benzene, formaldehyde, and other cancer-causing compounds. This is the reason that irradiation must be called a food additive.

> **The destruction of vitamins continues beyond the time of irradiation. Therefore, when irradiated food is stored, it will experience greater vitamin loss than food that has not been irradiated.**

Since the USDA's approval of irradiated meat in schools, many communities have joined together passing resolutions that ban irradiated foods from local school meal programs. The following Web site provides information on how to work with your school district to stop the purchase of irradiated foods: www.safelunch.org.

What else can you do?

Many communities have been able to influence local authorities to completely revamp their school lunch programs. The National Farm to School Program is a nonprofit organization that is committed to getting kids to eat healthier food. The organization connects farmers with nearby school cafeterias to provide produce, meats, and dairy products from local farmers. In 1997, only six local programs existed; in 2008 there were nearly two thousand programs in thirty-nine states.[375]

With the program, schools also provide students with experiential learning opportunities through farm visits, gardening, and recycling programs. By providing healthier options in school cafeterias and through education that connects the food in the cafeteria to farms and health, children learn how their food choices affect their own health—and how they affect the ability of local farmers to continue to provide nutritious food. Local farmers have access to a new market through schools and to connections with their community.

Berkeley, California, has become a model for how to make schools more sustainable. Students plant, grow, cook, and eat food that they grow in their school garden. This program has become so successful that many schools around the country now have their own gardens. As sustainability catches on around the country, more and more teachers, students, and parents are getting involved and demanding better quality lunches. It usually begins with one concerned parent who rallies other parents to change the way their schools think about food. How does a healthy school lunch campaign start? A few organizations of parents, teachers, and communities are listed in the sources section at the end of the chapter.

Vending machines

Many school districts now rely on vending machines to pay for computers, sports programs, and after-school activities. Unfortunately, most of the machines are packed with sugar and fat—and profits coming at the expense of student health. According to the National Conference of State Legislatures' Health Policy Tracking Service, many schools raise as much as $100,000 a year from vending contracts.[376] Some school districts have multimillion-dollar exclusivity contracts with vending companies. These contracts can include sales quotas. For example one contract required the sale of four thousand five hundred cases of soda a year—about fifty sodas per student. Schools have been known to violate federal and state laws because their contracts require that the vending machines operate all day, including the lunch hour. The issue has become so controversial that over twenty states are considering limits or total bans on vending machine products. About twenty states already restrict students' access to junk food until after lunch. As a parent, you can have an impact on what products are being sold in school vending machines.

PLAYGROUND EQUIPMENT

Much has been done to ensure that playground equipment is safe. Great effort has gone into design and durability. But what about the materials themselves?

Wood preservatives

Since the 1970s, most of the pressure-treated wood used in the United States for outdoor structures such as playground equipment, picnic tables, benches, and decks has been treated with the insecticide/preservative known as chromated copper arsenate (CCA). Chromium was used to bind arsenic and copper to the wood fibers, but it has been recently discovered that chromium is not as effective as originally thought. Studies show that CCA-treated wood continually leaches arsenic to the surface of the wood for long periods of time.

Arsenic is a potent skin, bladder, and lung carcinogen. It is also linked to immune system suppression, increased risk of high blood pressure, cardiovascular disease, hormone disruption, and diabetes. Recent studies have confirmed that high levels of arsenic can be released to children's hands by direct contact with arsenic-treated wood. Young children, in particular, are at risk of swallowing arsenic when they put their hands in their mouths after playing on CCA-treated wood.[377]

> **Never plant a vegetable garden in the vicinity of CCA-treated wood; never saw or sand this wood; and never burn it in the fireplace. Arsenic inhaled in sawdust or vapors from burning are even more toxic. If you decide to remove CCA-treated wood, it should be disposed of as hazardous waste.**

As of 2004, the EPA and the wood products industry agreed to stop the manufacture of CCA-treated wood for most residential uses. However, these wood playsets will remain in use for many years. California has mandated the sealing of CCA-treated wood on playground equipment with two coats of an oil-based stain which must be reapplied every year. Another option would be to use one of AMFs low-VOC sealants (see sources). To determine if wood is CCA-treated, simple test kits can be purchased for about $20 at www.safe2play.org.

PVC and other plastic

Other than wood, plastic is the most common material used in the construction of playground equipment. PVC is probably the most durable but it is also the most toxic and poses problems for the environment from the beginning of its life cycle to the end. PVC plastic contains phthalates used as softeners which are leached from the plastic—especially as temperatures rise. Phthalates can be absorbed through the skin, inhaled as fumes, or ingested. The EPA and the state of California have listed phthalates as carcinogens and possible reproductive toxins. You may want to work with your school to make sure that when playgrounds are planned, appropriate materials are used. If these materials are already present, their replacement should be a consideration.

 (see Chapter 5: PVC)

 (see Chapter 5: Phthalates)

School Bus Fumes

Children can spend anywhere from an hour to several hours a day on a bus when riding to and from school. Recent research has determined a variety of adverse health effects from breathing diesel exhaust. Buses built before 1990 release sixty times as much pollution as those built to 2007 standards. This research has led many states and school districts to upgrade buses with better pollution controls and cleaner fuels. However, about one-third of the nation's school buses still need renovation. This means that in many areas, children who ride busses every day are still at risk.

Diesel exhaust, which can build up inside buses, produces fine particles that penetrate deep into the lungs, triggering asthma attacks, aggravating bronchitis and other respiratory ailments. More than forty different compounds in diesel exhaust are classified as possible human carcinogens. Exhaust also includes compounds that contribute to smog and haze, acid rain, and global warming.

A study by the Natural Resources Defense Council (NRDC) found that levels of diesel exhaust on four Los Angeles school buses were eight and a half times higher than average levels found in California's smoggy air.[378] This was four times higher than the fumes from inside a car driven directly in front of the buses. Idling school buses are an additional problem. Idling for more than three minutes produces 66 percent more pollution than stopping and restarting the engine.

Parents should encourage school districts to adopt policies where idling is limited during loading of school children. Parents can also encourage school districts and legislative officials to set aside or seek funding to upgrade their bus fleets. Encourage your children who ride buses to sit at the front of the bus, where diesel fumes are considerably lower. Bus windows should also be kept open during rides, weather permitting.

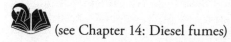 (see Chapter 14: Diesel fumes)

ATTENTION DEFICIT AND HYPERACTIVITY

Attention deficit disorder (ADD) and Attention deficit hyperactivity disorder (ADHD) are the most common behavioral disorders among school children. The National Institutes of Health estimate that from 3 to 5 percent of all American schoolchildren have been diagnosed with these disorders.

ADD and ADHD are at epidemic proportions along with the rise in asthma, allergies, chemical sensitivities, and autoimmune diseases—all connected in some way with environmental factors. But rather than treating the cause, ADD and ADHD are routinely suppressed with medications that have many long-term consequences.

> **I would allege to you that the ultimate pollution is pollution that affects the cognitive ability of future generations.**
>
> Dr. David Carpenter, MD, Dean,
> School of Public Health State University at Albany, New York

There is a complex body of information suggesting that ADHD may be a catch-all for neurological problems with a number of causal factors including those listed below.[379] Many of these are nutritional in origin and based on deficiencies in the American diet. Others are based on toxins in the environment. Research suggests that these same factors (listed below) during pregnancy predetermine a child's risk for ADD and ADHD:

- food and food additive allergies
- heavy metal toxicity and other environmental toxins
- low-protein, high-carbohydrate diets
- mineral imbalances
- essential fatty acid and phospholipid deficiencies
- amino acid deficiencies
- thyroid disorders
- B vitamin and phytonutrient deficiencies

Pharmaceutical influence in schools

Although there has been extensive discussion regarding the ethics of fast-food marketing within schools, there has been little discussion regarding the consequences of the pharmaceutical industry's infiltration of schools. Sadly, pharmaceutical companies have targeted teachers to play a primary role in diagnosing and medicating students with behavior and attention problems. Accepting medical treatment (drugs) is often the only way some children can receive specialized educational services.

The pharmaceutical industry's approach to educating teachers is similar to their approach to educating doctors. Drug manufacturers maintain educational Web sites which contain specific resources for teachers. On a page titled "If parents ask ...," one Web site suggests:

> *Make it clear to them that it is important for them—and their child—to understand and follow the doctor's medical advice about medication and other therapies for ADHD. ADHD is a serious condition that may require the child to be on medication and undergo counseling for a long duration.*[380]

The same Web page also contains the following advice:

> *There are a number of alterative therapies offered for the treatment of ADHD. However, there is no scientific proof of the effectiveness of the following in treating children with ADHD.*
>
> - *Restricted diet (mostly sugar, artificial coloring, and additives)*
> - *Allergy treatment*
> - *Megavitamins*
> - *Chiropractic adjustment and bone realignment*
> - *Treatment for yeast infections*
>
> *If parents ask about the above treatments, you should inform them that the most effective demonstrated treatment involves a combination of medication, psychotherapy, and support from caregivers, including parents, other family members, and you.*

Other school personnel are also targeted. In 1997, one pharmaceutical company collaborated with the National Association of School Nurses to run a nationwide campaign. School nurses were provided with a resource kit containing information on ADHD and its treatment. These methods are unethical and serve to increase the pressure on parents to medicate their children—all the while denying the dietary and environmental contributors to the problem.

Dietary and environmental factors in ADD and ADHD

The truth is, more often than not, ADHD can be controlled with diet and by removing the environmental factors that contribute to attention deficit and hyperactivity. Detoxification further supports these methods by reducing the burden of chemicals in the body. Much research has substantiated that dietary approaches to ADD and ADHD have significant merit. They are often at least as good as medication.

 (see Chapter 19: Detoxification)

Dietary changes, including the avoidance of sugar, food additives, colorings, and preservatives, show great promise.[381] In a study of 135 children in Jacksonville, Florida, children were required to drink four ounces of filtered water every hour (made using the Wellness filtration technology). The only other change in the school environment was the removal of soda and candy machines from the school. The students' grades and behavior were monitored, and at the end of the year only four of the thirty-four children who were originally taking mood-controlling drugs like Ritalin were still taking these medications. Behavior, attendance, and overall health were improved.[382]

In another study, it was discovered that the food coloring known as FD&C yellow No. 5 in excess of ten mg increased hyperactivity for a duration beyond twenty-four hours.[383] (Ten mg is the amount of food coloring that might be found in just a half-cup of Kool-Aid or in a serving of cake with bright yellow frosting.) A 2008 report released by the British Associate Parliamentary Food and Health Forum stated:

> *Tartrazine and sunset yellow [Yellow #5 and #6] are azo dyes and it is believed that they could be acting as chelating agents, binding the available blood zinc in the body to form complex metals, which are then excreted. Azo dyes inhibit gut enzyme activity and this can induce inadequate digestion. This could explain why many ADHD children are unable to absorb all the nutrients in the food they eat … ADHD children had relatively low levels of zinc. When the children were given the tartrazine containing solution their low levels of zinc became further depleted—they were excreting it at a higher rate through their urine than the control children, whose zinc levels were depleted*

less significantly and more slowly. [384] [Note: zinc levels were depleted by tartrazine in normal children as well.]

Research also exists showing that supplementation with essential fatty acids and antioxidants helps to improve focus and concentration in children with ADD and ADHD. The same British report stated:

> *A deficiency of omega-3 EFAs [Essential Fatty Acids] is associated with certain mental and behavioral disorders, such as ADHD, depression, dementia, dyspraxia, greater impulsivity and aggressive behavior*[385]

The Feingold diet is well known for helping to control ADD and ADHD. It is based on the elimination of food colorings, food preservatives, food additives such as MSG and aspartame, and on returning to a diet of whole foods. A wealth of information is available on the Feingold organization Web site: http://www.feingold.org/. Information on nutrient-dense whole foods is available at www.wyntersway.com

Besides dietary factors, other environmental contributors to attention and behavioral problems in children are lead contamination, cigarette smoke, pesticides, mercury toxicity, air pollutants, and EM fields—especially those radiated from older fluorescent lighting ballasts. Each of these and many more factors should be addressed before drugs are administered.

Ritalin

Ritalin (methylphenidate), also known as Concerta and Metadate, is the current drug of choice for children diagnosed with attention and hyperactivity disorders. Ritalin acts as a stimulant for adults and as a depressant for children before puberty. It has been used for more than two decades on children as young as six years old. Yet, recent manufacturer information states that "Sufficient data on safety and efficacy of long-term use in children are not yet available."[386]

> **Ritalin belongs to the group of drugs known as amphetamine-type drugs. It is classified as a Schedule II substance because of its high potential for addiction and abuse. Schedule II substances are the most heavily controlled substances for which a prescription can be written; they are in the same category as cocaine, morphine, and opium. If your child's school suggests the use of Ritalin, it is important for you and your child to seriously consider all the options.**

Because of the scarcity of safety data on this drug, a group of researchers at the University of Texas M. D. Anderson Cancer Center embarked on a preliminary study to determine the possible effects of the drug on DNA. After only three months on Ritalin, every one of the twelve children who participated in the study experienced a threefold increase in chromosome abnormalities, which are associated with increased cancer risk and other adverse health effects.[387]

Other research, conducted over the past twenty years, leads to the conclusion that Ritalin is one of the most dangerous and addictive substances that can be prescribed. The *Physician's Desk Reference* lists very serious adverse reactions and warnings about its use—including severe withdrawal symptoms and suicide. Ritalin can also cause neurological disorders, drug dependence, stunted growth, psychotic states, insomnia, nervousness, anorexia, nausea, dizziness, headache, and blood pressure changes. Between 1990 and 2000 there were 186 deaths from Ritalin reported to the FDA MedWatch program, which represents only about 10 percent of actual incidences. Despite the fact that the psychiatric industry is well aware of how dangerous Ritalin is, estimates currently place 4 to 6 million American children on Ritalin.

SOURCES (in the order they appear in the chapter):

Collaborative for High Performance Schools (CHPS):
http://www.chps.net/overview/index.htm

EMF protection:
Stetzer filters Stetzer Electric: www.stetzerelectric.com
LifeBEAT Products: sprays and Bio-wear for personal protection: www. wyntersway.com
BlockEMF: geo-magnetometers, EMF detection devices, personal protection, shielding devices, cell phone protection, whole home protection: http://www. blockemf.com/
EarthCalm EMF: personal and whole home protection: http://earthcalm.com/
Shield EMF: personal and cell phone protection: www.ShieldEMF.com
Energy Polarity EMF: personal protection and cell phone devices, appliance diodes and whole home harmonizers: www.energpolarit.com

Wood finishes:
AMF: www.afmsafecoat.com
AFM Safecoat wood sealant: www.afmsafecoat.com

Janitorial supplies:
Responsible Purchasing Network: http://www.responsiblepurchasing.org/index.php

Full spectrum lighting:
BlueMax: www.fullspectrumsolutions.com
Incandescent full spectrum: http://bluesbuster.com/

Alternate school lunch programs:
Appetite for a Change: Organic Consumers Association's nationwide campaign working to make school food programs healthy and sustainable: http://www.organicconsumers.org/sos.htm

Farm to School Program of the Community Food Security Coalition: Farm to School programs incorporating healthy, nutritious, produce into school lunches, snacks and salad bars. http://.www.foodsecurity.org/farm_to_school.html

Parents Action for Children: Organic Lunchbox Challenge, A resource and guide for parents who want to add organic food to children's diets: http://.www.drgreene.com/21_1432.html

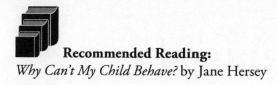

Recommended Reading:
Why Can't My Child Behave? by Jane Hersey

Chapter 18

WHAT TO DO WHEN YOU TRAVEL

✦

—and when you eat out

Mark Twain once said, "Nothing so liberalizes a man and expands the kindly instincts that nature put in him as travel and contact with many kinds of people." Today's travel, compared with travel in Mark Twain's day, is light-years apart, yet the allure and the benefits are the same. Travel can bring out the best or the worst—depending on how prepared you are. Being prepared to deal with the toxins you encounter when you travel can make all the difference.

The same factors you are concerned about in your home or workplace should be considered when you travel—and when you eat out. Air quality, water quality, food and food packaging, methods of cooking, electromagnetic radiation—each of these plays a role in your health, even if you are away for only a short period of time. If you travel on a regular basis, these factors can play a significant role in your ongoing health. This chapter discusses some of the ways you can prepare and protect yourself and your family when you travel and when you eat out.

AIR QUALITY
Recirculated air on airplanes

The quality of the air on airliners has been questioned many times—and for many good reasons. Airborne diseases transmitted during commercial air travel have become an important public health issue. In 2003, 120 travelers boarded Air China's flight 112 for the three-hour flight from Hong Kong to Beijing. Within eight days, twenty passengers and two flight attendants came down with the SARS virus. The incident raised many questions about air circulation on airliners. The Centers for Disease Control and the World Health Organization say you should only be concerned if you are sitting within two rows of someone who has an infection—and then only if you are sitting there for more than eight hours. But for Air China's flight 112, that proved that to be less than accurate. Some of the passengers on flight 112 who got sick were sitting as far as seven rows away from the man carrying the virus. Because you're in a confined space during air travel, you are at a greater risk.

A normal airplane cabin experiences changes of air more than fifteen times per hour. A typical office building changes air twelve times an hour. Yet several factors combine to make airplanes a more infectious space. One difficulty is the fact that cabin air is pressurized. Planes cycle air through their engines to pressurize it. This heats the air, which then has to be cooled. The process creates extremely dry air. The longer you fly, the drier your mucous membranes get; and the dryer they get, the more susceptible you are to infection. A second risk factor in airplanes is the higher concentration of people. Reduced oxygen and contamination with hydraulic fuels and engine oils adds to the problem. Even if you don't come down with an infection, you can experience the same kind of symptoms found in inadequately ventilated buildings: dizziness, lightheadedness, fatigue, and trouble breathing.

The documentary film *Welcome to Toxic Airlines* played at European film festivals in 2007. It exposed the link between contaminated aircraft air and a variety of symptoms experienced by passengers and crew members. The film specifically focused on engine oil and hydraulic fluid that are brought inside the plane during the pressurizing of the air. These contaminants cause stomach cramps, muscle pain, confusion, and fatigue. Depending on the condition of the engines and on the presence of possible leaks, the degree of contamination can be significant. The problem is well known in the airline industry but it has been kept from the public. According to Diana Fairechild, retired airline attendant and author of *Jet Smarter*, airline pilots can get ten times more oxygen than passengers.[388] Insufficient oxygen can cause many symptoms:

- impaired visual acuity
- difficulty concentrating
- clammy skin
- nausea (when there's no turbulence)
- headache

If the quality of the air on your flight causes any of the above symptoms, request your flight attendant to ask the pilot to provide passengers with less recirculated air and more fresh air. You'll know when this happens because you'll hear a louder whoosh from the plane's air-conditioning system. If you have trouble breathing, you can ask for an oxygen bottle. There are about twenty-five portable oxygen bottles on every 747.

> **Pilots often reduce the amount of fresh air in the cabin
> to conserve fuel. Their air (cockpit air) and cabin air (for
> passengers and crew) are separately controlled.**

For humidified breathing air, cover your nose with a water-saturated cotton bandana (folded on the diagonal with the ends wrapped around your ears). Leave it on as much as possible during the flight. It will also help to block the spread of germs. You may also want to close the vent just above your seat so that recirculated air is not forced into your breathing space. Another good idea is to use quality organic oil (almond, jojoba, or olive) to coat the lining of your nose before you take off. This will keep your nose from getting too dry during the flight and it will provide extra protection from germs. There are also personal air purifiers and air ionizers that hang around your neck and neutralize many toxins in your personal air space (see sources).

The very best thing you can do to prevent getting sick during air travel is to be healthy and well rested before you leave. Staying hydrated during the flight is also very important. Do whatever you can before you leave to minimize stress and lack of sleep. After landing, make a point to breathe some fresh air as soon as possible. Deep breathing during a brisk walk will get your circulation going, and it will help to detoxify your lungs. Take a hot bath and drink lots of water for several days to help detoxify your system.

Pesticides on international flights

Many countries require what is referred to as *disinsection* of international aircraft—the use of pesticides to control insects. The pesticides used are synthetic pyrethrin pesticides (pyrethroids), which in some countries have been banned from agricultural use. Pyrethroid pesticides are suspected carcinogens, with suspected liver and lung toxicity. According to a U.S. Department of Transportation memo, there are two methods of pesticide application:

1. Spray the aircraft cabin with an aerosol insecticide while passengers are on board.
2. Treat the aircraft's interior surfaces with a residual insecticide.[389]

During the first method, an applicator aims two cans of pesticide in opposite directions, pointed toward the narrow space between the overhead bins and the passengers' heads. Passengers are required to keep seatbelts fastened and the air conditioning is turned off. The pesticide label clearly states "avoid contact with skin and eyes" and "wash contaminated clothing separately from other laundry." No warning is offered to passengers when this occurs.

The second method of application takes place while an airplane is in the hanger between flights. The plane is sprayed with a "residual" pesticide which is applied every six to eight weeks. Residual pesticide lingers on the seats and on the interior of the aircraft for two months. More airlines are using this type of disinsection so passengers are not alarmed—but these planes are not restricted to foreign travel. Passengers may be exposed to residual pesticides even though they do not travel out of the country. More than one flight attendant has been medically grounded because of the repeated exposure to pesticides and because of contaminated air during air travel.

You can ask for an exemption to disinsection when you make your airline reservation. However, most airlines will require a note from your doctor saying you are allergic to pesticides, asthmatic, or pregnant. If you are successful in obtaining an exemption, you will need to remind the airline when you check in at the airport. If you do not have a note of exemption, ask if there is going to be pesticide sprayed on your flight. If so, be prepared to cover yourself with an airline blanket to reduce the amount of pesticide that you absorb through your skin or that you get on your clothes.

> **Pesticides have been reported in clothing that has been laundered several times.**

Air quality in hotels

Hotels deal with the same problems that home and apartment dwellers deal with when it comes to air quality. Mold, dust, VOCs, and especially tobacco smoke residue contaminate the air. You never know who has been in the room before you.

As travelers and workers demand clean air, hotels are finding new and innovative ways to provide it. Allergy friendly rooms, air purifiers, and smoke-free hotels are springing up in many areas. The Florida Green Lodging Program, established in 2004 by the Florida Department of Environmental Protection, recognizes environmentally conscientious lodging facilities in the state. The program requires each designated property to meet a minimum set of environmental standards including energy efficiency, water conservation, clean air practices, and waste reduction. More than two hundred properties, including bed and breakfasts and five star resorts, are currently listed on the Florida Green Lodging Web site. Until other states provide similar programs, the responsibility for having clean air in your hotel room lies with you. You may want to invest in a travel-size air purifier or air ionizer to take with you when you travel.

Small air purifiers or ionizers are now available for the traveler. Some of these have adapters that can be plugged into the car cigarette lighter or operated with batteries. They can be placed on the nightstand at hotels so that you can have better air quality during one of the most important times—your sleep (see sources).

WATER QUALITY

Water quality around the world is declining. Sources that used to be drinkable now are not—some of the sources you may have always considered safe never have been. One of those sources is the water on airplanes.

Water during air travel

There are no standards for commercial aircraft water tanks. A recent random sampling of airplane drinking water revealed that the water from one out of eight planes had harmful bacteria including coliform and E. coli.[390] With the new regulations that deny passengers the freedom to bring their own water on board, dehydration is a real issue.

Air travel is dehydrating. The humidity in the aircraft environment ranges from 10 to 20 percent. This can cause drying of skin, eyes, and airway passages. It can be especially problematic for people with asthma or allergies; the longer your flight, the greater the difficulty. You should drink at least one glass of water for every hour you are in flight. Rather than drink the soft drinks or fruit juices offered by airline attendants, ask for water during your flight—but only if it comes from a sealed container. If it comes from the aircraft water tank, supplied from a pitcher by the flight attendant, it is no better (and probably worse) than your tap water at home. The same goes for ice—you should pass. You should also pass on airline coffee and tea, which are made with the aircraft's water.

One way to work around the water dilemma is to bring a small bottle-size water filter. Bring it on empty and fill it once you get on board. The Swiss company, Katadyn, makes a bottle-size water purifier with three stages of filtration. It is the only EPA registered purification bottle that removes all types of organisms, including viruses. The Exstream filter treats up to twenty-six gallons (a hundred liters) per replacement cartridge—excellent for hikers, camping, and travel. It removes harmful organisms from any fresh water source (see sources).

Another bottle-size water purifier is called the Sport Berkey Portable Water Purifier (see sources). There are several others—just be sure they filter all organisms and other harmful contaminants. Investing in one of these personal water purifiers is a *must* for those who travel—especially if you travel internationally. It can also supply drinking water in hotels and throughout the day wherever you are.

In the absence of your own personal water filter, hydrogen peroxide will go a long way toward making drinking water safe. Add three drops per quart of water of a 3 percent food grade hydrogen peroxide solution. Make this by diluting a 17.5 percent food grade solution with purified water— five parts water to one part hydrogen peroxide (see sources). You can take a small dropper bottle on board an airplane (as long as it is no larger than two ounces) and add one drop to each glass of water.

Showering and bathing

When you travel, get used to taking a short shower. This will minimize the amount of chlorine or chloramine you absorb or breathe during your shower. If you like to bathe when you travel, take vitamin C tablets with you to neutralize chlorine or chloramine in the bathwater. One thousand mgs will neutralize up to one hundred gallons of water (see sources).

 (see Chapter 2: Bath filters)

FOOD

Everyone likes to dine out. The best part is that you don't have to prepare the food; you can relax and let someone else do the work. Unfortunately, when others don't have to eat the food they prepare, almost anything can happen. Depending on where or what you eat, this could be a problem.

Airline food

It's often hard to resist the airline meal when the aromatic cart comes rolling down the aisle. But you should learn to exercise resistance. Airline food is poor quality to start with—regardless of which famous chef has endorsed the menu. Airline food is loaded with preservatives and warmed up in microwave ovens. Neither will do you any good. These meals are also difficult to digest.

The circumstances inside an airliner simulate an altitude of eight thousand feet—a high-mountain altitude. Eating a protein meal at this altitude is hard to digest. Climbers who eat at high altitudes find carbohydrates much easier to assimilate. They also have the advantage of making a gradual adjustment to the altitude. Unless you have a very long, uninterrupted flight, you should consider bringing a few healthy, high-carbohydrate snacks of your own— then enjoy a real meal after you land.

> **Avoid eating food in airports, bus, and train stations. These places are the most likely to have irradiated food—whether it comes from a restaurant or from a vending machine.**
>
> (see Chapter 4: Irradiated food)

Restaurants

Americans eat out more than ever. They spend nearly half of their food dollar on food away from home, with many people handling the food along the way. People expect safe food at a restaurant. Yet according to the Centers for Disease Control, more than 76 million people in the United States become ill from contaminated food every year. Many of those instances occur from restaurant food. Among the most common infections that travelers can acquire from contaminated food are E. coli, shigellosis or bacillary dysentery, giardiasis, cryptosporidiosis, noroviruses, and hepatitis A. Parasitic infections are common—more common than most people think—and they are not limited to third-world countries.

Many of the rules that guide your food choices at home do not apply when you are away. For example, fresh, green salads are generally considered a good food choice. This is not necessarily the case in a restaurant, no matter what country you are in. Fresh fruits and vegetables may have been imported from anywhere; they may have been sprayed, irrigated, or washed with water containing fecal matter. You cannot be sure restaurant personnel have properly washed raw food items, so it is best to leave raw foods for consumption at home.

> **Human and animal waste is used as a fertilizer in many countries.**

There are several other problems with fresh salads in restaurants. Many salad ingredients, including lettuce, spinach, celery, and bell peppers, are on a list called the Dirty Dozen—the most heavily pesticided food crops in the country. Unless the restaurant serves organic food, salad is likely loaded with pesticides.

Sulfites are another reason to avoid the salad. These preservatives are used heavily in restaurants to prevent spoilage and food discoloration. They are frequently used in salad bars to keep foods looking fresh. Sulfites may also be found on fresh fruits, potatoes, cooked vegetables, and bakery products without informing the consumer.

 (see Chapter 4: Food preservatives)

The advice about raw food also applies to freshly squeezed juices sold by the glass. When the outer portion of a fruit is not washed before pressing or squeezing, parasites and other contaminants are consumed. Recently, a microbiology professor tested the lemon wedges served with a variety of drinks at twenty-one restaurants in New Jersey. Seventy percent had disease-causing bacteria—some had fecal bacteria.[391] In a restaurant, this could be because the fruit was not washed, but it could also be because the wedges were cut on the same cutting board as meat, or because an employee had bacteria on unwashed hands. Stick with cooked food when eating out, and make sure the food is still hot. When it comes to the lemon wedge with your drink, either ask for a whole lemon and wash it yourself—or pass on it. Many people take a small bottle of vegetable wash with them when they travel so they can wash and eat fresh fruits in their hotel room.

Harmful bacteria can also be found in raw or undercooked eggs. Some restaurants use uncooked eggs in foods like salad dressing, custard, and some sauces. Avoid foods that might contain raw or undercooked eggs.

And what about the meat? Meat is a prime host of bacteria, which can cause food poisoning. When eating out, your best choices are well-cooked, very hot entrees. When it is not possible to purchase organic meats, fish, and poultry, consider a vegetarian meal when you eat out—especially in the United States. Almost every other country rigorously tests meat for mad cow disease. There is little U.S. testing. Especially stay away from hamburgers and hot dogs.

 (see Chapter 4: Mad cow disease)

General guidelines for eating out

1. Drinks should come from a can or bottle—open them yourself. Use a straw that comes in an unopened wrapper. Skip the ice.
2. Wash your hands before eating. Carry a bottle of hand sanitizer—one without triclosan.
3. Unless you are in a restaurant where you know they have used a dishwasher with hot water, do not eat or drink from glasses or plates that appear damp from recent washing.
4. Avoid pre-prepared salad items.
5. Do not eat fresh fruits.
6. Eat vegetarian or well-cooked organic meat, fish, and poultry.
7. Do not eat undercooked eggs—no runny yolks.
8. Do not eat any cold foods, especially if they should be hot.
9. Ask for food to be prepared without MSG.

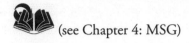 (see Chapter 4: MSG)

10. Raw seafood such as sushi should only be consumed in the most upscale restaurants—if at all.

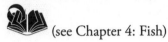 (see Chapter 4: Fish)

Nutritional supplements

Since five servings of fruits and vegetables rarely find their way into the daily traveler's diet, it is a good idea to find a convenient whole-food supplement you can take with you when you travel.

Gastrointestinal upset and food poisoning

If you do not handle spicy food well, travel with cayenne pepper and take two to three capsules with each meal. This will help your body to adjust to the spicy food without stomach upset. Cayenne pepper, taken with each meal, will also help your body to handle slightly contaminated food.

Food poisoning is more than stomach upset. It can be caused by food or drink that is contaminated with bacteria, viruses, chemicals, or toxins. Bacterial food poisoning is the most common. It is caused by:

1. undercooked food
2. food left too long at room temperature
3. cross-contamination from raw foods—especially meats
4. poor hygiene

Full recovery from the most common types of food poisoning usually occurs within twelve to forty-eight hours. However, there are several things you can do to get through it more quickly and safely. One of the most important things you can take with you when you travel is activated charcoal.

Activated charcoal is renowned for its ability to adsorb toxins. This is why it is used in most water filtration systems. It can also be taken internally to perform the same function in the gastrointestinal tract. It is sometimes used at poison centers and it is often used to combat food poisoning. Charcoal works by binding to irritating or toxic substances in the stomach and intestines. This prevents them from spreading throughout the body; they will be more easily and rapidly excreted in the stool without harm. Activated charcoal can be purchased in many drug stores as a tablet or as a powder.

If you end up with food poisoning, drink plenty of water to avoid dehydration. You will also need to replenish your electrolytes. Always have them with you (see sources). Don't eat solid foods until the diarrhea has passed, and avoid dairy, which can worsen diarrhea. Antibiotics do not help with food poisoning and can actually prolong diarrhea and keep the organism in your body longer. Get medical attention if:

- Diarrhea lasts for more than two to three days.
- There is blood in your stool.
- You have a fever over 101°F

ELECTROMAGNETIC RADIATION
In-flight ionizing radiation

Any air travel involves greater exposure to cosmic and solar radiation than staying on the ground. The intensity of in-flight radiation is a function of altitude and latitude. The air is thinner at high altitudes and provides less protection against radiation. Thus, flights at higher altitudes receive more radiation. (Radiation doubles every 6,500 feet.) Incoming radiation is also deflected by the earth's magnetic field. Strongest deflection takes place at the equator. At the same altitude, the radiation at high latitudes is two to three times greater.

 (see Chapter 3: Ionizing radiation)

> **During solar flares, radiation exposure can be up to one hundred times greater.**

Ionizing radiation penetrates an aircraft and exposes passengers. A one-way flight from New York to London exposes a person to about the same amount of radiation as a chest x-ray. In-flight radiation is more neutron-intensive, which is more damaging to cell structure than x-rays. This can harm a developing fetus, it can provoke cancer, and it can produce genetic mutations in human reproductive cells. Research into the risks of long, high-altitude flying is still limited, but several cancer studies among pilots have found increases in certain cancers that are associated with radiation.[392]

For most people, the radiation experienced on several flights a year is minimal and is not considered to be a problem. But for those who travel frequently, especially for those who travel transpolar routes, the danger is real. A passenger taking one round-trip flight a month via the transpolar route could easily surpass the maximum radiation dosage set by the Radiological

Protection Agency.[393] Pregnant women should minimize air travel as much as possible. If you are concerned about in-flight radiation, you can log onto the Space Environment Center for up-to-date information on solar flares, which can increase the amount of radiation by many times: www.sec.noaa.gov/

Exposure to ionizing radiation produces free radicals in human tissue. Antioxidant nutrients, such as vitamin E and selenium, are protective against the effects of radiation.[394, 395] Together or separately they can protect against the ionizing radiation incurred during flight. Anyone who supplements their diet with whole foods or antioxidants will have a higher concentration of antioxidants in their tissues. For additional protection before flying, take eight hundred micrograms (mcg) of selenium and up to one thousand IU of natural (not synthetic) vitamin E for several days before your flight.

CAUTION: Vitamin E naturally thins the blood. People who take blood-thinning medication should not take vitamin E supplements without medical supervision.

Electromagnetic pollution

Many silent sources of electromagnetic interference have entered our modern world. High-voltage power lines, cell phones, computers, microwave ovens, radio, television, cell phone towers, satellites, and countless other sources emit electromagnetic (EM) frequencies that are foreign to our biology. These invisible toxins create tremendous stress. When you are away from home, you are exposed to everything from electrical wiring near the bed in the hotel to television and clocks in close proximity. High-voltage power lines may also be a problem near your hotel. Having some form of personal EM protection is advisable when you travel. Devices like the Teslar watch can be worn. Others can be placed in the hotel room. (see sources in Chapter 3.)

JET LAG

More than 90 percent of long-distance travelers experience some degree of jet lag. Interestingly, people can suffer jet lag by crossing time zones, but they may not be affected by a north-south flight of the same distance. Crossing time zones seems to be the major factor. It plays havoc with your body clock.

> **Jet lag affects you physically, mentally, and emotionally. An example of a physical symptom is insomnia. A mental symptom is disorientation. An emotional symptom is anxiety.**

The body clock is programmed by regular cycles of daylight and darkness. It is also programmed by rhythms in the earth's frequencies. When these cycles are interrupted, we experience disorientation and insomnia. Depending on the number of time zones that have been crossed, it may take several days to restore natural rhythms. However, recent research indicates that jet lag can be reduced at the point of destination by standing barefoot on the earth for a minimum of fifteen minutes. This enables the electrical rhythm of the earth to reset hormonal clocks governing activity and sleep rhythms.[396] As soon as possible after reaching your destination, find a place where you can take off your shoes and socks and stand or walk barefoot.

It is also a good idea to avoid sleeping on the plane if it arrives at night. That way, you will be tired after landing and will be able to sleep. If your flight lands in the morning, however, do your best to get some sleep onboard so you can stay up until it is dark.

VACCINATIONS

Although many Web sites, including the Centers for Disease Control and the World Health Organization sites, have a long list of vaccinations that might *appear* to be required for international travel, the fact is that the only vaccination that is considered mandatory for a limited number of countries in Africa and South America is the yellow fever vaccine. Even this vaccine can be waived. Like other vaccines, those recommended for international travel have never been tested for efficacy, nor have they undergone long-term safety tests. Thousands of individuals travel worldwide every year without vaccination.

 (see Chapter 13: Vaccines)

According to Walene James in the book *Immunization: The Reality Behind the Myth*: The World Health Organization grants American travelers the right to refuse vaccinations when traveling internationally. The reason behind this is that when a person is vaccinated against his/her will, the agency must assume full responsibility for the consequences, both legal and medical. If an area you wish to enter is infected with yellow fever and you have not been vaccinated, you may be detained until the public health servant gives you the "go" (at his discretion).[397] For further information and for how to obtain a waiver, visit http://www.vaclib.org/index.htm.

SOURCES (in the order they appear in the chapter):

Air purifiers and air ionizers for travel:
Tools for Wellness: http://www.toolsforwellness.com/ionizers.html

Water filter bottles:
Berkey Sport water filter bottle: http://www.berkeyfilters.com/
Katadyn Exstream water filter bottle: http://www.katadyn.com/

Food grade hydrogen peroxide:
Natural Health Supply: http://www.naturalhealthsupply.com/servlet/Detail?no=142

Vitamin C tablets for dechlorination of bathwater:
http://vitacshower.com/FAQ.html

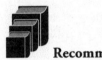 **Recommended Reading:**

Jet Smarter by Diana Fairechild

Chapter 19

DETOXIFICATION

What child hasn't been told, "Where there's a will, there's a way"? This statement applies to anything that requires resolve. When it comes to detoxification, if you have the will, there are *many* ways.

In our modern world, nearly every person carries a chemical burden made up of environmental toxins. As the earth becomes more and more polluted, our bodies inadvertently become a filter for those toxins. Many scientists believe environmental toxins are responsible for an entirely new group of disorders that involve multisystem symptoms. These include autoimmune and neurological diseases, food allergies, mood disorders, multiple chemical sensitivities, and a whole list of syndromes. There is no longer any doubt that environmental toxins are responsible for more than 90 percent of all cancers, and that toxins play a role in the severity of many other diseases. Each of these conditions results when a difficulty (deficiency, blockage, or overload) occurs in the body's detoxification pathways. When the burden becomes overwhelming, disease and other symptoms appear. Removing the toxic burden can restore these pathways. Detoxification is often accompanied by a reduction or complete elimination of symptoms. Many people have regained their health by reducing the toxic burden through detoxification.

Detoxification is the body's natural process of removing or neutralizing toxins by means of the liver, kidneys, colon, lungs, and skin. However, without sufficient energy and the nutritional resources to eliminate them, toxins end up being stored—tucked away where they are least likely to affect critical bodily functions. Toxins either accumulate in body fat and joints or they pass through and end up in the urine, stool, sweat, hair, nails, semen, and breast milk. Fat-soluble toxins (most environmental pollutants and pharmaceutical chemicals) have a high affinity for fatty tissues and cell membranes. This is why most toxins are stored in fat. It also explains why these toxins are difficult for the body to remove. The fact that many of these toxins are foreign substances adds to the problem because the body does not have designated pathways for their elimination. Toxins may be stored for years—even a lifetime—unless the circumstances are presented for their release and elimination.

Subtle indications that a person may need to detoxify:

- fatigue
- headaches
- rashes
- joint aches
- swollen glands
- difficulty concentrating
- dizziness
- restlessness
- irritability

Since toxic chemicals are in the air, water, food, and in thousands of consumer products, just removing the presence of many of these chemicals from your day-to-day environment can tip the scale in your favor—enough to allow your body to catch up and to be able to resume normal detoxification without interference. Many people have seen improvement just by removing toxic agents from their homes. For others, this is not enough.

Methods for helping the body to detoxify are based on providing the nutrients or the energy to release toxins and to eliminate them. Detoxification requires numerous vitamins and minerals, many that are missing from the modern diet. It also requires abundant, clean water. Detoxification further requires clear detoxification pathways. These three components are a prerequisite for safe, effective detoxification.

Detoxification is an extremely complicated subject, which is further complicated by each individual's personal circumstances. Whole books have been written on the subject. The intention of this chapter is to give you an overview of some of the basics and to provide enough information to help you get started. It is highly recommended that you work with a health professional when you decide to detoxify.

NUTRITION

A healthy, vibrant life lies in nutrient dense, regenerative foods. The food we eat either supplies the materials we need or it doesn't—it's that simple.

Unfortunately, the majority of the food on the planet today is deficient in some way. That's why food supplementation is a necessity. It is also one of the first things everyone should consider before they begin any kind of detoxification program. In fact, a good supplementation program is often all that is necessary to give the body the energy and resources its needs to unburden the system.

Nutrition is the most critical factor where detoxification is concerned. Like any of the body's functions, detoxification requires nutrients. If these nutrients are not present in sufficient quantity, detoxification is hindered or stalled completely. One reason many toxins are stored is because the nutrients are not available to complete the process. The other difficulty is that the number and amount of toxins are greater today than at any other time in human history. Between having more to detoxify and having fewer resources with which to accomplish the task, detoxification often has to take a backseat to more critical life-sustaining processes.

In many cases, toxins must be broken down before they can be carried from the body. Enzymes break down compounds. But enzymes require specific minerals to do their job. A deficiency in magnesium, zinc, selenium, copper, calcium, manganese, or other minerals will delay (sometimes indefinitely) the detoxification process.

Detoxification also requires antioxidants. This is because detoxification produces free radicals—unstable molecules that will tear electrons from healthy tissues if they are not stabilized. Unchecked free radicals are the cause of inflammation and pain. Free radicals are stabilized by antioxidants. Some antioxidants are produced in the body but most are meant to be supplied from the diet. Vitamin C, vitamin E, alpha-lipoic acid, glutathione, and other antioxidants are necessary for detoxification. Deficiencies in these nutrients will predispose the body to infection and free radical damage. Toxins themselves cause free radical damage.

> **Organic foods have 2 1/2 times the antioxidant power of conventionally produced produce.**
>
> (see Chapter 4: Organic food)

B vitamins are also consumed during any kind of stress. This is especially true during detoxification. During detoxification, taking extra vitamins, minerals, and antioxidants is a necessity. Whenever you can find these nutrients in whole-food supplements, you will be better off. When your body is in harmony, it cleanses itself remarkably well—even in a toxic world. This is the philosophy of Eastern medicine. Herbs and foods that nourish and cleanse your body on an ongoing basis will help you maintain that balance.

WATER

It is no secret that drinking more (and better) water can dramatically improve your health. Increasing the amount and the quality of the water you drink results in glowing skin, resistance to disease, better digestion, fewer aches and pains, weight loss, better concentration, and renewed vitality and energy. Nothing supports the body's cleansing and elimination like water. It is the ultimate detoxification tool. Whether by drinking it or soaking in it, water has been used to expel toxins and restore health since the beginning of time.

Releasing toxins without being able to flush them from the body accomplishes little. These toxins will be redeposited in other areas. During detoxification, wastes that have been stored in fatty tissue are dumped into the bloodstream and lymph—many are then sent to the liver and kidneys for processing and elimination. Water hydrates the blood and the lymph so that toxins can move rapidly through these pathways. Water is also a major component of the processes that take place in the liver and kidneys to neutralize and break down toxic compounds. And water is obviously important during the final stage of elimination, lubricating the intestines and providing the basis of urine.

Drinking more water during detoxification is a must. In fact, just as eliminating toxic exposure in your home or adding a quality food supplement to your diet, simply drinking more and better water may provide the energy you need to support normal detoxification. Certainly all three of these (elimination of toxins, nutritional supplementation, and enhanced water intake) should precede and accompany any program of detoxification.

DETOXIFICATION PATHWAYS

The next factor to consider before embarking on a detoxification program is whether or not your detoxification pathways are clear and functioning. If you release toxins but cannot eliminate them, you may create a bigger problem. Many people have intensified their symptoms by attempting to detoxify before clearing and supporting the detoxification pathways. Sluggish bowels, kidney infections, blocked bile ducts, and poor lymphatic drainage will stall the process and could be the source of the problem in the first place.

Although the toxicity of a chemical may vary, it is the responsibility of the liver to reduce toxins into compounds that the body can safely handle and eliminate. Some toxins must first pass through the liver to be broken down. Others may pass directly through the kidneys, the skin, the lungs, or the bowel. Maintaining these eliminative organs in good working order is essential. The following is a brief discussion of the detoxification pathways.

Liver-colon pathway

One of the liver's primary functions is to filter the blood. When working properly, the liver clears 99 percent of the bacteria and other toxins from the blood. However, when the liver is overworked, toxins may end up anywhere in the body. The liver also manufactures bile. Fat-soluble toxins removed from the blood are dissolved in bile—then moved into the intestines for excretion through the colon. In the intestines, the bile and its toxic load are absorbed by fiber and excreted. For most people, cleansing the colon—then the liver— is an important step prior to a more thorough detoxification program.

If the diet is low in fiber, toxins can actually be reabsorbed in the colon— another reason to eat whole foods. Eating fiber-rich, whole foods provides the necessary fiber so that toxins can be drawn from the body. There are two types of fiber necessary for detoxification: soluble and insoluble. Soluble fiber absorbs moisture. It becomes gel-like and entraps bile, toxins, and fats for removal. Insoluble fiber creates bulk, spacing food so that microbes can work to break down food more efficiently. Insoluble fiber also acts to dislodge materials adhering to the intestinal wall. It acts like a broom to sweep the walls of the intestine and colon. Make sure there is plenty of fiber in your diet during any detoxification program.

> **Fiber is the part of a plant that is not digested or broken down during normal digestion. A slice of whole wheat bread has four times the fiber of a slice of white bread. Fresh vegetables, fruits, seeds, and whole grains are the best sources of fiber.**

Colon cleansing

Colonic irrigation is one way to cleanse the large intestine of accumulated toxins and waste products. However, this method only reaches the lower colon and does not cleanse the entire intestinal tract. There are a variety of colon cleansing products on the market that will help to cleanse the entire tract. Recent oxygen-based products are gentler than herbal products and are easy to use. Oxygen-based colon cleanses soften and release the compacted mucoid plaque that builds up over time. They also oxidize harmful bacteria in the colon (see sources).

Following a colon cleanse, it is a good idea to replenish the natural flora of the intestinal tract with probiotics. Probiotics are healthy bacteria (flora) that inhabit the intestinal tract and aid in digestion and other functions. The modern diet, laden with sugar and refined carbohydrates, depletes the normal healthy flora in the intestinal tract. Anytime you take an antibiotic, you should replenish these organisms. It is also a good idea after a cleansing regimen. Most individuals benefit from regular use. A variety of probiotic products can be found in health food stores. Look for those with a blend of microorganisms—not simply acidophilus.

Liver cleansing

The most widely known liver cleanses are adaptations of Hulda Clark's work. Her liver flush has been used by thousands of individuals to remove liver stones that can block bile ducts and hinder normal detoxification. Most people—even seemingly healthy individuals—will flush hundreds of stones with a liver flush. The protocol is simple, costs little, takes only two days, and can be accomplished by almost anyone who has done the necessary preliminary preparation. The liver flush can be found online: http://www.drclark.net/en/cleanses_clean-ups/liver_cleanses.php.

Liver cleansing should be preceded and followed by nutritional support. Antioxidant vitamins like vitamin C, beta-carotene, and vitamin E protect the liver from free radical damage. B vitamins and minerals are also necessary. Whole foods with plenty of fiber also support the liver-colon detoxification pathway.

There are a number of herbs that support the liver. Milk thistle is the most impressive. It prevents damage to the liver through several mechanisms: by acting as an antioxidant, by increasing the synthesis of glutathione (a necessary antioxidant), and by increasing the rate of liver tissue regeneration. The protective effects of milk thistle against liver damage have been demonstrated in numerous studies. Ann Louise Gittleman's book *The Fast Track Detox Diet* identifies many herbs and foods that support the liver.

Kidney-bladder pathway

The main job of the kidneys is to remove wastes from the blood and to keep mineral salts and water in balance. The kidneys also maintain the pH of the blood. Wastes from the kidneys are passed to the bladder and eventually excreted in the urine. The kidneys can be overworked when excessive sugar is consumed. This is why diabetics often experience kidney failure. Excessive phosphates (from soft drinks, meat, and white bread) can cause kidney stones.

If you are not diabetic and have never had kidney stones, you can support your kidneys prior to further detoxification by drinking extra water and by taking one or more of the following herbs, available in most health food stores: cranberry, parsley, dandelion, and juniper berries. If you have ever had kidney stones, consider Hulda Clark's kidney flush, available online: http://www.drclark.net/en/cleanses_clean-ups/kidney_cleanses.php.

CAUTION: Sometimes people with serious kidney trouble may not have any symptoms. Under these circumstances, proceeding with a detoxification protocol may place too much strain on the kidneys and cause further damage. This is why it is a good idea to support the kidneys prior to detoxification.

Common Signs of Kidney Trouble:

- Rise in blood pressure
- Puffiness of the eyes, hands, and feet
- Passage of cloudy urine
- Presence of protein in the urine
- Foaming of the urine
- More frequent passing of urine during the night
- Difficulty passing urine
- Persistent, generalized itching

Skin-sweat pathway

Improving the condition of your skin supports all the other detoxification pathways. The skin is the largest eliminative organ. When combined, your skin's sweat glands can perform as much detoxification as both kidneys. Even heavy metals and other toxins can be released through the skin when you sweat. If the other detoxification organs are damaged, then helping the skin can "pick up the slack" and support other compromised organs. Selecting a method for detoxification that focuses on sweating may be a good option.

Understandably, it is important to support the skin during detoxification. Eliminate the use of any personal care products that may hinder the skin from breathing or that may contribute to toxic absorption through the skin. High-quality fats in the diet (olive oil, coconut oil, and others) and oils (including vitamin E) from natural sources in personal care products will nourish the skin.

Lung-breath pathway

The lungs remove volatile gases as we breathe. There is a tendency for most people to take short breaths of air—just enough to keep them alive. However, for effective cleansing of the lungs, you need to take long, deep breaths and to allow the air to be pulled in by your diaphragm rather than by your lungs. This simple process provides a more intense cleansing breath. Practice this consistently throughout the day to cleanse your lungs.

Exercise in the fresh air and sunshine is also a powerful detoxifying treatment for the lungs. It allows "dead air" normally trapped in the small alveoli of the lungs to be expelled. Brisk walking or rebounding on a trampoline is a wonderful way to cleanse the lungs and to stimulate the lymphatic system. Remember to inhale deeply and to move your arms and legs. You may also want to support your lungs with as many of the following antimucus foods as possible: onions and garlic, cayenne pepper, fresh ginger, and horseradish.

The lymphatic system

The lymphatic system has a dual purpose. It is a primary part of the immune system, manufacturing lymphocytes which break down bacteria and other invaders. It also acts as a garbage collection system, clearing the fluids that bathe every cell of your body. (There is more fluid in the lymphatic system than in the blood.) The lymphatic system is technically not an elimination pathway. It is more of a collection system that channels wastes to the elimination organs. However, when the lymphatic channels become sluggish, none of the detoxification pathways are able to function as they should.

Each day, water and solutes continually filter from capillary blood into the spaces between cells. Wastes collect in this fluid and are carried by tiny vessels to lymph nodes—filtering stations where bacteria, viruses, dead cells, and metabolic wastes are broken down. The filtered fluid is then returned to the bloodstream.

Although there is no pumping organ connected with the lymphatic system, lymph fluid steadily moves uphill from the lower regions of the body to the upper chest, where it is dumped back into the blood near the heart. Movement of the fluid is due to breathing and to skeletal muscle contractions. X-rays show that lymphatic fluid drains into central blood veins most rapidly at the peak of the in-breath (inspiration). Lymphatic flow is proportional to the depth of inspiration and to the contraction of skeletal muscles. During exercise, lymphatic flow may increase as much as ten to fifteen times.

Stagnant lymph fluid is a breeding ground for bacteria, parasites, and viruses. The best way to keep lymphatic fluid moving is to breathe deeply and to exercise regularly. Supporting the lymphatic system in this way supports all of the detoxification pathways.

METHODS OF DETOXIFICATION

Almost everyone needs detoxification—especially people who are exposed to industrial or environmental toxins in their profession. The degree of detoxification that may be necessary varies from person to person. A doctor can test your body's toxic burden, but these tests are expensive and not available to the general public. They are rarely performed. Tests for individual groups of toxins (like heavy metals) are less prohibitive. However, for most individuals, reducing symptoms and regaining a level of energetic vibrance is the goal. Testing may simply be validation of the results.

Many different approaches are effective, even though they address the problem in different ways or through different detoxification pathways. In many instances, more than one approach may be helpful—at different times or simultaneously. Since detoxification can reintroduce toxins into the body and bloodstream, it may be in your best interest to work with a health professional to determine which methods will best address your needs. Some of the most successful methods are discussed below.

Fasting

One of the simplest methods of detoxification is fasting. Any time your body is provided with extra energy, it will use the energy to "clean house." Fasting provides this extra energy because digestion is one of the largest energy drains on the body. This is why you often feel tired after a big meal. Eliminating food or eliminating the most difficult foods to digest provides the energy necessary for detoxification.

There are many kinds of fasts, including water and juice fasts. They all involve very little cost, and the results are usually worth the effort. There are fasting retreats and health spas in many areas that will guide you through a fast. For most people, a series of short (weekend) fasts is more convenient and much more realistic.

Water fasting uses fat (rather than food) for fuel. This releases stored toxins from body fat into the blood stream for elimination. You can begin a twenty-four to thirty-six-hour water fast on Friday with the elimination of the evening meal, or you can fast all day Saturday. During the fast, drink lots of pure water. This is one time when distilled water is recommended. Distilled water is more aggressive than water with minerals. It will attract and help to carry toxins from your body. Following a fast, be sure to replenish minerals (electrolytes) (see sources). During a water fast, it is recommended that you rest and do as little as possible.

Juice fasting is not as stringent as water fasting and provides nutrients while also providing the extra energy for the body to detoxify. It can be sustained for longer periods of time than a water fast and it may be more beneficial in the long run. During a juice fast you can often maintain a fairly normal routine, depending on your level of health. Juices are absorbed rapidly, and they contain a high vitamin, mineral, and enzyme content that can jump-start the immune system. Juices should be organic and diluted 1:1 with water because they are so concentrated. They should also be consumed immediately after juicing so that they don't lose their antioxidant capacity by combining with oxygen in the air. Between thirty-two and sixty-four ounces (one quart to a half-gallon) of juice is taken throughout the day. Typical fruits and vegetables include celery, carrot, kale, cabbage, apple, pineapple, cranberry, spinach, beet, and many greens. Citrus fruits are usually avoided during juice fasting.

Another well-known fast is often referred to as the Master Cleanse or the Lemonade fast. This fast consists of freshly squeezed organic lemons in purified water with organic maple syrup and cayenne pepper. This fast cleanses the eliminative organs, and supplies basic nutrition. It is often recommended prior to the liver flush. You can stay on the lemonade fast for several days or for longer periods of time up to ten days. The recipe below is taken throughout the day with water in between:

    2 Tbsp. freshly squeezed lemon or lime juice (approx. half a lemon)
    2 Tbsp. genuine organic maple syrup
    1/8 tsp. ground cayenne pepper (enhances circulation)
    10 to 14 ounces of pure water

It is important not to begin eating a normal diet after any type of fasting. Depending on the duration of your fast, it might take several days to build up to your normal diet by gradually introducing grains and animal protein.

Diets
Detoxification diets are vegetarian diets that help the body to eliminate toxins gently, over a period of time. Detoxification diets consist of fruits and vegetables (mostly vegetables), fresh sprouts, and whole seeds and grains. Detoxification diets also focus on eating in a relaxed environment and on chewing (thirty to fifty times per mouthful), both good habits to acquire. A natural, vegetarian diet includes the fiber needed for stimulating good bowel elimination. It also contains the vitamins, minerals, and enzymes that nourish the body. These diets eliminate all meat, dairy, refined sugar, and processed foods.

Herbal teas
Herbs and herbal teas have been used by cultures throughout history to stimulate and support detoxification. There are literally hundreds of herbal teas from a variety of sources that will support the detoxification process.

Moso bamboo
Bamboo leaf concentrate supports detoxification by clearing the detoxification channels of plaque, cholesterol, and other forms of build-up that hinder the waste removal process. It also works by balancing numerous systems and by

improving digestion, thus providing the necessary nutrients and antioxidants required for efficient detoxification. Moso bamboo supports detoxification in other ways as well. As a natural antibacterial and antimicrobial rich in chlorophyll, moso bamboo concentrate also helps bring many chronic infections under control so that deep healing can occur. It is frequently prescribed by Japanese dentists for gingival detoxification, which is one of the most difficult places to clear of infection.[398] Moso bamboo tea was provided for the survivors of the Hiroshima atomic bomb to help clear radiation toxins. For more information see www.wyntersway.com.

 (see Chapter 4: Food supplementation)

Chelation therapy

Chelation refers to a method of binding a substance to a chelating agent. In the case of chelation therapy, a synthetic amino acid known as EDTA is administered intravenously and binds to various toxic substances (specifically heavy metals) in the blood. The heavy metals lose their toxicity and are readily excreted by the kidneys. Though it has been used primarily to remove heavy metals, many doctors have found that chelation can remove the plaque present in the walls of arteries. It has become a widely used therapy for many patients with atherosclerosis. During chelation, the diet should be augmented with whole foods, extra vitamins, and minerals.

In 1958 a lengthy study was begun in Switzerland on more than two hundred adults who lived near a well-traveled highway. The population in that area had a higher rate of cancer and a higher incidence of nervous disorders, headaches, fatigue, gastrointestinal disorders, depression, and substance abuse. Researchers theorized that symptoms might be due to lead from automotive exhaust. Ten chelation treatments (to reduce lead toxicity) were administered to 59 of the participants; 172 participants received no treatment. After eighteen years, only one of the 59 treated patients died of cancer as compared to 30 deaths among the nontreated participants (a 90 percent reduction). Researchers also found that death from atherosclerosis was reduced among the treated patients.[399] Chelation therapy was the only significant difference between the control group and the treated patients.

Dr. Gary Gordon, MD, DO, MD(H), often referred to as the father of chelation therapy, has formulated an oral chelation supplement that includes a complete complement of vitamins, minerals, and other essential nutrients. The product, called Beyond Chelation Improved, is a great way to benefit on a long-term basis from chelation. His formulation, as the name suggests, goes beyond other oral chelation products offered today. It is available online (see sources).

Oil-pulling chelation

Another interesting form of chelation is an Ayurvedic technique referred to as Dr. Karach's oil therapy. Because toxic chemicals are fat-soluble, they are absorbed in oil. This natural chelation method draws toxins from the mucus membranes and circulating blood vessels traveling through the mouth. The average time required for blood to circulate from head to toe is approximately one minute; this technique absorbs toxic chemicals traveling in the blood from throughout the body.

In the morning before breakfast, on an empty stomach, place one tablespoon of sesame or sunflower oil in your mouth. Move the oil slowly as if rinsing or swishing your mouth. Dr. Karach recommends sucking it back and forth through your teeth. This activates the enzymes that draw toxins from the blood. As the process continues, the oil gets thinner and white. If the oil is still yellow, it has not been pulled/swished long enough. After fifteen to twenty minutes, spit it out, rinse your mouth thoroughly, and brush your teeth. Do not swallow the oil, which has picked up numerous toxins. Dr. Karach says this method has the potential to heal the entire organism— headaches, toothaches, eczema, ulcers, intestinal diseases, heart—and other maladies caused by chemicals and drugs.[400]

Hyperthermia (sweat therapy)

Heat gets your heart beating and your blood circulating. This helps your body to detoxify in unique ways. Physical sweating opens pores and allows the body to rid itself of heavy metals, excessive urea, toxic chemicals, and metabolic by-products. Sweating can also help to remove calcium deposits from blood vessels and to break down scar tissue. Anytime or any way you can find to increase sweating, you will enhance your body's detoxification processes.

Saunas and steam rooms are great for helping to remove toxins through the skin. As the heat increases, enzyme activity also increases. Besides mobilizing toxins from fat cells, it also stimulates the immune system and helps the body destroy virus and bacteria. The suggested protocol that follows for using a sauna is from Bill Akpinar's book, *No Sweat, Know Sweat*:[401]

1. Schedule an appropriate amount of time—don't rush. Focus on cleansing. Listen to healing music. Use appropriate essential oils.

    (see Chapter 16: Essential oils)

2. Relax and do some simple stretching for fifteen to twenty minutes before you get in the sauna. This stimulates the circulatory system to facilitate the detoxification process.

3. Drink warm water or hot tea. (Also drink two or three eight-ounce glasses of purified water before, during, and afterward to stay hydrated.)

4. Get into the sauna or sweat bath for ten to twenty minutes. Listen to your body—it's not a competition, it's a healing session.

5. When you leave the sauna or sweat bath, drink another two to three glasses of water.

6. Massage at this point is great—or do some massage for yourself (legs, arms, torso, scalp, ears) for ten to twenty minutes.

7. Get back into the heat for another ten to twenty minutes.

8. Drink more fluids, but don't over do it.

9. When you get out, don't rush to dress. Relax for another fifteen to twenty minutes. Sweating will continue after you leave for at least another fifteen to twenty minutes.

10. Shower and enjoy your day, or take a nap—or go to bed for the evening.

Dr. Akpinar suggests that the above protocol can be used five to seven times a week for detoxification with at least several sessions back-to-back. Then, use a sauna two to four times a week for maintenance.

Far infrared sauna (FIR)

There are two kinds of heat—convection and radiant heat. Convection heat uses air to carry warmth from the heat source to your body. Radiant heat uses a wavelength of light that resonates with water molecules. This wavelength is called far infrared (FIR). Unlike convection heat which, for the most part, just warms your skin, FIR heat penetrates several centimeters below the surface of the skin. Due to this deep-heating effect, FIR heat is able to warm the body much more quickly and much more deeply—producing more sweat with less heat. FIR is the same kind of heat that warms you in sunlight. FIR saunas use this kind of heat to produce a greater amount of sweat with a lower temperature. They are great for detoxification because a person can stay in the sauna longer without overheating.

Detoxification baths

The best way to really sweat, if you don't have access to a sauna, is to soak in a hot bath. Besides promoting profuse sweating, hot baths also stimulate the lymphatic and circulatory systems. They are another great way to open the channels that allow toxins to be eliminated through the skin. Sitting in water can actually help to pull the toxins through the skin.

By running a bath while sitting in the tub, most people can tolerate hotter water. The deeper you can immerse yourself, the better, so you may want to use duct tape to seal off the overflow in the tub and add more water. Additionally, if you can bring a portable heater into the bathroom to keep the whole room warm while you soak, you will have better results. Each of the following kinds of baths produces unique results.

Saltwater detox bath

Salt, especially sea salt or natural salt, draws toxins from the body. Epsom salts and baking soda also have therapeutic qualities and are known to draw (and hold) toxins so that they are not re-introduced back into the body. A gentle, detoxing bath recipe that you can use almost anytime includes the following: half a cup sea salt, one-quarter cup Epsom salts, and one-quarter cup of baking soda.

Essential oils detox bath

Essential oils have a powerful ability to draw toxins from the body. They also have the ability to soothe and relax—perfect for the bath. When using oils in your bath, wait until the bathtub is full before adding ten to thirty drops of your chosen oils. (Oils evaporate quickly—especially in hot water.) Avoid immersing yourself completely; oils should not come into contact with your eyes. Also avoid the use of soap in an essential oil bath. The soap may neutralize the action of the oils. Oils of rose, black pepper, cypress, juniper berry, fennel, coriander, parsley, sage, frankincense, carrot seed, and nutmeg are all known for their detoxifying properties. Citrus oils (grapefruit, bitter orange, and lemon) are also good for stimulating detoxification; however, they may not be good in a hot bath as they can irritate the skin. Test these sparingly before using them full strength.

Clay detox bath

Clay has been used for hundreds of years to help remove toxins from the body—both internally and externally. Its huge, charged surface area allows it to attach to toxins and pull them from the body. Soaking in a clay bath or clay foot bath can remove many toxins. LL's Magnetic Clay detox baths use proprietary blends of clay and herbs to gently pull lead, mercury, formaldehyde, arsenic, and other environmental toxins from the body while you soak. Their formulas are used in many spas and they are perfect for home use (see sources).

Foot baths

There are more sweat glands on your feet than anywhere else on your body. This information gives rise to the concept of detoxification using a foot bath—everything from simply soaking your feet in hot water to the use of salts, clay, essential oils, and bioelectric field enhancement. To take a detoxing foot bath, line a foot-sized basin or other container. Fill it with very warm water and your choice of salts, oils, or clay. Soak for thirty to forty-five minutes. Use two tablespoons of salts, ten to twelve drops of essential oil, or a half to one cup of LL's Magnetic Clay.

Detox foot spa

Detox foot spas are water ionizers. They consist of a power unit designed to place a tiny direct current into the water. The unit generates a complex waveform that interacts with the water in the body to provide a bioelectric boost to the cells. The absorption of this bioelectric charge increases the potential voltage across cell membranes and enhances cellular function. Detox foot spas recharge the cells, giving them the needed energy to perform all their functions—including the removal of wastes. Some toxins exit through sweat glands in the feet, others are taken to the blood to be carried out in the urine and stool. Because of the ability to optimize the body's bioelectric charge, many individuals use detox foot baths in their homes to detoxify as well as to increase vitality, speed recovery, reduce inflammation, and enhance metabolic function.

There are numerous different detox foot spas on the market—everything from manually operated units to completely computerized systems. The frequencies and waveforms used are unique to each unit. Some are more biocompatible than others. One company has performed the research to show that their unit releases heavy metals during the thirty-minute foot bath. Heavy metals were found in greater abundance in the water after a session; urine analysis showed fewer heavy metals in the urine after six sessions; and dry blood analysis showed the reduction of heavy metals following several sessions.[402] The best of these foot spas, a fully computerized and well-researched model, is made by Platinum Energy Systems in Canada (see sources).

Clay packs

Clay is an amazing substance formed from volcanic ash. Besides its use in baths, clay can be used in other ways to help detoxify. Taken internally, it adsorbs many toxins and food poisons from the gastrointestinal tract and carries them safely from the body. Stir one-half to one teaspoon of clay in a glass of water and drink. Some people prefer to let the clay settle and then drink the clay water from the top. Benefits seem to be similar either way. Make sure you get good-quality clay. Nature's Body Beautiful, Terramin, and Redmond Clay are good products (see sources).

Clay can also be used to draw toxins from specific areas of the body. To do this, a clay pack or poultice is used. To make a poultice, mix clay with enough filtered or purified water to form a gel, about the consistency of mustard. Apply it generously in a half-inch to three-quarters-inch layer directly on your skin; cover with cheese cloth and then with warm, moist towels. You can replace the warm towels every few minutes to keep the heat in. After twenty minutes, remove and discard the clay. This technique has been known to detoxify specific organs as well as to pull infection from swollen lymph glands and many other areas.

Homeopathic detoxification

Homeopathic remedies are unique. Unlike vitamins, foods, or herbs, they do not contain therapeutic components of a botanical nature. Homeopathy has proven useful for detoxification and can even remove the toxins caused by stress, mental imbalance, and hormonal changes. Homeopathy works not chemically, but vibrationally, to correct imbalances in the body. When it is combined with other energetic modalities, it can be extremely powerful, helping to eliminate food allergies and many other underlying causes of toxin build up. One company has created a whole line of detoxification formulas to address specific toxins and detoxification pathways. A homeopathic professional, trained in the use of these innovative formulas can be located by contacting Deseret Biologicals: info@deseretbio.com

DETOXIFICATION SUPPORT

Individuals can do a number of things to support the natural cleansing of the body. Methods of support include everything from body movement to cleansing foods, massage, and the use of technological advances that recharge cells and provide energetic nourishment.

Exercise and stretching

Brisk walking, jogging, dancing, rebounding, yoga, tai chi, pilates, and so on, all support detoxification. Exercise and stretching strengthen the respiratory, circulatory, lymphatic, and immune systems; they increase the circulation of nutrients throughout the body. By themselves, exercise and stretching will stimulate detoxification and should accompany any detoxification program.

Rebounding

Research has led some scientists to conclude that jumping on a mini-trampoline (rebounding) is possibly the most effective exercise yet devised—because of the effect rebounding has on the lymphatic system. The lymphatic system is totally dependent on physical exercise. Lymphatic channels have one-way valves so the lymph always moves in the same direction. The main lymph vessels run up the legs, up the arms, and up the torso. This is why the vertical up and down movement of rebounding is so effective. A mini-trampoline subjects the body to gravitational forces two to three times the force of gravity, depending on how high a person jumps. Unlike jogging and many other forms of exercise which put extreme stress on certain joints, rebounding affects every joint and every cell in the body equally. It is an ideal exercise for the home environment.

Pilates exercise

Pilates is another form of exercise that is well suited for almost everyone, including the elderly. It is a nonaerobic form of exercise and physical movement designed to stretch, strengthen, and balance the body. The pilates exercise system is gentle while giving your body a challenging workout. Many of the exercises are performed in reclining or sitting positions, and most are low impact and partially weight bearing. Pilates movements unlock stagnant energy, yielding numerous benefits. The following Web site offers a series of free videos on pilates exercises for beginners:
http://www.expertvillage.com/video-series/102_pilates.htm

Benefits of Pilates Exercise

1. **Provides a refreshing mind-body workout**: Pilates emphasizes proper breathing, correct spinal, and pelvic alignment, as well as complete concentration on smooth, flowing movement. A person becomes aware of his/her body and how to control its movement.
2. **Builds strength and flexibility**: Conventional workouts tend to build short, bulky muscles—the type most prone to injury. Pilates elongates and strengthens, improving muscle elasticity and joint mobility.
3. **Develops a strong core**: Pilates exercises develop a strong "core," which consists of the deep abdominal muscles along with the muscles closest to the spine.
4. **Creates an evenly conditioned body**: Pilates conditions the whole body. No muscle group is neglected. Your entire musculature is evenly balanced and conditioned, helping you to enjoy daily activities with greater ease and less chance of injury.
5. **Teaches efficient patterns of motion**: Pilates exercises train several muscle groups at once in smooth, continuous movements. You can retrain your body to move in safer, more efficient patterns of motion.

Skin brushing

Skin brushing is a simple way to promote the elimination of wastes through your skin and to stimulate the lymphatic system. It is a perfect compliment to a detoxification program. Before your shower or bath, take a couple of minutes and, starting at your feet, work your way upward toward your heart, brushing in little circles over your entire body. Brush from your extremities inward toward your torso. The best dry skin brushes are made of vegetable bristles that are neither too stiff nor too soft. They shouldn't scratch, but you should feel friction against your skin. These are available at many natural foods stores.

Massage

If your muscles are relaxed, then your body is likely to detoxify much better. But massage is not just about relaxation, although it is great for that purpose. Special detoxification massages can greatly support any cleansing program. This involves gentle compression and stretching of muscle tissues to mobilize toxins, to stimulate lymphatic flow, to improve circulation, and to improve the function of all the detoxification pathways. A massage therapist can focus on these systems and organs during your detoxification program. A massage two or three times a week is ideal.

Manual lymphatic drainage

Lymphatic massage, otherwise known as manual lymphatic drainage (MLD), is a highly specialized form of massage, which uses light, rhythmical, very precise hand movements, pressures, and sequences. The massage works at a skin level to influence the direction and speed of lymphatic flow to facilitate waste removal at a cellular level and to assist in the transportation of nutrients and oxygen. The aim of MLD is to restore equilibrium in the tissues. A treatment begins at the neck to make space for lymph to be brought there. Since lymph follows predetermined pathways and is continuous, if space is made at the top of the chain, fluid from lower down can move up. This is a very effective way to improve lymphatic flow and to support the detoxification process.

Psyllium husks

Many people can benefit from increasing the amount of fiber in their diet, especially during detoxification. Psyllium husks (purchased at any natural food store) are a source of fiber that can easily (and inexpensively) be incorporated in your diet. One tablespoon in a glass of water at the end of the day will absorb toxins and participate in the sweeping of the entire digestive system. Apple pectin, guar gum, oat bran, and rice bran are also good sources of fiber.

Essential oils

Essential oils can assist the body in detoxification, especially when used in conjunction with other natural cleansing processes. During detoxification, essential oils can be used in massage oil or in the bath.

 (see Chapter 16: Essential oils)

 (see Chapter 19: Essential oil detoxification bath)

Detoxifying Massage Oil

4 drops grapefruit oil
4 drops juniper oil
3 drops cypress oil
5 drops laurel oil
Mix the above essential oils with 2 Tbsp. of a carrier oil (sunflower, almond, or jojoba).

Detoxifying Bath Oil Blend

6–8 drops grapefruit oil
6–8 drops juniper oil
6 drops helichrysum oil
Mix essential oils with 1 cup natural salt and add to bath water.

Herbs

A variety of herbs have been used for centuries to assist in cleansing and detoxification. They can be taken as capsules or as teas to support your process. Below are some of the most widely used:

- Black cohosh loosens and expels mucous in the respiratory tract, and stimulates lymphatic, liver, and kidney function.
- Burdock root purifies the blood and improves liver function.
- Cayenne pepper purifies blood and increases fluid elimination and sweat.
- Cascara sagrada promotes peristaltic action in the colon but may be too harsh for some individuals.
- Dandelion stimulates liver detoxification and promotes healthy circulation.
- Echinacea improves lymphatic drainage and immune function.
- Garlic is a blood cleanser and natural antibiotic.
- Ginger root stimulates circulation and sweating and aids in cleansing of the bowels, kidney, and skin.
- Goldenseal cleanses blood, liver, kidney, and skin and stimulates detoxification. Never use for longer than two weeks.
- Horsetail tones the urinary tract and soothes the bladder, supports the skin.
- Licorice Root is a general detoxifier and mild laxative.
- Marshmallow root helps remove hardened mucous in the intestinal tract and lungs.
- Milk Thistle enhances liver function and helps rebuild the liver.
- Parsley flushes the kidneys.
- Peppermint brings oxygen to the blood and strengthens the bowels.
- Yellow dock root cleanses skin, blood, and liver.

Light Beam Generator

The Light Beam Generator (LBG), made by the same company that makes the Teslar watch, stimulates lymphatic drainage and the movement of waste material to the organs responsible for their disposal. The LBG emits photons (units of light) and utilizes scalar wave technology to correct the electromagnetic charge on cells. This often breaks up hardened lymphatic deposits and releases wastes that have built up over long periods of time. The energy also helps to restore the natural cellular electromagnetic signature. It can be a powerful tool, not just to support detoxification but to maintain overall cellular health. LBG light sources are placed on the body for forty-five minutes to an hour at a time several times a week. This method is used by many practitioners but can also be used in the home (see sources).

Quantron Resonance System (QRS)

The Quantron Resonance System (QRS) was developed by a team of international scientists in conjunction with the Russian space program. It has been used in many clinics, practitioner's offices, and private homes. The QRS supports detoxification and all the functions of the body. It helps normalize cellular metabolism by recharging every cell and by helping the body to regenerate healthy cells. Once charged, cells are able to take in more oxygen and nutrients to purge more wastes. Besides being a complement to detoxification, the QRS is something that many people can use in their homes to support ongoing cellular regeneration and improved health. The QRS takes only eight minutes every day. Treatment is received by lying on a mat that sends a variety of biocompatible frequencies that are utilized by the body to energize and regenerate (see sources).

Energy Enhancement System (EES)

The Energy Enhancement System (EES) is a computerized system that sets up an enhanced energetic environment. When the body is exposed to the energy, multiple bioactive fields generated by the device raise the cell membrane potential and return cells to their original healthy energy levels. This encourages cellular cleansing. It also improves immune function, provides relief from pain, elevates moods, assists in balancing right and left hemispheres of the brain, and promotes cellular regeneration.[403] Clinical trials and a variety of case studies have demonstrated remarkable cleansing and healing benefits.[404]

The EES creates an array of beneficial wave forms, which include scalar waves. The resulting energy field cancels out the detrimental effects of sixty-cycle current and provides a virtual cocoon of biologically supportive wave forms in which regeneration can occur. The technology may also amplify intention and manifestation because it balances the entire electromagnetic field that surrounds the body. Exposure to the EES energy field can vary from twenty minutes to all night. Although most systems are available in a professional setting, many individuals have purchased their own system for private use (see sources).

CAUTIONS WITH DETOXIFICATION:

- Before you begin a detoxification program, make sure you are well enough to undertake the protocol. It is important to choose cleansing techniques that are not too extreme for your circumstances. Begin slowly and first focus on nourishment, water, and on the elimination of toxins in your living environment. Next, incorporate breathing, stretching, and exercise. Be comfortable at each level of preparation before you move on to more vigorous action. Detoxification is not a contest; neither is it something you do once and think you're done.
- Sometimes when you begin to detoxify, you may experience what is known as a "Herxheimer reaction" or healing crisis. This occurs when toxins are released faster than your body can eliminate them. When this occurs, you may experience headaches, nausea, fatigue, and malaise—headaches are the most common. If this occurs, it is an indication to either slow the process or stop and begin again later, more slowly.
- It is not advisable for pregnant or nursing mothers to embark on a detoxification program. Detoxification releases toxins that can end up being transferred to your baby if they are not efficiently eliminated. If you are nursing, toxins will end up in your breast milk. It is better to wait until after you have finished nursing before you contemplate a vigorous detoxification protocol. In the meantime, nourishment and a healthy lifestyle are important. Ideally, detoxification a year before becoming pregnant is recommended.

DETOXIFICATION FOR SPECIFIC PROBLEMS
Parasites
According to Hulda Clark, parasites are a cofactor in almost every illness, including cancer.[405] Parasites are so common that today, most people are likely to have one or more different types. If you have pets; if you eat out regularly; if you eat rare meat; or if you have children in daycare centers, your chances of having some form of parasite are nearly 100 percent.

Like any other type of infection, parasites are an opportunistic infection. If you are healthy and if your immune system is strong, parasites usually cannot get a foothold. But everyone goes through periods of stress when they are more vulnerable. And since parasites are so prevalent, there are few individuals in our day that are not affected. A parasite cleanse is highly recommended for everyone. Even if you have no apparent symptoms (this is often the case), you may be surprised to find that you have more energy, that you sleep better, that cravings are reduced, or that you have fewer food intolerances once you have completed a parasite cleanse.

Three herbs can rid you of more than a hundred types of parasites, including liver flukes, pinworms, threadworms, hookworms, round worms, and tapeworms. Used together, these three herbs have helped thousands of people to rid themselves of parasitic infections and a host of accompanying symptoms.

Three Herbs Used to Eliminate Parasites:

1. Black walnut hulls (from the black walnut tree)
2. Wormwood (from the Artemisia shrub)
3. Common cloves

These herbs must be used together as a single treatment to eradicate both adult and egg stages of parasites. The complete parasite protocol takes three weeks and can be found online: http://www.herbalparasitecleanse.com/. It is recommended that a family do the cleanse together to avoid reinfecting each other. Following the cleanse, regular maintenance doses are necessary to prevent reinfection.

Mercury detoxification

The body is capable of eliminating small amounts of mercury—just as it is capable of removing small amounts of other toxins. The problem begins when the body becomes overwhelmed. Long-term exposure to mercury (especially when mercury amalgam fillings are present) depletes the body of the antioxidants and minerals that are required for the task. Supplying the building blocks for these antioxidants is critical for a successful program.

Glutathione is perhaps the most potent antioxidant in the body. It is used up rapidly during the detoxification of mercury. Anyone with amalgam fillings is likely depleted of glutathione—and simply taking glutathione supplements does not seem to help improve glutathione levels. Glutathione is made of three amino acids: cysteine, glutamic acid, and glycine. Cysteine is the limiting factor. Supplying cysteine in the form of N-acetyl cysteine (NAC) is an essential part of a mercury detoxification program. Other essential factors in a mercury detox program are:

- Alpha-lipoic acid, which binds with mercury to carry it from the body.

- Free-form amino acids. These supply the building blocks for glutathione and other antioxidants and enzymes required for mercury detoxification.
- MSM (methylsulfonylmethane) which is a form of bioavailable sulfur that acts on cell membranes to help eliminate mercury.
- Vitamin C.
- Milk thistle, which provides support for the liver.

In addition to the above supplements, there are several foods that will help to draw mercury from the body. These include sea vegetables (chlorella, spirulina, and blue green algae), cilantro, and garlic. Extra fiber during mercury detoxification is also a good idea to help move debris through the intestines.

Sea vegetables (especially chlorella) bind to mercury to pull it from the body. The Kyoto brand, available in most natural food stores, is a good brand.

CAUTION: Roughly 25 to 30 percent of people cannot tolerate chlorella. Start slow, and if you experience any kind of reaction, eliminate this product from your detoxification program.

Cilantro helps to mobilize mercury, but it may not be strong enough to actually pull the mercury from your body. It should be used only in conjunction with the other herbs and vitamins mentioned here. Cilantro is an herb that is widely available in the produce section in grocery stores. Chop it and eat it in soups, salads, and sandwiches every day. It is a delicious addition to a freshly juiced vegetable cocktail.

Garlic can be incorporated into your diet or taken as capsules. The Kyolic brand is highly reputable.

Approximately 80 to 90 percent of the mercury in our bodies is eliminated through the liver-colon pathway.[406] In 1991, Swedish researchers placed one small mercury filling in an eleven-year-old girl with no history of cavities or fillings. They then measured her stool for the next three days. In comparison to a control group, the excretion of mercury was enormous—four hundred micrograms—on the third day.[407] (World Health Organization maximum acceptable level of mercury intake is forty-five micrograms in a twenty-four-hour period.) This study illustrates that there is a critical time to support the detoxification of mercury after amalgam fillings are removed. The five-day period immediately after removal is critical.[408] However, following a mercury detoxification protocol for several months is important.

 (see Chapter 12: Mercury amalgam fillings)

Tom McGuire's book *Mercury Detoxification: The Natural Way to Remove Mercury From Your Body* is another excellent resource. His protocol does not require a pharmaceutical chelating agent and focuses on rebuilding and repairing the damage done by mercury; www.dentalwellness4u.com

Dr. Mercola has a detailed mercury detoxification protocol available online which you may want to read and consider. His recommendations include a pharmaceutical chelating agent:
http://www.mercola.com/article/mercury/detox_protocol.htm

Detoxification and autism

It is well known that there is a genetic disposition to autism. Many autistic children also show genetic evidence of a diminished ability to perform the functions of detoxification. Parents and physicians have reported extremely good results in improving the health and behavior of autistic children when the mercury was removed from children's bodies using a variety of detoxification protocols. Many physicians who have specialized in the treatment of autistic children report that no other treatment has brought about the improvement that the removal of mercury has brought.[409] This is further evidence that mercury is a primary factor for some children with autism. There are many routes by which children can receive toxic doses of mercury (vaccines, dental fillings, dietary fish, and from the mother while in the womb).

(see Chapter 13: Vaccines)

(see Chapter 12: Mercury amalgam fillings)

Diet is high on the list of important concerns for parents of autistic children. Many, if not most, autistic children suffer from some degree of intestinal permeability and nutritional deficit, each of which must be corrected prior to any attempt at detoxification. Supporting the detoxification process is also a major concern.

In 2001, the Autism Research Institute enlisted a group of scientists and physicians from around the world to seek answers. They surveyed more than twenty-three thousand parents of autistic children who rated seventy-seven biomedical interventions. Mercury detoxification received a far higher rating than any drug, supplement, or special diet. Mercury detoxification was rated helpful by 73 percent of parents. A gluten/casein-free diet was next with 63 percent.[410] In 2005, this group convened to review a variety of mercury detoxification protocols. The paper that resulted, Treatment Options for

Mercury/Metal Toxicity in Autism and Related Developmental Disabilities: Consensus Position, is available online: http://autism.asu.edu/TreatmentOptions.pdf. The paper focuses on physician-administered chelation but addresses several other methods. Dr. Mercola's comments are also found online and worth reading: http://articles.mercola.com/sites/articles/archive/2001/06/02/mercury-autism2.aspx

SOURCES (in the order they appear in the chapter):

Colon Cleanse:
ColonTone: www.swansonvitamins.com

Oral Chelation:
Beyond Chelation Plus: http://longevityplus.com/

Clay detox formulas:
LL's Magnetic Clay Baths: http://www.magneticclay.com/

Clay for internal and external use:
Terramin: http://terramin.com/
Nature's Body Beautiful: http://www.naturesbodybeautiful.com/
Redmond clay: http://www.redmondclay.com/

Detox foot bath:
Platinum energy systems: www.platinumenergysystems.ca

Homeopathic detox formulas:
Deseret Biologicals: http://www.desbio.com/

Light Beam Generator:
http://www.teslartech.com

Quantron Resonance system (QRS):
www.QRSforhealth.com

Energy Enhancement System (EES):
http://www.eesystem.com

Parasite cleanse:
http://www.drclark.com/

 Recommended Reading:

The Fast Track Detox Diet by Ann Louise Gittleman
Mercury Detoxification: The Natural Way to Remove Mercury from Your Body by Tom McGuire, DDS

Chapter 20

CONCLUSION AND CALL TO ACTION

The previous nineteen chapters have hopefully enlightened you—enough for you to begin to understand the huge impact that chemicals and other toxins have had on our environment and on our well-being. Perhaps you have already made shifts in your thinking and in your purchasing decisions. If this is the case, then our purpose in writing this book has been met. We believe that as more people begin to insist on unadulterated food and on nontoxic products and services, the safer alternatives will become increasingly available and accessible.

The foregoing chapters may have also illustrated how seriously we have damaged the earth—the wonderful garden that has sustained and supported life for millions of years. This is a travesty that will take many generations to fully overcome. However, the sooner we begin, the sooner the earth will be able to provide safe food, air, and water for our children and grandchildren. Everyone makes a contribution, for good or ill. The greater the number of people who are committed to making conscious choices and to taking conscious action, the faster the process can proceed.

Perhaps you have also become aware that detoxifying and living a toxin-free life opens many doorways that seem to be closing all around us. Removing the toxins from your body and living in a toxin-free environment are the keys to vibrant health and vitality, but they are also the keys to mental clarity, balanced emotions, enhanced creativity, and inner peace. As the lower vibrations of chemicals and other toxins are removed, we are able to hold the higher vibrations of harmony and love that are so lacking in today's world. We may ultimately discover that eliminating toxins goes a long way toward the reduction of many common problems that are on the rise, including road rage and school violence. We may also discover that the elimination of toxins will help us to reestablish a vital connection with the earth—with the water, with the plants, and with the animals that have always been linked with our sustenance.

Choosing *nontoxic* when given the choice will help you to be all that you were meant to be. It may also help you to reestablish a connection with the earth. But choosing nontoxic must happen on a much larger scale if we are to truly make a difference. We hope you have come to realize that you cannot count on the FDA or any regulatory agency to provide fair guidance about what is safe. The nation's toxic regulatory laws are some of the weakest in the world. They are in drastic need of reform. As long as our politicians and regulatory agencies are allowed to be *influenced* with pharmaceutical and corporate funds, the American people (and the rest of the world) will suffer. Choosing nontoxic on a larger scale means supporting political leaders with the integrity to stand up to corporate America—leaders who will help us to take back our government from the huge corporations that have controlled it for years. Perhaps the only way to keep corporate funds out of politics and government is to support reforms that change the way political campaigns are financed. When our politicians are no longer funded by corporate America, they will cease to be obliged to their wishes. We encourage you to initiate and support these kinds of reform.

As a human race, we are at a critical juncture. The decisions our generation makes will determine the fate of the next generations, just as the decisions of the past (made mostly in ignorance) have placed us in this precarious position. The knowledge that previous generations did not have is surfacing—albeit slowly. Now, we must get beyond knowing better and be willing to spend the time and resources to make a difference. It is time we rediscovered respect for all life. It is time we relearned to live from our hearts, and it is time we remembered how to live in gratitude rather than in the greed that has governed this planet for too many years. We encourage you to:

Live in gratitude; be open to the bounty all around; enjoy the journey; take action; make a difference.

Sharyn Wynters, ND and Burton Goldberg, LHD

Endnotes

1   U.S. EPA *Respiratory Health Effects of Passive Smoking: Lung Cancer and other Disorders,* Dec. 1992.

2   Dept. of Health and Human Science—Agency for Toxic Substances and Disease Registry. *Toxicological Profile for Benzene.* Aug. 2007.

3   U.S. EPA Survey of Perchloroethylene Emission sources. EPA-450/3-85-021 Office of Air Quality Planning Standards 1985.

4   Dept. of Health and Human Science—Agency for Toxic Substances and Disease Registry. *Toxicological Profile for Toluene,* Sept. 2000.

5   Dept. of Health and Human Science—Agency for Toxic Substances and Disease Registry. *Toxicological Profile for Xylene.* Aug. 2000.

6   Ma, X, et al., Critical Windows of Exposure to Household Pesticides and Risk of Childhood Leukemia. *Environmental Health Perspectives 2002 110:955–960.* Available online: http://www.ourstolenfuture.org/NEWSCIENCE/human/cancer/2002-08maetal.htm

7   Dept. of Health and Human Science—Agency for Toxic Substances and Disease Registry. *Toxicological Profile for Formaldehyde* July 1999.

8   University of Texas at Austin News, Inadequate air cleaning ability, production of harmful ozone plague ion-generating products sold as air cleaners. Sept. 15, 2005. Available online: http://www.utexas.edu/news/2005/09/15/engineering/

9   Agency for Toxic Substances and Disease Registry. 2006. Public health statement for lead. Available online: http://www.atsdr.gov./ToxProfiles/tp.asp?id=96&tid=22.

10   American Academy of Pediatrics Committees on Environmental Hazards and Committee on Accident and Poison Prevention.

Statement on childhood lead poisoning. *Pediatrics.* 1987; 79:457–465.

11 Nriagu, J. Some candles with lead wicks emit lead into the air, University of Michigan News Release, Oct. 6, 1999(5). Available online: http://www.umich.edu/~newsinfo/Releases/1999/Oct99/r100699.html

12 U.S. EPA *Assessment of Risks from Radon in Homes* (EPA 402-R-03-003) 1999.

13 National Academy of Sciences *Health Effects of Exposure to Radon.* Committee on Health Risks of Exposure to Radon (BEIR VI) 1999.

14 Llope, W. J. Radiation and Radon from Natural Stone, Rice University, Houston, TX May 27, 2008. Available online: http://wjllope.rice.edu/saxumsubluceo/LLOPE_StoneRadRn.pdf

15 U.S. Environmental Protection Agency, Office of Air and Radiation. *Indoor Air Facts No. 4: Sick Building Syndrome,* revised, 1991.

16 Lipton, B. *Biology of Belief* Mountain of Love /Elite Books. 205.

17 University of Texas at Austin News, Inadequate air cleaning ability, production of harmful ozone plague ion-generating products sold as air cleaners. Sept. 15, 2005. Available online: http://www.utexas.edu/news/2005/09/15/engineering/

18 Soyka, F. *The Ion Effect* Lester and Orpen Limited, 1977, pp. 57–58.

19 Windsor, T et al. Biological Effects of Ionized Air in Man, *Am. J. Physical Med.* 37:83 1958.

20 Palti, Yoram et al. The effect of atmospheric ions on the respiratory systems of infants, *Pediatrics* Vol. 38 No. 3 September 1966, pp. 405–411.

21 http://web.mac.com/jimadison/OCRainbow/OCMAAAH.html

22 Carson, C. F. et al. Susceptibility of methicillin-resistant Staphylococcus aureus to the essential oil of Melaleuca alternifolia. *Antimicrobial Chemother.* 1995; 35: pp. 421–424.

23 Settineri, R. et al. Antimicrobial effects of plant-derived essential oil formulations on pathogenic bacteria, *JANA,* Vol. 6 No. 3, Summer 2003 pp. 27–31.

24   Hendel, Barbara & Ferreira, Peter, *Water and Salt: The Essence of Life*, Natural Resources, pp. 184.

25   B. C. Wolverton, Anne Johnson, and Keith Bounds, "Interior Landscape Plants for Indoor Air Pollution Abatement, Final Report—September 15, 1989." Stennis Space Center, Mississippi: NASA.

26   Hal Levin Building Ecology Research Group. *Can House Plants Solve Indoor Air Quality Problems?*

27   Batmanghelidj, F. *Water: For Health for Healing for Life—You're Not Sick You're Thirsty.* Warner Books, Inc. New York, NY 2003.

28   Jhon, M.S. *The Water Puzzle and the Hexagonal Key.* Uplifting Press, 2004.

29   Institute of Medicine. *Dietary Reference Intakes: Water, Potassium, Sodium, Chloride, and Sulfate.* Feb 11, 2004.

30   Groundwater Cleanup-Cross-Program Task Force Available online: http://www.epa.gov/oswer/onecleanupprogram/init1-GW.htm.

31   Environmental Working Group, National Tap Water Quality Database, Dec. 20, 2005. Available online: http://www.ewg.org/tapwater/findings.php.

32   Price, Joseph M. *Coronaries/Cholesterol/Chlorine* Jove Book, Alta Enterprises, 1969.

33   Villanueva, C. M. et al. *Bladder cancer and exposure to water disinfection by-products through ingestion, bathing, showering, and swimming in pools.* Am J Epidemiol. 2007 Jan 15;165(2):148–156. Epub 2006 Nov.

34   Plewa, M. J., E.D. et al. Chemical and biological characterization of newly discovered iodo-acid drinking water disinfection byproducts. (2004) *Environ. Sci. Tech.* 38:4713–4722.

35   San Francisco Water Quality Bureau bench test lab results, memo issued July 18, 2004. Available online: http://www.lmtf.org/FoLM/Plans/Water/PUCreports/LMJuly6ltrwattachments.pdf

36   Christopher Bryson. *The Fluoride Deception*, Seven Stories Press, New York, NY, 2004.

37   http://www.cyber-nook.com/water/tbl_afl.html A list of scientific articles and abstracts on the problems with fluoridation.

38   *Newsweek Magazine.* Don't Drink the Water, Feb. 5, 1990.

39   Michaud, C. & Slovak, R. Unpublished report released at the 2009 annual Water Quality Association convention.

40   Dept of Energy, Non-Chemical Technologies for Scale and Hardness Control, 1998, DOE/EE 0162. Available online: http://www.etpwater.com/Reports/FTA/FTA.pdf

41   Environment News Service (ENS), Associated Press, *Pharmaceuticals Again Found in U.S. Drinking Water,* March 10, 2008. Available online: http://www.ens-newswire.com/ens/mar2008/2008-03-10-099.asp

42   Ibid.

43   Ibid.

44   Houston Chronicle. *Tap Water at Risk.* Available online: http://www.chron.com/content/houston/interactive/special/water/06/water/series.html

45   Steven J. Spindler, S. J. and Spindler, G. A. *Evaluation of a stabilized chlorine dioxide paste-rinse combination regimen vs. a phenol related rinse regimen.* 1998. Available online: http://www.halitosis-research.com/articles/Evaluation_of_Chlorine_Dioxide_Toothpaste_and_Rinse.pdf

46   Dr. William Marcus' Internal EPA Memo, Fluoride Conference to Review the NTP Draft Fluoride Report, May 1, 1990, http://fluoridealert.org/health/cancer/ntp/marcus-memo.html

47   Graham, J. R., Burk, O., and Morin, P. 1987. A current restatement and continuing reappraisal concerning demographic variables in American time-trend studies and water fluoridation and human cancer. *Proc Pennsylvania Academy of Sci.* 61:138–146.

48   Bruce Siegel, MD, PhD. *An Epidemiologic Report on Drinking Water and Fluoridation,* 1992, New Jersey Dept. of Health. Available online: http://www.fluoridealert.org/health/cancer/cohn-1992.pdf

49   WHO Guidelines for Drinking-water Quality. Aug. 2004.

50   Kozisek, F. *Health Risks from Drinking Demineralized Water.* National Institute of Public Health Czech Republic. 2005.

Available online: http://www.who.int/water_sanitation_health/dwq/nutrientsindw/en/

51 Ibid.

52 Pangman, M. J., *Dancing with Water* 2011, pp 77–79.

53 Cousens, Gabriel, *Spiritual Nutrition,* North Atlantic Books 1986, 2005. p. 478.

54 Cousens, Gabriel, *Spiritual Nutrition,* North Atlantic Books 1986, 2005. p. 477.

55 Oschman, J. L. *Energy Medicine in Therapeutics and Human Performance*, Elsevier Limited 2003. p. 61.

56 Ibid. pp. 98–99.

57 Pangman, M. J. *Hexagonal Water, The Ultimate Solution, revised edition,* Uplifting Press, Inc. 2007, pp. 22–41.

58 Water Connoisseur Newsletter, Antimony, (Sb) in PET bottles. April, 2006. Available online: http://www.finewaters.com/Newsletter/April_2006/Antimony_Sb_in_PET_Bottles.asp

59 Rust, S., *JS Online* 20 years of research on bisphenol A studied. Available online: http://www.jsonline.com/watchdog/watchdogewports/34431194.html

60 NRDC Petition to the FDA, Mar. 1999, *Bottled Water: Pure Drink or Pure Hype,* Available online: http://www.nrdc.org/water/drinking/bw/bwinx.asp

61 Environmental working Group Web site. Bottled water contains disinfection byproducts, fertilizer residue, and pain medication. 2008. http://www.ewg.org/reports/bottledwater

62 Cherry, N. Evidence that electromagnetic fields from high voltage powerlines and in buildings are hazardous to human health, especially to young children. Environmental Management and Design Division, Lincoln University, New Zealand, April, 2001.

63 Cherry, N. Evidence that Electromagnetic Radiation is Genotoxic: The implications for the epidemiology of cancer and cardiac, neurological and reproductive effects. Available online: http://www.neilcherry.com/documents/90_m2_EMR_Evidence_That_EMR-EMF_is_genotoxic.pdf

64 Michrowski, Andrew, PhD. Electromagnetic Pollution, Consumer Health Organization of Canada, 1991, Available

online: http://www.consumerhealth.org/articles/display. cfm?ID=19990303163909.

65   Havas, M. Biological effects of non-ionizing electromagnetic energy: A critical review of the reports by the US National Research Council and the US National Institute of Environmental Health Sciences as they relate to the broad realm of EMF bioeffects. *Environ Rev.* 2000, 8:173–253.

66   Wever, R. Autonomous circadian rhythms in man. *Naturwissenschaften*, Sept.1975, Vol. 62 No. 9.

67   Cherry, N. 2003, Human intelligence: The brain, an electromagnetic system synchronised by the Schumann Resonance signal, *Medical Hypotheses* 60(60):843–844.

68   Ghaly, M. and Teplitz, D. The biologic effects of grounding the human body during sleep as measured by cortisol levels and subjective reporting of sleep, pain and stress. *Journal of Alternative and Complementary Medicine* 2004 Vol. 10, No. 5 pp. 767–776.

69   Ibid.

70   Chevalier, G. et al. The effect of earthing (grounding) on human physiology. *European Biology and Bioelectromagnetics* 31/01/2006, pp. 600–621.

71   Amalu, W. Medical Thermography Case Studies. Available online: http://www.earthinginstitute.net/studies/thermograph ic_histories_2004.pdf

72   Don Maisch, Mobile Phone Use: It's time to take precautions. *Journal of Australasian College of Nutritional & Environmental Medicine* Vol. 20 No. 1; April 2001 pp. 3–10. Available online: http://www.buergerwelle.de/assets/files

73   ABC News story, *Cell Phone War,* a YouTube video available at: http://www.youtube.com/watch?v=sEqCkwPmQ_w.

74   Hope, J. Men who use mobile phones face increased risk of infertility, *Daily Mail* Oct 2006, Available online: http://www. dailymail.co.uk/pages/live/articles/news/news.html?in_article_ id=412179&in_page_id=1770

75   Salford, L. et al. Nerve Cell Damage in Mammalian Brain after Exposure to Microwaves from GSM Mobile Phones, *Environmental Health Perspectives* Vol. 111, No. 7, June 2003. Available online: http://www.ncbi.nlm.nih.gov/pmc/articles/PMC1241519/

76   Khurana, V. G. Mobile Phones and Brain Tumours—A Public Health Concern. 2008. Available online: http://www.brain-surgery.us/mobilephone.html#abst

77   Yates, J and Borenstein, S. Pittsburgh cancer center warns of cell phone risks, *The Associated Press*. 2008. Available online: http://www.physorg.com/news136083905.html

78   Mortazavi, S. M., et al. Mercury release from dental amalgam restorations after magnetic resonance imaging and following mobile phone use. *Pak J Biol Sci*. 2008 Apr 15;11(8):1142–1146.

79   Goldhaber , M. et al. The risk of miscarriage and birth defects among women who use visual display terminals during pregnancy, *American Journal of Industrial Medicine*, 1988, Vol. 13:695–706.

80   EMF RAPID Program. Electromagnetic Health Hazard Control. NIH98-3981 (pp. 180, 182), August 1998.

81   Breakspear Hospital Web site: http://www.breakspearmedical.com/

82   Environmental Health Center Web site: http://www.ehcd.com/

83   Ho, Mae-Wan. *The Rainbow and the Worm: The Physics of Organisms*. World Scientific 1998.

84   Chevalier, G., et al. The effect of earthing (grounding) on human physiology. *European Biology and Bioelectromagnetics* 31/01/2006, pp. 600–621.

85   Oschman, J. L. Can Electrons Act as Antioxidants? A Review and Commentary, *The Journal of Alternative and Complementary Medicine,* Vol. 13 No. 9 2007 pp. 955–967.

86   Huang, D. et al. The Chemistry behind Antioxidant Capacity Assays, *J. Agric. Food Chem.* 2005, 53(6), pp. 1841–1856. Abstract available online: http://pubs.acs.org/doi/abs/10.1021/jf03723c.

87   Ibid.

88   Mitelman F, et al. Database of chromosome aberrations in cancer. *Cancer Genome Anatomy Project*, 2007. Available online: http://cgap.nci.nih.gov/Chromosomes/Mitelman

89   Kaltsas, H. *X-rayed to Death* unpublished manuscript. 2008.

90   Brenner, D. et al. Computed Tomography—An increasing source of radiation exposure. *NEJM,* Nov. 2007, #22. Vol. 357:2277–

2284. Available online: http://content.nejm.org/cgi/content/full/357/22/2277#R25

91   Kaltsas, H. *X-rayed to Death* unpublished manuscript. 2008

92   Health risks from exposure to low levels of ionizing radiation—BEIR VII. Washington, DC: National Academies Press, 2005.

93   Brenner, D. et al. Computed Tomography—An increasing source of radiation exposure. *NEJM,* Nov. 2007, #22. Vol. 357:2277–2284. Available online: http://content.nejm.org/cgi/content/full/357/22/2277#R25

94   Gofman, J. *X-Rays, Health Effects of Common Exams* Sierra Club Books, San Francisco, 1985 p. 23.

95   Gofman, J. *Radiation and Human Health.* Pantheon Books, New York, 1983. pp. 411–414.

96   Interview with John Gofman *Mother Earth News,* March/April 1981. Available online: http://www.ratical.org/radiation/CNR/PlowboyIntrv.html

97   Gofman, J. *X-Rays, Health Effects of Common Exams.* Sierra Club Books, San Francisco, 1985, pp. 352–353.

98   International Commission on Radiological Protection. Managing patient doses in digital radiology. Amsterdam: Elsevier, 2005.

99   Reiner B. I, et al. Effect of filmless imaging on the utilization of radiologic services. *Radiology* 2000;215: 163–167. Available online: http://radiology.rsnajnls.org/cgi/content/abstract/215/1/163

100   Rogers, Sherry A. *Detoxify or Die.* Sand Key Company, Inc., Sarasota, FL, 2002, p. 33.

101   Rapp, Doris J. *Our Toxic World: A Wake Up Call.* Environmental Medical Research Foundation, Buffalo, NY, 2004, back cover

102   Rogers, Sherry A. *Detoxify or Die.* Sand Key Company, Inc., Sarasota, FL, 2002, p. 30.

103   Curl, Cynthia L. et al. Organophosphorus Pesticide Exposure of Urban and Suburban Preschool Children with Organic and Conventional Diets, *Environmental Health Perspectives*, Vol. 111 No. 3, Mar 2003.

104   Bergelson, J. et al. Promiscuity in transgenic plants. *Nature* 1998, Sept. 3, 395:25.

105 Health Freedom USA.org GM Files: Horrifying New Disease Contains Identical Material to GM "Food" Available online: http://www.healthfreedomusa.org:80/index.php?p=599

106 Ho, Mae-Wan & Cummins, J. Agrobacterium & Morgellons Disease, A GM Connection? ISIS Press Release 28/04/08. Available online: http://www.i-sis.org.uk:80/agrobacteriumAndMorgellons.php

107 Louria, D. R. PhD. Expert testimony: Congressional Hearings into Food Irradiation: House Committee on Energy and Commerce Subcommittee on Health and the Environment, June 19, 1987. Available online: http://www.ccnr.org/food_irradiation.html

108 Srikantia, S. G. Expert testimony: U.S. Congressional Hearings into Food Irradiation: House Committee on Energy and Commerce Subcommittee on Health and the Environment, June 19, 1987. Available online: http://www.ccnr.org/food_irradiation.html

109 Fallon, S. Caustic Commentary-Cold Pasteurization. *Wise Traditions*. Vol. #3, #1 Spring 2002, pp. 9–10.

110 Pauling, Linus. U.S. Senate Doc. 264, 74th Congress, 2nd Session, 1936.

111 FDA,USDA. Food Safety System, *Precaution in U.S. Food Safety Decisionmaking: Annex II to the United States' National Food Safety System Paper*, March 3, 2000.

112 Oprah Winfrey, Television program, *Dangerous Food*. April 16, 1996.

113 Lasky, Tamar, et al., Mean Total Arsenic Concentrations in Chicken 1989–2000 and Estimated Exposures for Consumers of Chicken. *Environmental Health Perspectives* Vol. 112, No. 1, January 2004.

114 Gibbs, Gary. *Deadly Dining: The Food that would Last Forever*. Avery Penguin Putnam, 1993.

115 Food Code: 2005 Recommendations of the U.S. Public Health Service Food and Drug Administration U.S. FDA 2005. Available online: www.cfsan.fda.gov.

116 Diaz, K. Juicy Debate: What is fresh meat's true color? *Minneapolis Star Tribune*, Nov. 14, 2007.

117 Manuelidis, E., et al. Suggested Links Between Different Types of Dementias: Creutzfeldt-Jakob Disease, Alzheimer Disease, and Retroviral CNS Infections. *Alzheimer Disease and Associated Disorders* 2 (1989): 100–110.

118 Lyman, H. F., and Merzer, G. *Mad Cowboy: Plain Truth from the Cattle Rancher Who Won't Eat Meat.* Scribner, 2001.

119 Fallon, S. *Nourishing Traditions,*2nd ed. New Trends Publishing, Inc., Washington DC, 1999, p. 258.

120 Burros, M. Tests find hazardous levels of mercury in [bluefin] tuna sushi in New York,
New York Times, January 22, 2008.

121 Ibid. p. 35.

122 Daniel, K. *The Whole Soy Story: The Dark Side of America's Favorite Health Food.* 2005

123 Irvine, C., et al. "The Potential Adverse Effects of Soybean Phytoestrogens in Infant Feeding." *New Zealand Medical Journal,* May 24, 1995, p. 318.

124 Klein, K.O. Isoflavones, Soy-based Infant Formulas and Relevance to Endocrine Function. *Nutrition Reviews,* July 1998, Vol. 56, No. 7, pp. 193–204.

125 Hersey, J. *Why Can't My Child Behave?* Pear Tree Press, 1996.

126 http://www.macrobiotics.co.uk/sugar.htm Sugar: It's Effects on the Body and Mind. 2007

127 Field, Meira 2001. "Wise Traditions in Food, Farming and the Healing Arts" Weston A. Price Foundation.

128 Hull, J.S. *SweetPoison.com* http://www.sweetpoison.com/

129 Frazer, R. Diet Sodas and Cancer, Oct. 13, 2007. Available online: http://cancer.suite101.com/article.cfm/diet_sodas_and_cancer

130 Earles, J. Sugar-free Blues. *Wise Traditions,* Vol. 4 #4, 2003, pp. 21–23.

131 Ibid.

132 Mohamed, B. et al. Splenda alters gut microflora and increases intestinal P-glycoprotein and cytochrome P-450 in male rats. *Journal of Toxicology and Environmental Health* Part A 2008. Vol.71 Issue 21 pp. 1415–1429. Available online: http://www.informaworld.com/smpp/content-content=a902553409~db=all~jumptype=rss

133 Earles, J. Sugar-free Blues. *Wise Traditions*, Vol. 4 #4, 2003, pp. 21–23.

134 PR-GB.com. *Stevia the All Natural Sweetener*, Jan 2008.

135 Alles, M. S., et al. Fate of fructo-oligosaccharides in the human intestine. *British Journal of Nutrition*, 1996; 76(2):211–221.

136 Briet, F., et al. Symptomatic response to varying levels of fructo-oligosaccharides consumed occasionally or regularly. *Eur J Clin Nutr* 1995; 49(7):501–507.

137 Ten Bruggencate S.J., et al. Dietary fructooligosaccharides affect intestinal barrier function in healthy men. *J. Nutr.* 2006 Jan;136(1):70–4.

138 Erb, J. *The Slow Poisoning of America*. Paladins Press, 2003.

139 Benarde, M. A. *The Chemicals We Eat*. New York: American Heritage Press, 1971.

140 Djazayery A, et al. The use of gold-thioglucose and monosodium glutamate to induce obesity in mice. *Proc Nutr Soc.* 1973 May; 32(1):30A–31A.

141 OSHA Web site: http://www.osha.gov/dsg/guidance/diacetyl-guidance.html

142 Feingold, Ben, *Why Your Child is Hyperactive?* Random House

143 Schab, D. W.,et al. Do Artificial Food Colors Promote Hyperactivity in Children with Hyperactive syndromes? *Journal of Developmental & Behavioral Pediatrics* (2004). 25(6) 423–434 Available online: http://www.fabresearch.org/view_item.aspx?item_id=789.

144 Lindgren, D. Artificial Food and Cosmetic Coloring: A Hidden Source of Toxic Metals. *Townsend Letter*, Nov. 2007. Available online: http://www.townsendletter.com/Nov2007/artfood1107.htm

145 Ibid.

146 Holden, Robert A. et al. Dietary salt intake and blood pressure, *Journal of the American Medical Association*, Jul 15, 1983, 250:356–369.

147 McCance, R. A. Experimental Sodium Chloride Deficiency in Man, *Nutrition Reviews*, Mar 1990, 48:145–147.

148 Bieler, Henry, MD. *Food Is Your Best Medicine*, Random House, 1965.

149 Hendel, B. and Ferreira, P. *Water and Salt the Essence of Life,* Natural Resources. p. 103.

150 Fallon, S. and Enig, M., Why Butter Is Better, Available online: http://www.westonaprice.org/food-features/why-butter-is-better.

151 Cousens, G. *Spiritual Nutrition,* North Atlantic Books, 1986, 2005, pp. 289–304.

152 Bhargava, A., et al. Bamboo parts and seeds for additional source of nutrition. *Journal of Food Science and Technology.* 1996 33(2): pp. 145–146.

153 A. Kobayashi,et al. Antioxidant activity of bamboo leaf. 17th International Congress of Nutrition, 2001.

154 Person communication with Linda Harris co-founder of Great Basin International. Sep. 24, 2009.

155 Duty, S. M., et al. The relationship between environmental exposures to phthalates and DNA damage in human sperm using the neutral comet assay. *Environmental Health Perspect.* 2005. 111(9):1164–1169.

156 Lovekamp-Swan, T., Davis, B. A. Mechanisms of phthalate ester toxicity in the female reproductive system. *Environmental Health.* 2003.

157 Bornehag, C. G. The Association between Asthma and Allergic Symptoms in Children and Phthalates in House Dust: A Nested Case-Control Study; *Environmental Health Perspectives* Volume 112, Number 14, October 2004, Available online: http://www. ehponline.org/docs/2004/7187/abstract.html.

158 Is It In Us? Chemical Contamination in our Bodies. A report from the Body Burden Work Group and Commonwealth Biomonitoring Resource Center. April 2007. Available online: http://www.isitinus.org/documents/Is%20It%20In%20Us%20 Report.pdf

159 Nelson, C. Carcinogens At 10,000,000 Times FDA Limits. *Options* May 2000. Published by People Against Cancer.

160 Lyons, G. Bisphenol-A A Known Endocrine Disruptor, A WWF European Toxics Program Report, 2000.

161 Sugiura-Ogasawara, M. et al. Exposure to bisphenol A is associated with recurrent miscarriage. *Human Reproduction.* 2005. 20:2325–2329.

162 Newsmax.com Heating Baby and Plastic Bottles Releases Gender-Bending Chemical, Jan 30, 2008.
Available online: http://www.newsmax.com/health/heating_releases_chemical/2008/01/30/68609.html

163 Environmental Working Group Web site, Bisphenol A: Toxic Plastics Chemical in Canned Food, Available online: http://www.ewg.org/reports/bisphenola

164 Rogers, Sherry A. *Detoxify or Die,* Prestige Publishing 2002. p. 98.

165 Webb, D. *New York Times*, Eating Well, Dec. 12, 1990. Available online: http://query.nytimes.com/gst/fullpage.html?res=9C0CE3 D91531F931A25751C1A966958260&sec=&spon=&pagewanted=all

166 Graziano, J. H. et al. A human in vivo model for the determination of lead bioavailability using stable isotope dilution. *Environ Health Perspect.* 1996. February; 104(2): 176–179.

167 Watson, T. Coated Pots and Pans Can Present Health Hazards. *Seattle Times.* August 10, 2007.

168 Fromme, H. Perfluorooctane sulphonate (PFOS) and perfluorooctanoic acid (PFOA) in human breast milk: Results of a pilot study. *Int J Hyg Environ Health* 2007 Vol. 211 pp. 440–446. Available online: http://www.molecularstation.com/research/perfluorooctane-sulphonate-pfos-and-perfluorooctanoic-acid-pfoa-in-human-breast-milk-results-of-a-pilot-study-17870667.html#abstract

169 Quan, Richard MD et al. Effects of Microwave Radiation on Anti-infective Factors in Human Milk. *Pediatrics*, 1992, Vol. 89, No. 4.

170 Lee, Lita, *Microwaves and Microwave Ovens,* available online: http://www.litalee.com/shopexd.asp?id=182

171 Cancer project Web site. http://www.cancerproject.org/media/news/fiveworstfoodsreport.php

172 The Connecticut Agricultural Experiment Station http://www.ct.gov/caes/cwp/view.asp?a=2815&q=376676

173 Zhang, Zhi-Yong et al. Effects of home preparation on pesticide residues in cabbage. *Food Control* Dec. 2007, Vol. 18 No. 12, pp. 1484–1487.

174 Baillie-Hamilton, P. *Toxic Overload, A Doctor's Plan for Combating the Illnesses Caused by Chemicals in Our Foods, Our Homes, and Our Medicine Cabinets*. Avery Publishing-Penguin Group, New York, 2005.

175 Wilkenfeld, I. R. Patient Education: Scents Make No Sense. *The Environmental Physician*. Fall, 1991.

176 Oldenberg, D, Home Is Where The Toxins Are; *The Washington Post*, Tuesday, April 14, 1987.

177 Campaign for Safe Cosmetics, http://SafeCosmetics.org 2004.

178 Ginsberg, G. & Toal, B. *What's Toxic, What's Not*. The Berkley Publishing Group, New York, New York, 2006, p. 156.

179 WWF & Greenpeace. *A Present for Life, Hazardous Chemicals in Umbilical Cord Blood,* Sept. 2005. Available online: http://www.greenpeace.org/eu-unit/en/Publications/2009-and-earlier/a-present-for-life/

180 Malkan, Stacy. *Not Just a Pretty Face*. New Society Publishers, Gabrioloa Island, Canada, 2007.

181 *Lindgren, D.* Artificial Food and Cosmetic Coloring: A Hidden Source of Toxic Metals. *Townsend Letter* Nov. 2007. Available at http://www.townsendletter.com/Nov2007/artfood1107.htm

182 1,4-Dioxane (1,4-Diethyleneoxide). Hazard Summary—Created in April 1992; Revised in January 2000. U.S. Environmental Protection Agency. Available online: http://www.epa.gov/ttn/atw/hlthef/dioxane.html.

183 Dept. of Health and Human Science—Agency for Toxic Substances and Disease Registry. Toxicological Profile for Formaldehyde July 1999.

184 Office of Environment, Health, and Safety, Univ. of CA, Berkeley Web site: http://www.ehs.ucsb.edu/units/labsfty/labrsc/factsheets/phenol.pdf

185 Greater Boston Physicians for Social Responsibility. In Harm's Way: Toxic Threats to Child Development—Fluoride, May 2000. Available online http://psr.igc.org.

186 Graves, A.B., et al. The association between aluminum-containing products and Alzheimer's disease. *J Clin Epidemiol,* 1990;43(1):35–44.

187 Vince, G. Beware of Paraben Preservatives in Body Care Products, New Scientist.com news service, 12:24 12 January 04. Available online: http://www.organicconsumers.org/bodycare/paraben011304.cfm.

188 Food and Drug Administration (FDA) AHAs and UV sensitivity: Results of new FDA-sponsored studies. Office of Cosmetics and Color Fact Sheet. March 2, 2000 referenced in: http://www.cosmeticsinfo.org/HBI/12

189 Soref, A. Bright ideas for dry eyes: red, tired, dry eyes can make anyone want to cry. *Better Nutrition,* Oct. 2006.

190 Hamel, C. Dry Eye: Omega-3 nutraceuticals helps dry eye. *Eye World.* Available online: *http://www.eyeworld.org/article. php?sid=4000.*

191 The Environmental Working Group's Skin Deep Cosmetic Safety Database. Available online http://www.cosmeticsdatabase.com/browse.php?sunscreens=1&best=1

192 Ibid.

193 http://www.environmentalhealth.ca/spring03hazards.html

194 Environmental News Service, Mosquito Repellant DEET Linked to Neurological Damage, May 10, 2002. Available online: http://www.dirtdoctor.com/view_org_research.php?id=127

195 http://www.environmentalhealth.ca/spring03hazards.html

196 Goldberg, B. *Alternative Medicine The Definitive Guide 2nd Edition.* Celestial Arts, Berkeley, California 2002. p. 1011.

197 Holton, A, et al. Nasal mucociliary clearance in hairdressers: correlation to exposure to hair spray, Clinical Otolaryngology, 1984, 9 (6), 329–339. Abstract available online: http://www.ncbi.nlm.nih.gov/pubmed/6532604.

198 Berthold-Bond, A. To Dye or Not To Dye? Permanent Hair Dyes. *Green Living Healthy Solutions,* available online: http://www.care2.com/greenliving/permanent-hair-dye-dangers.html.

199 Zheng, Y. et al. Hair-coloring Product Use and Risk of Non-Hodgkin's Lymphoma: A Population-based Case-Control Study

in Connecticut; *American Journal of Epidemiology*, Jan. 15, 2004; Vol. 159: pp. 148–154. Abstract available online: http://aje. oxfordjournals.org/cgi/content/abstract/159/2/148.

200 SWikipedia Web site: http://en.wikipedia.org/wiki/Lead%28II %29_acetate.

201 American Hair Loss Council Web site: http://www.ahlc.org/ causes-m.htm

202 Freyschmidt-Paul, P. et al. Alopecia Areata: Treatment of Today and Tomorrow. *Journal of Investigative Dermatology Symposium Proceedings* 2003, 8, pp.12–17. Available online: http://www. nature.com/jidsp/journal/v8/n1/full/5640084a.html

203 Appleby, J; Head-Lice Drug Tied to Health Risks, *USA Today*, 1-31-08.

204 Sen. Edward Kennedy, Sept 10, 1997 hearings on the FDA reform Bill (HR 1411).

205 Malkan, S; *Not Just a Pretty Face*. New Society Publishers, Gabriola Island, BC Canada, 2007. p. 60.

206 Derbyshire, D/ Warning on long-term side-effects of Botox, *Telegraph.co.UK*, 21/11/2002. available online: http://www. telegraph.co.uk/news/main.jhtml?xml=/news/2002/11/22/ nbtox22.xml

207 Associated Press, FDA warns of Botox side effects, deaths. Feb 8, 2008. Available online: CSNWashington.com http://www.csnwashington.com/pages/mobile_landing?blockI D=121425&tagID=29037

208 Oliveria, S. A. et al. Sun exposure and risk of melanoma, *Archives of Disease in Childhood* 2006; 91:131–138. Abstract available online: http://adc.bmj.com/cgi/content/abstract/91/2/131?ct.

209 EPA National Center for Environmental Assessment, Guidelines for Carcinogen Risk Assessment (2005). Available at: http:// www.epa.gov/ttn/atw/cancer_guidelines_final_3-25-05.pdf.

210 Environmental Working Group. EWG's Guide to Infant Formula: BPA in baby bottles: http://www.ewg.org/node/25572.

211 Environmental Working Group, Bisphenol A: Toxic Plastics Chemical in Canned Food, Mar 5, 2007, Available online: http:// www.ewg.org/reports/bisphenola.

212 Lu, Chensheng et al. Dietary Intake and its Contribution to Longitudinal Organophosphorus Pesticide Exposure in

Urban/Suburban Children. *Environmental Health Perspectives,* 2006,Vol. 114 No. 2. Available online: http://www.ehponline. org/docs/2008/10912/abstract.pdf.

213 Takao, Y. et al. Fast screening for Bisphenol A in environmental water and in food by solid-phase microextraction. 1999. *Journal of Health Science* 45:39. Summary available online http://www. sciencenews.org/pages/sn_arc99/7_24_99/food.htm.

214 Sathyanarayana, S. et al. Baby Care Products: Possible Sources of Infant Phthalate Exposure. *Pediatrics,* Vol. 121 No. 2 February 2008, pp. e260-e268. Abstract available online: http://pediatrics. aappublications.org/cgi/content/abstract/121/2/e260

215 Washington Post.com, Study Sees Hazards in Baby Powder and Lotion, Feb 4, 2008.

216 EWG Cosmetics database, 2-Bromo-2-Nitropropane-1,3-Diol Available online: http://www.cosmeticsdatabase.com/ingredient. php?ingred06=700019&nothanks=1

217 *Mothering Magazine,* Disposable Diapers Linked to Asthma Issue 98, January/February 2000. Available online: http://moth-ering.com/green-living/disposable-diapers-linked-to-asthma.

218 EPA, Pollution Prevention and Toxics, Polybrominated diphenylethers (PBDEs), Available online: http://www.epa.gov/ oppt/pbde/.

219 Birnbaum, L.S. et al. Brominated Flame Retardants: Cause for Concern? *Environmental Health Perspectives* Vol. 112, No. 1, January 2004. Available online: http://www.ncbi.nih.gov/ pmc/articles/PMC1241790/.

220 Ecology Center. Lead, Cadmium, and Other Harmful Chemicals Found in Popular Children's Toys—Leading Environmental Health Groups Release Testing Results Today at www. HealthyToys.org Dec. 5, 2007. Available online: http://www. ecocenter.org/press-release/2007/lead-cadmium-and-other-harm-ful-chemicals-found-popular-children%E2%80%99s-toys-%E 2%80%99s-toys-%E2%80%93-leading-

221 Greenpeace Press Release, PVC Toys and Heavy Metals, Oct. 9, 1997. Available online: http://home.scarlet.be/chlorophiles/Eng/ answ/PVCToys2.html.

222 Ecology Center, The Consumer Guide to Toxic Chemicals in Cars, 2006/2007 Guide to Child Car Seats, May 2007, Available online:

http://www.healthycar.org/documents/healthycarseatguide07.pdf.

223 American Academy of Pediatrics Committees on Environmental Hazards and Committee on Accident and Poison Prevention. Statement on childhood lead poisoning. *Pediatrics.* 1987; 79:457–465.

224 Agency for Toxic Substances and Disease Registry. 2006. Public health statement for lead. Available online: http://www.atsdr.cdc.gov/toxprofiles/phs13.html#bookmark06.

225 Blanc, Paul, MD. *How Everyday Products Make People Sick*, University of California Press, Ltd. Berkeley, CA. 2007. pp; 154–170.

226 Ibid.

227 Greenpeace Investigative Report. Toxic Childrenswear by Disney – A Worldwide Investigation of Hazardous Chemicals in Disney Clothes. Available online: http://archive.greenpeace.org/docs/disney.pdf

228 Gloria Gilbère. The "Fabric" of Allergic Responses. Available online: http://www.yourhealthdetective.com/2009/12/the-fabric-of-allergic-responses.html

229 Toxic-Free Legacy Coalition, Pollution in People; Toxic Chemicals in Washingtonians, Available online: http://www.pollutioninpeople.org/results/report/executive-summary.

230 EPA, Pollution Prevention and Toxics, Polybrominated diphenylethers (PBDEs), Available online: http://www.epa.gov/oppt/pbde/.

231 Birnbaum, L. S. et al. Brominated Flame Retardants: Cause for Concern? *Environmental Health Perspectives* Vol. 112, No. 1, January 2004. Available online: http://www.ehponline.org/members/2003/6559/6559.html.

232 Environmental Oncology News, THE PROBLEM: Toxic flame retardants in furniture threaten the health of humans, the environment, and wildlife, Oct, 17, 2007, Available online: http://www.environmentaloncology.org/FAQsFlameRet.htm.

233 Environmental Working Group, Toxic Fire Retardants (PBDEs) in Human Breast Milk, Available online: http://www.ewg.org/reports/mothersmilk/

234 Raloff, J. Formaldehyde: Some surprises at home—many common products contain formaldehyde, *Science News*, Jan 9, 1999. Available online: http://findarticles.com/p/articles/mi_m1200/is_2_155/ai_53630864.

235 Green Seal's Report on carpet, Dec. 2001. Available online: www.greenseal.org/resources/reports/CGR_carpet.pdf

236 Air Resources Board, Indoor Emissions of Formaldehyde and Toluene Diisocyanate, Research Note 979. August 1997. Available online: http://www.arb.ca.gov/research/resnotes/notes/97-9.htm

237 Thornton, Joe, Environmental Impacts of Polyvinyl Chloride (PVC) Building Materials, A briefing paper for the Healthy Building Network http://www.healthybuilding.net/pvc/ThorntonPVCSummary.html.

238 Ibid.

239 Lipinski, L. et al. Repair of oxidative DNA base lesions induced by fluorescent light is defective in xeroderma pigmentosum group A cells. *Nucleic Acids Research* Vol. 27, No. 15 pp. 3153–3158. Available online: http://nar.oxfordjournals.org/cgi/content/full/27/15/3153.

240 Aucott, Michael, et al. Release of mercury from broken fluorescent bulbs. (Technical Paper). *Journal of the Air & Waste Management Association*, Feb. 2003. Available online: http://www.entrepreneur.com/tradejournals/article/98012373.html.

241 Lamp Recycling Outreach Project – funded by the EPA, A Message for All, 2002. Available online: http://www.almr.org/support_files/messageforall.htm

242 Environmental Working Group website Green Lighting Guide: http://www.ewg.org/node/27221

243 Rea, Mark, Light- Much More Than Vision, Light and Human Health: EPRI/LRO 5th International Lighting Research Symposium: Palo Alto, CA: The Lighting Research Office of the Electric Power Research Institute (2002): 1–15.

244 Ott, J. The Effect of Color and Light, Part 3 *International Journal of Biosocial Research* 9 1987 71–107.

245 Czarry, C. *Twenty-Minute Feng Shui*. Wind and Water Publishing, 2006, p. 7.

246 Montenegro, M. Feng Shui: New Dimensions in Design. Available online: http://www.equip.org/articles/feng-shui-decorating.

247 Wright,. Machaelle, *Perelandra Garden Workbook*. Perelandra Ltd. 1993. http://www.perelandra-ltd.com/index.cfm

248 Porter, W. Do pesticides affect learning and behavior? The neuro-endocrine-immuune connection. *Pesticides and You*, Vol. 24, No. 1, 2004. Available online: http://www.beyondpesticides.org/lawn/activist/PorterLearningBehavior.pdf

249 Guillette, E. et al. An anthropological approach to the evaluation of preschool children exposed to pesticides in Mexico. *Environmental Health Perspectives* 1998, 106(6): 347–353.

250 Porter, W. Do pesticides affect learning and behavior? The neuro-endocrine-immuune connection. *Pesticides and You*, Vol. 24, No. 1, 2004. Available online: http://www.beyondpesticides.org/lawn/activist/PorterLearningBehavior.pdf

251 Hayes, Howard M. et al, Case-Control Study of Canine Malignant Lymphoma: Positive Association With Dog Owner's Use of 2,4-Dichlorophenoxyacetic Acid Herbicides. *Journal of the National Cancer Institute* Vol. 83, Sept. 1991, pp. 1226–1231.

252 Nishioka, M. et al. Distribution of 2,4-D in Air and on Surfaces Inside Residences after Lawn Applications. *Environmental Health Perspectives* 2001, 109, pp. 1185–1191.

253 U.S. Patent Application 0040091514, Biological Pesticide, Steven Tvedten. Available online: http://www.safesolutionsinc.com/Tvedten_Biological_Pesticide_Patent.pdf

254 Goodman, N. *Benjamin Rush*. Philadelphia: University of Pennsylvania Press, 1934, p. 235.

255 McGuire, T. *Poisons in Your Teeth*. The Dental Wellness Institute, Sebastopol, CA, 2008, p. 75.

256 WHO Environmental Health Criteria Geneva Switzerland, Vol. 118, 1991, Inorganic Mercury, p. 61.

257 International Academy of Oral Medicine and Toxicology online video. Available at: http://iaomt.org/.

258 Williams, Louisa L. *Radical Medicine*. International Medical Arts Publishing, 2007, p. 80.

259 Lorscheiner, F. L. et al. Mercury exposure from "silver" tooth fillings: emerging evidence questions a traditional dental paradigm. *FASEB J.* 1995, 9: pp. 504–508.

260 Hahn, L. J. et al. Dental "silver" tooth fillings: a source of mercury exposure revealed by whole body scan and tissue analysis, *FASEB J.* 1989, 3: pp. 2641–2646.

261 Aposhian, H. V., et al. Urinary Mercury after Administration of 2, 3-dimercaptopropane-1-sulfonic acid: Correlation with Dental Amalgam Score, *FASEB J.* 1992, 6: pp. 2472–2476.

262 Vimy, M. J. et al. Maternal-fetal distribution of mercury (203Hg) released from dental amalgam fillings, *Am. J. Physiol.* 1990, 258 (Regulatory Integrative Comp. *Physiol.* 27): R939–R945.

263 Hultman, P, et al. Adverse immunological effects and autoimmunity induced by dental amalgam and alloy in mice, *FASEB J.* 1994, 8(14): pp. 1183–1190.

264 Boyd, N. D. et al. Mercury From Dental "Silver" Tooth Fillings Impairs Sheep Kidney Function, *Am .J. Physiol.* 1991 p 261, Regulatory Integrative Comp. *Physiol.* 30: R1010–R1014.

265 Summers, A. O. et al. Mercury released from dental "silver" fillings provokes an increase in mercury and antibiotic resistant bacteria in primates oral and intestinal flora., *Antimicrobial Agents and Chemotherapy* 1993, Vol. 37, pp. 825–834.

266 Gerhard, I. et al. Heavy Metals and Fertility. *Journal of Toxicology and Environmental Health*, Part, A, 1998, 54: pp. 593–611.

267 The International Academy of Oral Medicine and Toxicology, The Scientific Case Against Amalgam Available online: http://iaomt.org/articles/files/files193/The%20Case%20Against%20Amalgam.pdf

268 Williams, Louisa L. *Radical Medicine*, International Medical Arts Publishing, 2007, p. 514.

269 Ibid. p. 87.

270 The International Academy of Oral Medicine and Toxicology, The Scientific Case Against Amalgam Available online: http://iaomt.org/articles/files/files193/The%20Case%20Against%20Amalgam.pdf

271 McGuire, T. *Poisons in Your Teeth*, The Dental Wellness Institute, Sebastopol, CA, 2008, p. 59.

272 Gerhard, I. et al. Heavy Metals and Fertility, *Journal of Toxicology and Environmental Health*, 1998; Part A, 54(8), pp. 593–611.

273 Gerhard I., et al. Impact of heavy metals on hormonal and immunological factors in women with repeated miscarriages. *Human Reproductive Update* 1998; 4(3), pp. 301–309.

274 CDC, National Center for Environmental Health , National Report on Human Exposure to Environmental Chemicals, 2001. Available online: http://www.cdc.gov/exposurereport/

275 Holmes J: Clinical reversal of root caries using ozone, double-blind, randomized, controlled 18-month trial. *Gerodontol* 2003: 20 (2): 106–114.

276 Domingo H and Holmes J: Reduction in treatment time with combined air abrasion and ozone compared to traditional "Drill & Fill." *IADR* abstract 2004.

277 Stockton, S. Dangers of Dental Anesthetics (From Letters to the Editor), Issue #1 of Cavitations Plus Quarterly newsletter 2004. Available online: http://www.healthcarealternatives.net/dangers.html.

278 Meinig, G. *Root Canal Cover-Up*. Ojai, California: Bion Publishing, 1994, p.3.

279 Williams, Louisa L. *Radical Medicine*, International Medical Arts Publishing, 2007, p. 505.

280 Ibid. p. 506.

281 Pulgar, R. et al. Determination of Bisphenol-A and Related Aromatic Compounds Released from Bis-GMA-based Composites and Sealants by High Performance Liquid Chromatography. *Environmental Health Perspectives* Vol. 108, No. 1, Jan 2000.

282 Ibid.

283 Chemicals known to cause contact dermatitis. http://www.haz-map.com/allergic.htm

284 Leggat, P. et al. Toxicity of cyanoacrylate adhesives and their occupational impacts for dental staff. *Industrial Health*, 2004, 42, pp 207–211. Available online: http://www.jniosh.go.jp/en/indu_hel/pdf/42-2-14.pdf.

285 Ibid.

286 Ibid.

287 Animated-teeth.com Safety concerns associated with tray-based at-home teeth whitening products. http://www.animated-teeth. com/teeth_whitening/t5_whitening_teeth.htm

288 Hasson H. et al. Home-based chemically-induced whitening of teeth in adults. *Cochrane Database of Systematic Reviews* 2006, Issue 4. Art. No.: CD006202. DOI: 10.1002/14651858. CD006202. Available online: http://mrw.interscience.wiley.com/ cochrane/clsysrev/articles/CD006202/frame.html

289 Goldberg, B. *Alternative Medicine The Definitive Guide second edition,* Celestial Arts, Berkeley, CA, 2002, pp. 1054.

290 Eisenstein, M. *Don't Vaccinate Before You Educate*, revised edition. CMI Press, 2008. pg. xiii.

291 Think Twice Global Vaccine Institute. http://thinktwice.com/ secret.htm

292 Illinois Vaccine Awareness. http://www.vaccineawareness.org/ facts.htm

293 Williams, L. L. *Radical Medicine.* International Medical Arts Publishing, 2007, p. 672.

294 Minutes of the Simpsonwood Retreat—Scientific Review of Vaccine Safety, June 7, 8, 2000, Available online: http://www. safeminds.org/legislation/foia/Simpsonwood_Transcript.pdf

295 Illinois Vaccine Awareness. http://www.vaccineawareness.org/ facts.htm

296 Torch WC. Diphtheria-pertussis-tetanus (DPT) immunization: a potential cause of the sudden infant death syndrome (SIDS). *Neurology* 1982; 32(4).

297 Null, G. et al. Vaccination: an analysis of the health risks—part III, *Townsend Letter for Doctors and Patients,* Dec, 2003.

298 Mendelsohn, R. MD. The Medical Time Bomb of Immunization Against Disease. *East West Journal* Nov. 1984. Available online: http://whale.to/vaccines/mendelsohn.html

299 Levy, Thomas E. *Vitamin C, Infectious Diseases, & Toxins— Curing the Incurable.* Xlibris Corp., 2002.

300 Yeh, S. H. ,et al. Safety and immunogenicity of a pentavalent diphtheria, tetanus, pertussis, hepatitis B and polio combination vaccine in infants. *Ped Inf. Dis. J.* 2001;20:973–980.

301 Vaccine awareness.com http://www.vaccineawareness.org/ concerns.htm#07

302 Bridges, A. FDA: Rotavirus Vaccine May Harm Infants, *Associated Press,* Washington, Feb. 13, 2007. Available online: http://www. cbsnews.com/stories/2007/02/13/ap/health/mainD8N932LO0. shtml

303 *FDA News* Feb. 3 2006, FDA Approves New Vaccine to Prevent Rotavirus Gastroenteritis in Infants. http://www.fda.gov/bbs/ topics/news/2006/NEW01307.html

304 Tenpenny, S., U.S. Adults Need Booster Shot of Diphtheria, Tetanus, Available online: http://www.vran.org/vaccines/dpt/ vaccine-tetanus.htm

305 Vaccination Risk Awareness Network, Article available online: http://www.vran.org/vaccines/dpt/pentacel-dpt.htm.

306 *Vaccinations: A Thoughtful Parent's Guide*; pp. 81–82. What Your Doctor May Not Tell You About Children's Vaccinations; p. 151.

307 Williams, L. *Radical Medicine.* International Medical Arts Publishing, 2007, p. 696.

308 FEAT daily Newsletter. CDC Data: Vaccines Cause Diabetes— Public Health House of Cards Falling? September 20, 2000. Available online: http://www.whale.to/v/classen2.html

309 Miller, N. *Vaccines: Are They Really Safe and Effective?* pp. 14– 17.

310 Williams, L. *Radical Medicine*, International Medical Arts Publishing, 2007, p. 706.

311 *The Seattle Times,* Thursday, Jun 19, 1993, p. A1.

312 Jefferson, T. Influenza vaccination: policy versus evidence, BMJ 2006;333:912–915 (28 October). Available online: http:// www.bmj.com/cgi/content/full/333/7574/912

313 Gardner, A. Study Questions Value of Flu Shots. *Health Reporter* Oct. 26, 2006.Available online: http://www.healthscout.com/ news/1/535746/main.html.

314 In: Vaccine Action Letter. Available online: http://www. vaccineactionletter.blogspot.com/

315 Cannell, J. et al. Epidemic Influenza and Vitamin D. *Epidemiol Infect.* 2006 Sep 7;1–12. Available online: http://www.medicalnewstoday.com/articles/51913.php

316 Morley, D. The public health problem created by measles in the developing countries, *Archives of Virology,* Vol. 16, Nos. 1–5, February, 1965, pp. 19–26. Available online: *http://www.springerlink.com/content/x220k8108j0419m0/*

317 Mendelsohn, R. The Medical Time Bomb of Immunization Against Disease. *East West Journal,* Nov. 1984. Available online: http://whale.to/vaccines/mendelsohn.html

318 Hussey, G. D. and Klein, M. A randomized, controlled trial of vitamin A in children with severe measles, *New England Journal of Medicine,* 323(3):160–4, 1990 Jul 19.

319 Kawasaki Y, et al. The efficacy of oral vitamin A supplementation for measles and respiratory syncytial virus (RSV) infection. *The Journal of the Japanese Association for Infectious Disease* 1999 Feb;73(2):104–9. Abstract available online: http://www.ncbi.nlm.nih.gov/pubmed/10213986?dopt=Abstract

320 Yazbak, F. E. et al. Adverse Outcomes Associated with Postpartum Rubella or MMR Vaccines, Available online: http://www.vran.org/vaccines/mmr/yazbak-lang-mmr.htm

321 Fiecke, S. Chickenpox strikes G-E-T schoolchildren. *Winona Daily News,* January 20, 2006.

322 Annals of Internal Medicine website: http://www.annals.org/cgi/content/full/0000605-200711200-00187v1

323 *Ozark's Real News,* Merck gets caught in their own web of lies. Feb, 20, 2007. Available online: http://ozarksrealnews.blogspot.com/2007/02/merck-gets-caught-in-their-own-web-of.html

324 Letter to the Editor, Varicella Vaccine and Shingles. *Journal of the American Medical Association*, Vol. 287 No. 17, May 1, 2002. Introduction available online: http://jama.ama-assn.org/cgi/content/extract/287/17/2211

325 Zwillich, T. FDA Approves First Shingles Vaccine. *WebMD Health News,* Available online: http://www.webmd.com/skin-problems-and-treatments/shingles/news/20060526/fda-approves-shingles-vaccine

326 Product Information Leaflet Arepanrix™ H1N1 AS03-Adjuvanted H1N1 Pandemic Influenza Vaccine. Available online: http://www.hc-sc.gc.ca/dhp-mps/alt_formats/pdf/prodpharma/legislation/interimorders-arretesurgence/prodinfo-vaccin-eng.pdf

327 Vaccine Action Letter. Available online: www.vaccineactionletter.blogspot.com

328 Williams, L. *Radical Medicine*. International Medical Arts Publishing, 2007, p. 731.

329 Ibid.

330 Ibid. p 727.

331 U.S. Department of Energy, Energy Efficiency and Renewable Energy, Alternative Fuels and Advanced Vehicles Data Center, Available online: http://www.eere.energy.gov/afdc/incentives_laws_security.html

332 Brown, J., Brutoco, J., and Cusumano, J. *Freedom from Mid-East Oil*. World Business Academy, 2007., p. 312.

333 Ibid.

334 Brown, S., and Cheng, . Volatile Organic Compounds (VOCs) in New Car Interiors Presented at the 15th International Clean Air & Environment Conference Sydney, Nov. 2000, CASANZ 464-8 26–30. Available online: http://www.mindfully.org/Plastic/New-Car-Interior-VOCs30nov00.htm

335 Ibid.

336 EPA, Pollution Prevention and Toxics, Polybrominated diphenylethers (PBDEs). Available online: http://www.epa.gov/oppt/pbde/.

337 Birnbaum, L. S. et al. Brominated Flame Retardants: Cause for Concern? *Environmental Health Perspectives*. Vol. 112, No. 1, January 2004. Available online: http://www.ehponline.org/members/2003/6559/6559.html.

338 Toxic at Any Speed: Chemicals in Cars & the Need for Safe Alternatives. Ecology Center, 2006. Summary Available online: http://www.consumeraffairs.com/news04/2006/01/car_chemicals.html

339 Motavalli, J. New car smell: It's not so sweet, www.emagazine.com, Jan/Feb. 2006, p2.

340 Borm, P. et al. Diesel Exhaust Inhalation Stresses Your Brain. *Particle and Fibre Toxicology* March 13, 2008. Available online: http://www.sciencedaily.com /releases/2008/03/080311075339. htm

341 University of Edinburgh, Diesel Exhaust May Increase Risk in Patients with Heart Disease. 2007 *ScienceDaily*. Available online: http://www.sciencedaily.com/releases/2007/09/070912190002. htm

342 Brown, J,, Brutoco, J., and Cusumano, J. *Freedom from Mid-East Oil*. World Business Academy, 2007. p. 149.

343 Wald, M. A Plastic Wrapper Today Could be Fuel Tomorrow. *New York Times,* April 9, 2007. Available online: http://www. nytimes.com/2007/04/09/business/09plastic.html

344 Brown, J,, Brutoco, J., and Cusumano, J. *Freedom from Mid-East Oil*. World Business Academy, 2007. p. 407.

345 Honda.com Feb 6, 2007, http://corporate.honda.com/ environment/fuel_cells.aspx?id=fuel_cells_fcx

346 Sullivan, M. World's First Air-Powered Car: Zero Emissions by Next Summer. *PopularMechanics*, June 2007. http://www. popularmechanics.com/automotive/new_cars/4217016.html

347 Green Earth Technologies: http://www.getg.com/products/ products.php?CategoryID=1&ProductID=1

348 Young, B. Best motor oil to use to aid the environment. Available online: http://www.helium.com/items/787420-motor-market-environment-argument

349 Martin, A. *Food Pets Die For*. New Sage Press, Troutdale, OR 2003, p. 153

350 Lyman, H. F., and Merzer, G. *Mad Cowboy: Plain Truth from the Cattle Rancher Who Won't Eat Meat*. Scribner, 2001, p. 12.

351 Pasternak, H. *Healing Pets With Nature's Miracle Cures*. Highlands Veterinary Hospital 2001, p. 11.

352 Hofve, J. Mad Cow Disease and Your Pets. Available online: http://www.littlebigcat.com/index.php?action=library&act=sho w&item=madcowdiseaseandyourpets

353 Pottenger, F. *Pottenger's Cats: A Study in Nutrition, second edition*. Price-Pottenger Nutrition Foundation, 1995.

354 *Pets Need Wholesome Foods Also, 1996. Available free online:* http://pet-grub.com/

355 Ibid.

356 Natural Resources Defense Council Report: *Poisons on Pets Health Hazards from Flea and Tick Products.* Nov. 2000. Available online: http://www.nrdc.org/health/effects/pets/execsum.asp

357 Farrel, S. The Green Pet *The Green Guide #24,* Saturday, June 30, 2007. Available online: http://healthychild.org/resources/article/the_green_pet/

358 Science Lab MSDS – Fenbendazole. http://www.sciencelab.com/xMSDS-Fenbendazole-9924023

359 Oh, S. et al. Ecological hazard assessment of major veterinary benzimidazoles : Acute and chronic toxicities to aquatic microbes and invertebrates, *Environ.Toxicol.Chem,* 2006, vol. 25, No. 8, pp. 2221–2226.

360 Hayes, H. et al. Case-control study of canine malignant lymphoma: positive association with dog owner's use of 2,4-D, *J. of Nat. Cancer Inst.* 1991, 83(17) pp. 1226–1231.

361 Schultz, R., and Phillips, T. *Kirk's Current Veterinary Therapy XI.* 1992.

362 Twark L, Dodds WJ. Clinical application of serum parvovirus and distemper virus antibody titers for determining revaccination strategies in healthy dogs. *J Am Vet Med* Assoc 217:1021-1024, 2000.

363 Lipton, B. H. *The Biology of Belief.* Mountain of Love/Elite Books, Santa Rosa, CA, 2005.

364 Ibid, p. 344.

365 ⁴ Rein, Glen and McCraty, Rollin, Local and Non-local Effects of Coherent Heart Frequencies on Conformational Changes of DNA. Institute of HeartMath, 2001. Available online: http://appreciativeinquiry.case.edu/uploads/HeartMath%20article.pdf

366 Pert, C. *Molecules of Emotion*: *The Science Behind Mind-Body Medicine.* Touchstone Publishing, New York, 1997.

367 Mein, C. *Releasing Emotional Patterns with Essential Oils.* fifth edition, VisionWare Press, 2004. p. 5.

368 Simmons, R. and Ahsian, N. *The Book of Stones* Heaven and Earth Publishing, 2005.

369 Melody, *Love is in the Earth: A Kaleidoscope of Crystals* Earth Love Publishing, 1995.

370 Barnett, C. Statement to U.S. Senate Environmental and Public Works Committee Hearing, May 15, 2007.

371 Havas, M. et al. Power quality affects teacher well-being and student behavior in three Minnesota schools. *Sci total Environ.* 2008 doi: 10.1016.

372 Ott, J. The Effect of Color and Light, Part 3. *International Journal of Biosocial Research* 9 1987 71–107.

373 Hathaway, W. Effects of School Lighting on Physical Development and School Performance. *Journal of Educational Research*, Mar-Apr 1995, Vol. 88 no. 4, pp. 228–242.

374 Louria, D. R. Expert testimony: Congressional Hearings into Food Irradiation: House Committee on Energy and Commerce Subcommittee on Health and the Environment, June 19, 1987. Available online: http://www.ccnr.org/food_irradiation.html

375 Muzaurieta, A. Farm to School Lunch Table: A New Program Offers Farm-Fresh Foods to Kids, Helping Local Farmers Too, *The Daily Green Newsletter*, 3-28-2008. Available online: http://www.thedailygreen.com/healthy-eating/eat-safe/farm-to-school-44032808

376 Chang, A. Schools Across U.S. Target Vending Machines in Obesity Controversy, *Associated Press*, February 26, 2004. Available online: http://www.organicconsumers.org/school/obesity031904.cfm

377 U.S. EPA, A probabilistic risk assessment for children who contact CCA-treated playsets and decks.

378 Able, K., School Bus Diesel Fumes Fueling Kids' Cancer Risk? Family Education.com: http://life.familyeducation.com/health-and-safety/school-safety-month/36307.html.

379 Harding K. et al. Outcome-based Comparison of Ritalin versus Food-supplement Treated Children with ADHD, *Alternative Medicine Review*, 2003, 8 (3): 319–330.

380 Novartis, ADHDinfo.com: http://www.adhdinfo.com/info/school/caring/sch_if_parents_ask.jsp.

381 Harding K. et al. Outcome-based Comparison of Ritalin versus Food-supplement Treated Children with ADHD, *Alternative Medicine Review,* 2003, 8 (3): 319–330.

382 Sea Coast Academy Wellness Filter Hydration Study, 2007. Available online: https://www.wellnessfilter.com/about/seacoast.asp

383 Beseler L. Effects on Behavior and Cognition: Diet and Artificial Colors, Flavors, and Preservatives *International Pediatrics,* Volume 14, No. 1, 1999. Availoable online: http://www.feingold.org/Research/adhd.html#Banerjee2007

384 Report of the British Associate Parliamentary Food and Health Forum, The Links Between Diet and Behavior: The influence of nutrition on mental health, January 2008. Available online: http://www.feingold.org/healthforum.html.

385 Ibid.

386 Ritalin product insert.

387 El-Zein,R. et al. Cytogenetic effects in children treated with methylphenidate. *Cancer Letters,* Vol. 230, Issue 2, December 2005, pp. 284–291.

388 Fairechild, D. *Jet Smarter: The Air Traveler's RX.* 2003. http://www.flyana.com/

389 Aviation Policy, U.S. Dept. of Transportation., http://ostpxweb.dot.gov/policy/safety/disin.htm

390 Fairechild, D. *Jet Smarter: The Air Traveler's RX,* 2003. http://www.flyana.com/

391 Loving, A. Microbial flora in restaurant beverage lemon slices. *Journal of Environmental Health,* Dec. 1, 2007. Available online: http://www.pccc.edu/uploads/Xu/1x/Xu1xPvHvoXeYex8Gf1Uh0Q/JEH_Dec_07_with_Copyright.pdf

392 Band P. R. et al. Cohort study of Air Canada pilots: Mortality, cancer incidence, and leukemia risk. *American Journal of Epidemiology* 143(2):137–143; 1996.

393 Crampton, T. Flying on Top of the World: A Radiation Risk. *International Herald Tribune, Global edition of the New York Times,* May 24, 2001. Available online: http://www.iht.com/articles/2001/05/24/radiate_ed3__0.php

394 Weiss J. et al. Protection against ionizing radiation by antioxidant nutrients and phytochemicals, *Toxicolog,* 2003 Jul 15;189(1–2) pp. 1–20.

395 Noaman, E. et al. Vitamin E and selenium administration as a modulator of antioxidant defense system, *Biological Trace Element Research,* Vol. 86, No. 1, April, 2002, pp. 55–64. Abstract available online: http://www.springerlink.com/content/bq14j86684735l14/

396 Oschman, J. Assume a Spherical Cow: The role of free or mobile electrons in bodywork, energetic and movement therapies. *Journal of Bodywork and Movement Therapies,* 2008, vol. 12, 40–57.

397 James, W. *Immunization: The Reality Behind the Myth.* Second edition. Bergin & Garvey, 1995, p. 226.

398 Sato, T. et al. The use in periodontal therapy of a bamboo leaf extract solution. *Nippon Shishubyo Gakkai Kaishi.* 1986 Jun;28(2):752–757.

399 Blumer W., et al. Leaded gasoline—a cause of cancer. *Environmental International,* 1980; 3: pp. 465–471.

400 Karach Pulling Oil, *Journal of World Teletherapy Association.* June 1992. Available online: http://www.oilpulling.org/wp-content/uploads/2009/09/Pulling_Oil_Karach_Article.pdf

401 Akpinar, B. *No Sweat Know Sweat: The Definitive Guide to Reclaim Your Health.* 2007, pp. 205–206.

402 Detox Foot Spa System Comparison Guide, Available from Platinum Energy Systems www.platinumenergysystems.ca

403 Transcript of an interview with Sandra Rose Michaels. Technology Hour, American Freedom Network, Jan. 3, 2004. Available online: http://www.alphaomegamex.com/dgen/album/1253667547.pdf

404 Marcial-Vega, V. A. Energy Enhancement System Initial Clinical Study, 2001. Available online: http://eesystem.com/docs/EES_ClinicalStudies.pdf

405 Clark, H. *The Cure for All Diseases.* New Century Press, Chula Vista, CA, 1995.

406 Ibid.

407 Williams, L. *Radical Medicine.* International Medical Arts Publishing, San Francisco, CA, 2007, p. 136.

408 Ibid.

409 Autism Research Institute Press Release, February 12, 2001. Available online: http://www.whale.to/m/ari.html

410 Autism Research Institute, Treatment Options for Mercury/ Metal Toxicity in Autism and Related Developmental Disabilities: Consensus Position Paper, Feb. 2005. Available online: http:// www.autism.com/triggers/vaccine/heavymetals.pdf

Index

plastic warnings, 366
radon safety guides, 19
safety issue exposure, xix
school air quality, 356
treated wood product restrictions, 365
epinephrine, 278
epoxy, 63
Epsom salts, 400
Equal, 114
erythritol, 119
essential oils
air cleaners, 30
air freshener alternatives, 159
antibiotic alternatives, 30, 284–285
bacteria neutralizers, 13–14
detoxification methods using, 400, 405–406
dispersal methods for, 30–31
energetic tools, 350
insect repellants, 189
perfume alternatives, 190
warnings, 30, 31, 284
estrogen
chemicals mimicking, 64, 110, 173, 174, 176, 182, 204, 223, 233, 280
as growth hormones in meat products, 100
plant-based, in soy products, 110
Eternity, 190
ethanol, 6, 168
ethanol (E85), 319
ethoxylated nonyl phenol, 155
ethoxylation, 172, 173, 174, 177, 178
ethoxyquin (E), 328
ethyl alcohol, 5–6, 180
ethylene glycol, 165, 167, 323, 328
ethylene oxide, 155, 174
ETS (environmental tobacco smoke), 2c, 3, 278
European Chemical Bureau, 218
European Commission, 192
European Union, 42, 94, 103, 108, 111, 172, 219

Evenflo, 208
E vitamins, 111, 384
EWG. *See* Environmental Working Group
excitotoxins, 115, 120–121
exercise, 348, 393–394, 402–404
exfoliants, 183–184
Exstream water filters, 378
eye drops, 185–186
eye health and disease, 251–252
eye movement desensitization and reprocessing (EMDR), 344

fabrics and clothing. *See also* fabric treatments
bedding and décor, 9, 216–217, 235–236
dry cleaning, 6–7, 232–233
fabric softeners, 162–163, 215
fair trade certification, 234–235
for infants, 212–214
laundering, 6, 164, 214–215, 377
natural, 214, 226–230
organic, 214, 227, 228
overview, 222
resources for, 237
seminatural, 225–226
static eliminators, 215
synthetic, 212–213, 222–225
undergarments, 233–234
fabric softeners, 162–163
fabric treatments. *See also* fire retardants
dyes, 232
no-iron/wrinkle-resistance/ permanent-press, 7, 9–10, 213, 216, 227, 230–231, 235
stain resistance, 227, 230–231
factory-farming, 103
Fairechild, Diana, 375
fair trade certification, 234–235
falcon studies, 232
far infrared saunas (FIRs), 399
Farm Security and Rural Investment Act, 101
fasting, 395–396

macular degeneration, 252

mad cow disease, 101, 103–105, 328

made from natural (labeling terminology), 132

made with (labeling terminology), 132

made with organic ingredients (labeling terminology), 89

magnesium, 21, 43, 59

magnesium oxide, 43, 59

magnetic resonance imaging (MRIs), 73

magnetic water conditioners, 40, 44, 165

malathion, 194, 262–263

malnutrition, 97, 98

mammograms, 84, 85, 86

Manhattan Project, 84

manual lymphatic drainage (MLD), 405

maple syrup, 118

Marcus, William, 51

margarine, 126

markers, felt-tipped, 357

Markovitz, David, 305

marshmallow, 406

Martin, Ann, 325

Martini, Betty, 115

mascaras, 196

massage, 404, 405

Master Cleanse, 396

Material Safety Data Sheet (MSDS), 282, 334

mattresses, 13, 216–217, 235–236

mattress foundations, 216, 236

Max Planck Institute for Behavioral Physiology, 68

Maybelline, 196

McDonald, Marguerite, 185

McGuire, Tom, 273, 411

MCS (multiple chemical sensitivity), 21–22, 79–80, 154, 225, 236

MDF (medium-density fiberboard), 239–240

MDI (methyl diisocyanate), 240

MEA (monoethanolamine), 155–156, 179, 210

measles, mumps, rubella (MMR) vaccines, 299–300

measles vaccines, 299–301

meat

alkaline water washes, 150

antibiotics, 100

barbecuing, 148–149

diseases due to contaminated, 103–105, 328

environmental costs of, 105

growth hormones, 100

irradiated, 101–102, 363

organic, 105

overview, 99

packaging techniques, 102–103

in pet foods, 326–327

preservatives used in, 112

restaurant dining and contaminated, 381

meat by-products, 326–327

meat meal, 326

medical radiology, 83–86

Medical Sciences Bulletin, 188

medications, 46–47, 64, 348–349, 368–369, 370–371

medium-density fiberboard (MDF), 239–240

Meinig, George, 279

melamine, 108–109

Mendelsohn, Robert, 301

meningitis, 297

menstrual cups, 197

Mercer Island study, 207

Mercola, Joseph, 411, 412

mercury

Alzheimer's disease and, 273

amalgam fillings with, 270–272, 274–275

cell phone usage and, 73

in children's toys, 218

clean-up methods, 17

in coloring agents, 122, 174

detoxification methods for, 409–412

fetus development and, 273–274

fish diets and, 106

MSDS (Material Safety Data Sheet), 282, 334

MSG (monosodium glutamate), 120–121, 291–292

MSM (methylsulfonylmethane), 410

MTA (mineral trioxide aggregate), 280

MTBE (methyl tertiary-butyl ether), 46

multiple chemical sensitivity (MCS), 21–22, 79–80, 154, 225, 236

mumps vaccines, 299–300, 302

muscle testing, 342, 344

mutagens, 177

Myobloc, 199

myoglobin, 102

NAC (N-acetyl cysteine), 409

Naled, 332

NanoClean, 150

naphthalene, 156, 160, 168, 233

National Academy of Sciences, 359

National Association of School Nurses, 368–369

National Cancer Institute, 79

National Center for Toxicological Research, 138

National Childhood Vaccine Injury Act, 288

National Electrical Safety Code, 76

National Ethanol Vehicle Coalition, 319

National Farm to School Program, 363–364

National Institute for Occupational Safety and Health, U.S., 7, 121, 155

National Institute of Environmental Health Sciences, 21

National Medical Library, 42, 179

National Radon Proficiency Program, 19

National Research Council, 91

National Resources Defense Council, 64

National School Lunch Program, 362, 363

National Vaccine Information Center, 304–305, 306

National Vaccine Injury Compensation Program, 288

natto, 110

natural (labeling terminology), 100, 131–132, 171

Natural Resources Defense Council (NRDC), 331, 366

Nature (magazine), 94

NatureFlex, 142

Navy, U.S., 68

negativity, 338, 345–347, 350

Nelson, Claire, 138

Neomycin, 294

Neotame, 116

neuro-emotional technique (NET), 344

neuro-linguistic programming (NLP), 343

neurotoxins. *See also* aluminum; fluoride; formaldehyde; mercury
 cleaning agents, 154, 155, 163, 164, 165, 167
 cosmetics, 195
 dental hygiene products, 179
 dentistry procedures, 73, 270
 dry cleaning fluid, 233
 food additives and flavorings, 120, 123
 personal care products, 182
 pesticides, 261
 synthetic fabrics, 223
 vaccines, 290

New England Journal of Medicine, 301

Newsweek (magazine), 42

New York Times (newspaper), 106

New Zealand, 53, 94

Nickel, Alfred, 277, 278

nickel oxide, 126

nipple cracking, 206

nipples, baby bottle, 208

nitrates/nitrites, 43, 112, 156, 158

nitrobenzene, 163

nitrogen dioxides, 2c, 4

nitrogen oxides, 316–317

About the Authors

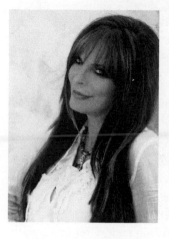

Sharyn Wynters, ND

Sharyn Wynters is a naturopath with more than thirty years experience in health and wellness. Her commitment to helping people change their lives through nontoxic living came as the result of her own personal health challenges. Years ago, by modifying her diet, by changing the products she routinely used in her home and in her personal care, and even by reviewing the thought patterns in her life, she was able to cure herself of degenerative disease. With regained health, she immersed herself in the world of wellness. She studied dozens of disciplines and obtained a degree as a naturopath from the Clayton School of Natural Healing. Since then, she has been able to help thousands of individuals on the pathway to a more vibrant life.

Sharyn was not always focused on health and nutrition. Throughout her life she has enjoyed success in a variety of adventures. At the age of seventeen, she became Miss Pennsylvania in the Miss World competition. Later, she became a top fashion model for Oleg Cassini, the famed dress designer for Jacqueline Kennedy. The first major role of her acting career was as Cat Girl on the original Batman TV series. She later appeared in a number of films such as *Odd Couple*, *Hook, Line & Sinker*, and *West World*.

Today, Sharyn is internationally recognized for the regenerative program she advocates based on a lifestyle that includes raw, whole-food nutrition and a toxin-free living environment. She is on the faculty of the Institute for Integrative Medicine in San Diego, CA, and is the author of two other books: *Ah Raw Veda* and *How to be a Successful Thinker: Creating the Life of Your Dreams*. She has received numerous awards and honors including Naturopathic Doctor of the Year (2011) awarded by the Qi Gong Congress, and the Lifetime Achievement award (2011) from the Amazing Women Organization. Sharyn lives in Tarzana, California. She is fully committed to the empowerment of others, and she is dedicated to being a healing influence on as many lives as possible. Visit her Web site: www.wyntersway.com

Burton Goldberg, LHD

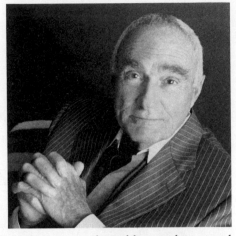

Known as the *Voice of Alternative Medicine*, Burton Goldberg is a self-made businessman and an internationally recognized expert in the field of alternative medicine. Having spent more than thirty years carefully researching every aspect of holistic and integrative medicine—visiting leading health clinics throughout the United States, as well as Europe, Israel, Mexico, and Russia—he has for more than a decade been in the forefront of the movement to educate and empower the public to take control of their health. He is committed to helping forge profound, positive changes in health care.

Burton Goldberg is the founder and former publisher of *Alternative Medicine* magazine. He is also the author of a series of eighteen books that provide in-depth information on some of our nation's most serious health conditions. His landmark book, *Alternative Medicine: The Definitive Guide*—a 1,250 page reference work—has been hailed as *the bible of alternative medicine*. Equally broad in its scope is his book *An Alternative Medicine Definitive Guide to Cancer*. In recognition of his expertise on this subject, Burton Goldberg was invited, in June 2000, to testify before the U.S. House of Representatives Committee on Government Reform during the hearing on Integrative Oncology—Cancer Care for the New Millennium. In 2004, in recognition of Dr. Goldberg's commitment and numerous contributions to the field of alternative and integrative medicine, he was awarded an honorary Doctor of Humanities degree by Capital University of Integrated Medicine, in Washington DC.

Today, Burton Goldberg lives in Tiburon, California. He continues to broaden his outreach to the public as a filmmaker and producer and as a health consultant specializing in the field of integrative cancer care. He has produced three feature-length DVDs: *Cancer Conquest: The Best of Conventional and Alternative Medicine; Curing Depression, Anxiety and Panic Disorder;* and *Ethical Stem Cells Now*. Visit his Web site: www.burtongoldberg.com